D1709050

Movement Disorders in Children

Medicine and Sport Science

Vol. 36

Series Editors
M. Hebbelinck, Brussels
R.J. Shephard, Toronto, Ont.

Founder and Editor from 1969 to 1984
E. Jokl, Lexington, Ky.

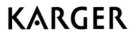

Basel · Freiburg · Paris · London · New York · New Delhi · Singapore · Tokyo · Sydney

International Sven Jerring Symposium, Stockholm, August 25–29, 1991

Movement Disorders in Children

Volume Editors
H. Forssberg, Stockholm
H. Hirschfeld, Stockholm

53 figures and 11 tables, 1992

KARGER

Basel · Freiburg · Paris · London · New York · New Delhi · Singapore · Tokyo · Sydney

Medicine and Sport Science

Published on behalf of the
International Council of Sport Science and Physical Education

Library of Congress Cataloging-in-Publication Data
International Sven Jerring Symposium (1991: Stockholm, Sweden)
Movement disorders in children: proceedings of the International Sven Jerring Symposium,
Stockholm, August 25–29, 1991/volume editors, H. Forssberg, H. Hirschfeld.
(Medicine and sport science; vol. 36)
"Published on behalf of the International Council of Sport Science and Physical Education"
Includes bibliographical references and index.
1. Movement disorders in children – Congresses.   2. Gait disorders in children – Congresses.
3. Cerebral palsied children – Congresses.
I. Forssberg, Hans, 1949–   . II. Hirschfeld, H. (Helga)
III. International Council of Sport Science and Physical Education.   IV Title.   V. Series.
[DNLM: 1. Movement Disorders – in infancy & childhood – congresses.
W1 ME6490 v. 36]
ISBN 3–8055-5556-3 (alk. paper)

Drug Dosage
The authors and the publisher have exerted every effort to ensure that drug selection and dosage
set forth in this text are in accord with current recommendations and practice at the time of
publication. However, in view of ongoing research, changes in government regulations, and the
constant flow of information relating to drug therapy and drug reactions, the reader is urged to
check the package insert for each drug for any change in indications and dosage and for added
warnings and precautions. This is particularly important when the recommended agent is a new
and/or infrequently employed drug.

© Copyright 1992 by S. Karger AG, P.O. Box, CH-4009 Basel (Switzerland)
Printed in Switzerland on acid-free paper by Thür AG Offsetdruck, Pratteln
ISBN 3–8055–5556–3

Contents

IV. Control of Locomotion, Posture and Spasticity

V. Measurement of Motor Performance

Preface

Movement disorders of children with neurological disorders were earlier considered to mainly be an orthopedic problem with the goal to correct secondary musculoskeletal malformations with surgery and orthoses. When physical therapy for children emerged it was still within this framework, to train the muscle strength of individual muscles and to prevent contractures. Gradually, and partly from the work with post-poliomyelitic children in the middle of this century, the focus was directed towards the central nervous system and the original cause of the impairment. Occupational therapy has later become an important tool in the habilitation of young children with motor handicaps but from a different and maybe less dogmatic and more functional standpoint.

The physiotherapy was initially based on certain theories and techniques. Examples of such treatment, widely used in western Europe, were the schools of Bobath (or NDT), Vojta and Sensory Integration. These therapies were often developed from clinical experience and were later equipped with neurophysiological theories. At that time neurophysiology was mainly dealing with different reflexes and the movements were believed to be controlled by different sets of reflexes, triggered by various sensory stimuli. Hence, an important concern was the influence on various reflexes. However, while some schools emphasized the inhibition of pathological reflexes in their treatment and handling, other schools utilized the induction of other reflexes to produce movements. During the last decades the knowledge of the neural mechanisms controlling the movements have expanded immensely and the reflexes are no longer believed to play a major role. It is now time to transfer the new knowledge of basic neurobiological mechanisms into clinical practice and to develop new therapeutic concepts.

In addition to outdated theoretical concepts there is an absence of controlled studies documenting the positive effect of the treatment, common for most physical and occupational therapies. Although some methods have been modified since the beginning, the treatment of children with movement disorders is an underdeveloped field based on old theories and without scientific documentation of the effect.

The poor scientific development in this area reflects the absence of a research tradition in many of the professions dealing with children with motor handicaps. For example, the education of physical and occupational therapy does not occur at the university level in most countries in Europe. However, more and more therapists are now receiving a research training and starting their own academic career. Particularly, this happens in North America, but also in some European countries. This progress will influence the field in several directions. One is that therapists with a clinical background will learn more about how the central nervous system is organized and what mechanisms are failing in children with movement disorders. From this, they may form the basis for new strategies and treatments. Research experience will also allow therapists to design proper studies to evaluate the effect of their training programs.

The present book is one step in the development of an active research focusing on the treatment of children with movement disorders. It covers several aspects from current basic neuroscience to the influence of the movement disorders at a society level. Some of the more traditional schools have also described their current concepts and methods. The individual chapters have been written by the authors participating in the International Sven Jerring Symposium in Stockholm in August 1991. We are very grateful to the Sven Jerring Foundation for making the symposium and this book possible. The symposium had a unique constellation of contributors from different fields, such as basic neuroscientists, therapists with research background as well as clinicians from most professions dealing with movement disorders in handicapped children. Intense and vivid discussions followed the lectures, and these are reviewed and commented on in the discussion chapters by task forces made up of Swedish therapists.

Stockholm, December 1991

Hans Forssberg

I. Therapeutic Concepts

Forssberg H, Hirschfeld H (eds): Movement Disorders in Children.
Med Sport Sci. Basel, Karger, 1992, vol 36, pp 1–6

The Bobath Concept – Evolution and Application[1]

Margaret J. Mayston
The Bobath Centre, London, UK

Since Dr. and Mrs. Bobath commenced their work in the 1940's, the treatment has undergone many changes but the basic concept has not changed. The most important aspect of the Bobath Concept is the clinician's ability to observe and analyse the client's functional skills. The treatment is given according to this detailed analysis and is tailored to the individual. The techniques of treatment are merely tools. The Bobath Concept is primarily a way of thinking – this presents a challenge to the therapist and also enables specific intervention to be provided. The aim of treatment is to *prepare* for specific function by handling which utilises specific techniques of inhibition, facilitation and stimulation of more normal movement patterns to give the foundation for functional skills. This preparation is then carried over by working *in the functional activity* which has been prepared for.

Basis of the Concept

The concept has always described the problems of co-ordination in relation to the normal postural reactions or central postural control mechanism [1]. This gives the prerequisites for automatic and voluntary activity as follows:

(1) Normal postural tone. Postural tone is used in preference to muscle tone as this emphasises the fact that the central nervous system activates muscles in groups for the maintenance of posture and execution of movements. Postural tone must be high enough to withstand gravity but low enough to allow for movement.

---

[1] Dedicated to the late Dr. and Mrs. Bobath.

(2) Normal reciprocal interaction of muscles for: (a) synergic fixation proximally to allow for mobility distally; (b) automatic adaptation of muscles for postural changes; (c) graded control of agonist and antagonist, i.e. normal co-contraction for timing, grading and direction of movement.

(3) The automatic movement patterns which form a background against which all movements take place, mainly postural adjustment.

All upper motor neurone lesions can be described as a disturbance of this mechanism, resulting in abnormal postural tone (spasticity, hypotonia, fluctuating tone), disordered reciprocal interaction of muscles (over-fixation, lack of grading) and a disturbed automatic background of activity on which skills can be performed.

The Bobaths recognised that inhibition is a major factor in the control of movement and posture. It is considered to be important in the development of selective and graded movement for function. Inhibition is active at every level of the central nervous system (CNS) [1]. It is the balanced activity of excitation and inhibition during a movement which controls the speed, range and direction.

Inhibition therefore modifies and controls action by acting on excitation to change and mould it for the purpose of co-ordination.

All of the clients we see are considered to have a lack of inhibition. For example, the athetoid with fluctuating tone and involuntary movements has primarily a lesion of the basal ganglia which we know are important for the inhibition of excitation from the cerebral cortex [2]. The child with ataxia has a lesion of the cerebellum with resultant decreased stretch reflex activity and uncoordinated movement. The cerebellum also has a major role to play in inhibition [3]. The cerebral cortex is instrumental in driving the inhibitory reticular formation and a lesion there will result in hypertonia because of increased stretch reflex activity [6].

Inhibition then has always been considered an important part of the treatment, the best inhibition being seen to be the client's own *more* normal activity. Over the years the treatment has become more dynamic and more functional in its approach. The following discussion will attempt to explain this evolution.

Evolution of the Concept

In the early days the motor patterns of the child with hypertonus were described in terms of the release of a few tonic reflexes, including the tonic neck and tonic labyrinthine reflexes. It was realised that these reflexes did not explain the abnormal patterns of activity seen in the child with hypertonus or dystonia. It is more useful to analyse the *patterns* of activity and to assess how these interfere with movement and function rather than assessing reflexes.

The emphasis on reflexes in the early years has also led to many misinterpretations of the Bobath concept. I still hear therapists talking about the inhibition of tonic reflexes which they consider to be responsible for the patterns of hypertonus seen in a particular child. This approach to management is not part of the Bobath concept in the 1990s. The Bobaths have recognised this in recent publications [4, 5].

Another important modification has been the change from the use of 'reflex-inhibiting postures' to the more dynamic 'reflex-inhibiting patterns'. Although the 'postures' inhibited spasticity by modifying its patterns, they were seen to be too passive and prevented movement. This did not allow for any carry-over into movement and function. The reflex-inhibiting patterns allowed the control of movement from key-points of control where techniques of inhibition, stimulation and facilitation could be applied. In this way, the child could be more active, the pattern and quality of movements could be guided and controlled and whole sequences of movement could be facilitated without the influence of hypertonus.

There was much concentration on facilitation of the automatic righting, equilibrium and protective reactions in the hope that these would provide the basis for functional and voluntary movements. It, however, proved to be inadequate because the child needed to be able to control movements himself. This necessitated a less 'hands on' approach to allow the child to control his own balance reactions and movements. This approach also required more interaction between therapist and client, with the client's reactions guiding the therapist's handling.

The next step was developed as a result of closely studying the development of movement in normal babies. The approach had been to facilitate the child through the sequence of rolling, creeping, sitting, side-sitting, kneeling, half-kneeling, crawling and then finally standing. It was recognised that a child prepares for these activities through the development of a sequence of basic motor patterns of co-ordination which at one stage make possible the performance of a particular skill [7]. This adherence to a rigid developmental sequence is also an aspect of the Bobath concept which is outdated but still utilised by many so-called Bobath therapists. This has also led to confusion and misinterpretation of the Bobath concept.

The most recent stage, and one which is still developing, was the recognition that the approach needed to be more functional to enable carry-over into daily life. This attitude changed not only the approach to treatment but also to assessment. The child was no longer immediately undressed and placed on the floor, but instead a problem solving approach to the child's abilities and inabilities was adopted.

Application of the Concept

The basic concept has not changed, i.e. that we work to specifically prepare for a specific function. Through the use of techniques of handling and through guiding the client's movements with carefully graded stimulation, we aim to give a more normal sensation of active movement which is translated into function. It may be useful to give an example of how this is put into practice by considering a child with spastic diplegia.

This child may be able to walk but falls often due to a lack of reliable balance reactions, and may have difficulty using his hands in sitting because of associated reactions in his legs which increase hypertonus and interfere with balance reactions in sitting. In order for this child to function more efficiently there needs to be a better level of background activity which can be achieved through techniques of inhibition and facilitation, i.e. preparation. The positions in which the client functions also need to be taken into consideration.

To enable more normal function we need to achieve:

(a) More normal postural tone especially in his legs to provide a better basis for more normal activity and to reduce associated reactions.

(b) Work for better control of standing on one leg to enable better balance and therefore better gait, and in some cases better speech (with less associated reactions in his arms and orofacial muscles). It is also important to consider the use of the child's arms as he may need good arm support not only for balance but also to use equipment as an aid to locomotion.

(c) Work for the patterns of activity which will give the basis for this. Work for control against gravity and for variety of movement patterns to overcome the problem of the client's use of flexion for function and being pulled into flexion by gravity. Exclude crawling until the client has good control in standing which is in accordance with how the normal child develops. This counteracts the danger of flexor contractures which occur due to a predominance of flexion. In this we note Milani-Comparetti's concept of the 'competition of patterns' which is valuable in understanding the need to work for many activities at one time instead of perfecting one activity before going onto the next.

(d) Encourage use of his hands in standing rather than sitting or if working in sitting arrange the activity at an angle to inhibit pull into flexion and adduction with resultant increased hypertonus in the legs.

(e) Counteract the influence of repetition (which through effort can increase hypertonus) by inhibition as required to maintain the quality of function.

In order to achieve carry-over into all aspects of the child's life it is essential that the child, parents and caregivers participate in the activities, working towards specific goals which will lead to a realistic outcome for the child.

Whilst our main aim is to prevent and minimise the need for surgery, we also need to recognise the part surgery has to play in the management of the child with cerebral palsy. The most important aspects to realise here are the part that treatment has to play in preparing the child for surgical intervention, the timing of the procedure and the ongoing management after the procedure.

Again the concept of preparation for function is an important one, to ensure that the quality of outcome is the best possible. Just as the normal child prepares for function so we with our client's prepare for function.

The Bobath Concept in the Future

We are still working to achieve a more functional application of the concept, through systematic preparation for skills, thorough parent training and liaison with other professionals involved in the management of each child.

The basis of the Bobath Concept has always been hypothetical. We are now actively engaging in research to try and find quantitative evidence to support what we feel to be successful qualitative results.

We are currently involved in various studies. My own area of research [8] is investigating the occurrence and measurement of normal co-contraction as a basis for a quantitative measure of spasticity (which is viewed as exaggerated co-contraction).

We are also involved in the development of a reliable assessment tool as well as carrying out single case studies and are carrying out a retrospective study of the orthopaedic status of clients who have been on regular treatment at the Bobath Centre over the last 10 years. In addition, we are collaborating with other medical professionals in various studies. One such study is of associated movements (mirror movements) which can give information regarding the plasticity of central motor pathways in children [9]. The other project is investigating reflex mechanisms controlling upper limb function in normal children and in children with cerebral palsy through the study of cutaneous reflexes [10].

Conclusion

The Bobath concept will not change although the application of it will continue to develop over time as we learn more both clinically and theoretically. The essence of the concept will always be:

(1) The emphasis on quality of movement.
(2) Geared towards function with regard to quality.
(3) Forward looking: consideration of long-term outcome especially regarding orthopaedic intervention.
(4) Individual treatment/programme planning.
(5) Non-selective: able to treat any disorder of motor control.
(6) The client is seen as a whole.
(7) Parent (helper) training is essential.
(8) Multidisciplinary approach with an emphasis on teamwork.

Every client, whether a child or an adult, has the potential for more normal activity and function. Our responsibility as therapists is to discover the best way for our clients to achieve their best potential.

References

1   Bobath B: Adult Hemiplegia. London, Heinemann Medical Books, 1990.
2   Brooks V: The Neural Basis of Motor Control. Oxford, Oxford University Press, 1986.
3   Rothwell J: Control of Human Voluntary Movement. London, Croom Helm, 1986.
4   Bobath K, Bobath B: The neurodevelopmental treatment; in Scrutton D (ed): Management of the Motor Disorders of Cerebral Palsy. Clinics in Developmental Medicine, No 90. London, SIMP with Heinemann Medical, 1984.
5   Bobath B: Abnormal Postural Activity Caused by Lesions of the Brain. London, Heinemann Medical Books, 1985.
6   Oke L: Bobath Course lecture notes, Melbourne, Australia, 1990.
7   Bobath K, Bobath B: Motor Development in the Different Types of Cerebral Palsy. London, Heinemann Medical Books, 1975.
8   Mayston MJ, Newham DJ: Activation of human knee flexors and extensors during active and passive extension. J Physiology 1991; in press.
9   Farmer SF, Harrison LM, Ingram DA, Stephens JA: Evidence of plasticity of central motor pathways in children with hemiplegic cerebral palsy. 17th Int Study Group on Child Neurology and Cerebral Palsy, 1990.
10 Evans AEL, Harrison L, Stephens JA: Cutaneous reflexes recorded from the first dorsal interosseous muscle of children with cerebral palsy. Dev Med Child Neurol 1990;33.

Margaret J. Mayston, MSc; BAppSc., The Bobath Centre,
5 Netherhall Gardens, London, NW3 5RN (UK)

Forssberg H, Hirschfeld H (eds): Movement Disorders in Children.
Med Sport Sci. Basel, Karger, 1992, vol 36, pp 7–15

Vojta: A Neurophysiological Treatment

Dorit von Aufschnaiter[1]
Bremen, FRG

We are used to seeing the time of birth as the beginning of movement development. In fact, 9 months have already passed – and with them also 9 months of movement development.

As the fantastic films of Prof. Prechtl (Groningen) show, the fetus can already turn for example the head, roll the eye-balls, move arms and legs and even rotates around the body axis – all basic movement patterns of later life are already present in utero [1]!

During birth the child is 'thrown' into a totally changed, unknown surrounding and it must slowly rediscover its movement abilities under changed sensory stimulation and the influence of gravity. This happens and thereby the central nervous system – due to the basics of proprioceptive, tactile and vestibular stimulations and muscular activities – is able to register, to recognize similarities to earlier, premature movements, e.g. head movements!

But not only do muscular, vestibular, and proprioceptive processes have to adapt to new conditions, the visual and auditory systems also develop in parallel and rapidly (the central nervous system is a highly specialized parallel stimulation-processing system) [2, 3].

The newborn already disposes over a certain 'maturity' of his motor development. This pre-stage of his ontogenesis of locomotion development enables specific activities, which are seen in its postural control, uprighting mechanisms and phasic movements.

---

[1] The editors have urged the author to explain the terminology used in a manner understandable for non-Vojta specialists and also to support the statements with scientific references. Despite lack of compliance, we have included this chapter since the Vojta method was presented and vividly discussed during the meeting and is frequently referred to in the discussion chapters.

Thus, the baby learns to interpret visual stimulation in connection with head movements. The visual orientation in particular is the *most* motivating factor for head movements. The child itself connects action and perception and so organizes the neuronal structures in the central nervous system *on its own* [4, 5].

We, the medical and therapeutic observers, notice in a child with a *primary* conspicuous movement that the ability for action is impaired, that movements are 'wrong' and we therefore conclude that the neuronal structures must be faulty. We, the observers, have a relatively clear idea how movements of infants within the first year of life should look like. We are the ones who talk of ideal, abnormal or pathological movement patterns. The child itself does not know anything of right or wrong movements!

A child with progressive differentiation of muscular function[2] presents itself to us as being able to satisfy its immediate interests (for example to watch a moving ball or grasp a toy) which leads to progressive realisation. Competence of performance always develops from simple to complex.

An ideal therapy for developmentally impaired children would be such a form of therapy which comes as near as possible to the well-known healthy developmental patterns or even is identical with them.

Dr. Vaclav Vojta, a Czechoslovakian-born neurologist and neuropediatrician, who has been living in Germany since 1968, is engaged intensely in the sensorimotor development of healthy infants as well as in the diagnosis and therapy of cerebral palsy, from the early fifties onwards. In an empirical way, he was able to discover the complexes of *'reflex locomotion'*[3] [6].

This is a form of global and automatic locomotion provoked by external stimuli. This locomotion shows great similarities in coordination and differentiation of muscle function in regard to the automatic control of posture, the uprighting mechanisms against gravity, so equilibrium reactions as highly differentiated phasic and the onward striding phasic movements as well as to the spontaneous locomotion patterns of the first year of life of healthy children [7, 8].

It is possible to provoke reflex locomotion with its different complexes of coordination – the so-called 'reflex creeping' and 'reflex turning' – in any human, be it newborn or adult.

---

[2] Differentiation of muscular function means more and more muscle chains become able to coordinate in various forms of contraction. Changing points of support outside the support base make it possible to move the body axis, *as the point mobile!*

[3] Dr. Vojta uses the term *'reflex locomotion'* although it has no connection with our usual understanding of a reflex like PSR or ASR!

That means that the neuronal structures involved in eliciting these patterns of reflex locomotion must be organized in utero (in fact, the child already completed 9 months of motor development) or must be genetically determined or both.

In any case, these coordination complexes are inborn, already present at birth and recallable from delivery onwards.

The provocation of these patterns of reflex locomotion only functions when: (1) the patient lies in a certain position (and if necessary must be held there); (2) the stimuli are given on clearly defined body points – we call them 'zones'; (3) these stimuli must have been experienced by the infant pre-natally.

There are approximately 20 different starting positions – many of them just variations of the 3 original positions, which are prone, side-lying and supine. During the reflex locomotion the body always moves from a certain starting position into an end position – this dynamic way means passing of many movement sequences, which in their turn could be starting positions again.

There are 9 zones where stimulation can be given to provoke the patterns of reflex locomotion. The stimulation of these points shows *mainly* an effect on the proprioceptors and the periost. Pressure given is always three-dimensional and varies in intensity from patient to patient. Each stimuli on the appropriate zone can be combined with other stimuli on other zones, so we have more than 10,000 combinations to elicit the whole complex of reflex locomotion.

In cases of healthy infants reflex locomotion patterns are provokable from 1 zone with its stimuli – these patterns in which the whole body is involved occur immediately and completely – in case of infantile cerebral palsy (ICP) children, we need more than 1 zone and stimuli summation concerning time is necessary, because the development of the expected Vojta pattern takes longer.

But to get these motoric responses in therapy quicker and more complete, certain movements of reflex locomotion must be resisted totally. Through that isotonic contractions will change into isometric contractions.

Besides 'functional reversal' in all muscle chains is generated; under *'functional reversal'* we understand the ability to change the direction of effect of muscle action, it means to change the mobile point with the fix point in the muscle chains. This ability is absolutely necessary and partly responsible for each kind of locomotion. Otherwise, neither posture control nor equilibrium reactions are possible. I want to elucidate with the following two examples the fact that the patterns of reflex locomotion contain certain parts of normal movement patterns of healthy children:

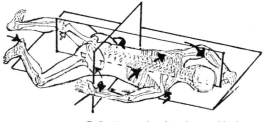

Reflexlocomotion (starting position)
Levels and Trigger Points

Fig. 1. Starting position of reflex locomotion – creeping – with 9 zones and the 3 dimensional levels.

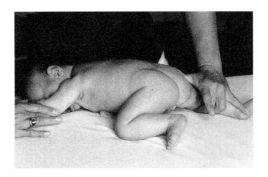

Fig. 2. Reflex-creeping: this 10-day-old baby is pulling – by forearm-elbow support – and pushing away – from the contralateral foot – its body forward, sideways and in a vertical direction into a locomotion.

(1) *'Reflex creeping'* (fig. 1 and 2): From the 9 zones I choose for example the one on the epicondylus medialis humeri, both on the facial side, and the tuber calcanei on the nonfacial side.

If three-dimensional pressure on both zones is given, direction and intensity are adjusted to the reactions of the patient, the response to the stimuli will be comparable and nearly the same in each patient:

(a) The face sided elbow moves into extension in the shoulder joint.

This extension is given a total resistance in order for the body to be *pulled* (through the supporting elbow) dynamically in a cranial, lateral and vertical direction. Now reversal of muscle function can be seen [9]! As the reflex locomotions are provocable in the *healthy* neonate, as in the ICP child, this indicates a common neuronal structure; with Vojta therapy the ICP child is able to experience these normal patterns!

(b) The shouldergirdle becomes stabilized on the trunk and uprighting antigravity action appears: the body is pulled forward in an ideal way. This skill resembles creeping which is part of healthy spontanous locomotion (at the age of 7 or 8 months).

(c) The face turns to the other side due to the contractions of dorsal and ventral neck muscles, in an optimal way. The ventrally positioned muscle group is never in function in the case of a spastic child!

(d) The nonfacial arm moves with more and more abduction and external rotation in the shoulder joint and totally unfolding the hand in a cranial direction. Something similar can be observed in the spontaneous motor development on the transition between the second to third trimenon (a trimenon means the term of 3 months).

(e) The nonfacial leg extends. There again total resistance is given, so that the heel becomes the point of fixation and the body is *pushed* away; the second way to move the center of gravity of the body into locomotion; during locomotion the fixpoint slides from heel to forefoot. In the articulus talocruralis extension, in the articulus talocalcanearis inversion are to be seen. The toe joints show flexion. In the spontaneous locomotion of healthy children this 'pushing' can be observed in the third or fourth trimenon.

(f) The facial leg shows more and more external rotation and abduction in the hip joint, an increasing flexion in a cranial direction in the knee joint, an eversion in the fore foot and extension with abduction in the toes. This 'stepping motion' is meant to imitate the step taken when crawling or walking [10].

(g) The vertebral column moves segment by segment from an asymmetrical starting position into a symmetrical extension.

(h) The center of gravity is actively shifted into a cranial, lateral and vertical direction.

Just remember, all these elicited physiological movements are actively done by the patient, and are never seen in children with ICP without Vojta therapy. The therapist only gives stimulation on the zones in certain positions and resistance to the visible locomotion movements.

(2) *'Reflex turning'* (fig. 3 and 4): A turning pattern can be elicited by applying pressure between the seventh and eighth rib in the supine position.

You can easily recognize the different kinesiological component seen in normal motor development:

(a) Both legs are flexed in a physiological way with slight external rotation and marked abduction in the hip joints. The feet find – regardless

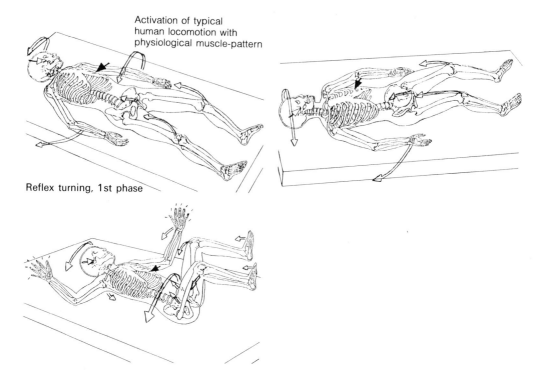

Activation of typical human locomotion with physiological muscle-pattern

Reflex turning, 1st phase

Fig. 3a–c. The dynamic of reflex turning first phase (situation during therapy).

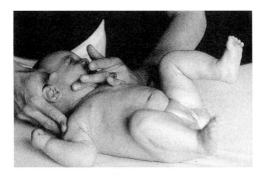

Fig. 4. Reflex turning; 1st phase (10-day-old baby).

of their original position – the orthograde neutral position, the pelvis extends and begins rotation, whereas the upper trunk and back of the head are the basis of support.

(b) The center of gravity is shifted in a clearly visible way cranially and later in a lateral direction.

This pattern of turning contains the physiological movement abilities of automatic postural control, verticalisation mechanisms and phasic abilities of a healthy child in the second trimenon.

We understand under automatic postural control the unconsious adjustment of the whole body to internal changes of body postures as well as the adjustment of the whole body to forces which come from external surroundings. This adjustment happens automatically, and is termed 'postural actability' by Vojta. The origin of this automatic adaption of the body can be seen shortly after birth:

Firstly, the healthy infant can control the prone position so well that it usually does not tilt. Secondly, we can check the adjustment of posture through passively changing the body positions with the help of 'postural reactions' – here they are termed 'postural *re*actability'. The *impaired* postural actability is observed in all cases of later ICPs!

Uprighting mechanisms against gravity means the establishment of points of support outside of the body center, so that dynamic shifting of the center of gravity in a cranial, lateral and vertical direction becomes possible. Healthy *human locomotion* always occurs in three-dimensional motion planes – opposite to the locomotion of ICP children: they are not able to find reciprocal supporting points in the periphery for moving the body foreward, sideward *and* against gravity *simultaneous*! In therapy, as well as in spontaneous motor development of healthy infants, active points of support are continuously used to control the body against gravity and to *pull* or *push* it away from its spot. Coordinated locomotion *without* adequate body control and erection mechanisms is not possible in human locomotion development!

The third element in human locomotion ontogenesis are first the highest form of phasic movements: the equilibrium reactions and second the step-taking, coordinated and goal-aimed movements of arms and legs. Both depend on the postural ability – and on the changing points of support *during* locomotion.

Whoever can dynamically 'steer' the body center in the correct way might be able to style phasic movments in an ideal way.

In sequel of the therapy we observe the alteration of pathological patterns due to the alteration of the physiological quality of movements. The field of action enlarges due to the lesser pathological and more economical and successful movements, respectively, due to the differentiation of muscle function [11].

Kinds of locomotion like turning, crawling and walking are *never* trained with ICP children! The mentally agile child treated with reflex locomotion discovers *its* locomotion itself.

The fact that *the central nervous system through use of reflex locomotion is able to do a natural movement complex* may be elucidated with an example. If a hypotonic child with hyperabducted legs is elicited through stimulating the zone on the chest, it will move like a spastic child into a turning pattern: the one child 'closes' its legs, the other one 'opens' them.

Decisive for the success of Vojta therapy is the fact that the infant must integrate the movements made during therapy into his spontanous movement repertoire and needs to repeat them frequently. In addition to these motor alterations, we can also see effects on the autonomic nervous system as well as changes within the sensitive and sensory changes [12, 13]. Due to all these effects the improved motor activity shows us that muscle tone and body scheme must have normalized.

In therapy, the locomotion tendency is prevented and resistance is given to the forwards, sideways and upwards movement of the body so that the patterns of reflex locomotion can fully unfurl and the proprioceptive stimulation of the central nervous system becomes intensified [14].

But it also means that the infant tries to overcome the given resistance and must work very hard – this is sometimes a reason for crying. If the external pressure on the zones and the simultaneous fixation of the body in defined physiological positions ceases, the crying stops immediately. If these phases of great exertion of the performing child are limited to three to four times a day and to 7 or maximally 25 min a session, the child is sure to be neither physically nor psychically overstrained or permanently damaged [15].

Conclusion

The Vojta method is a facilitation system which makes it possible to provoke normal sensorimotoric behavior and to reproduce it as often as wished. These elicited muscular activities of the reflex locomotions coincides with inborn physiological abilities; the patterns of reflex locomotion contend all the necessary differentiations of muscle function for human locomotion ontogenesis.

Because the product of provocation is always a physiological and complex movement pattern and its context is known in great detail, this therapy is suitable for all patients with neuromuscular disorders and not just for cerebral palsied infants, as is so often wrongly assumed.

References

1   Prechtl HFR: The optimality concept. Early Hum Dev 1980;4:201.

2   von Aufschnaiter S, Fischer HE, Schwedes H: Kinder konstruieren Welten, Perspektiven einer konstruktivistischen Physikdidaktik; in Schmidt SJ (Hrsg): Kognition und Gesellschaft. Der Diskurs des radikalen Konstruktivismus, Band II. Frankfurt, Suhrkamp, 1992.

3   Maturana HR, Varela FJ: Der Baum der Erkenntnis. How to Create the World by our Own Perception – The Biological Roots of Human Recognisation, ed 3. Bern, Scherz, 1987.

4   Schmidt SJ (Hrsg): Gedächtnis. Frankfurt, Suhrkamp, 1991.

5   Schmidt SJ (Hrsg): Der Diskurs des radikalen Konstruktivismus. Frankfurt, Suhrkamp, 1987.

6   Vojta V: Die Zerebralen Bewegungsstörungen im Säuglingsalter. Frühdiagnose und Frühtherapie, 5. Ed. Stuttgart, Enke, 1989.

7   von Aufschnaiter D: Technik und Wirkung der Reflex-Lokomotion nach Vojta. Conference Report of International Symposium, Ennepetal, 1987; in: Funktions-Krankheiten des Bewegungsapparates. Stuttgart, Fischer, 1988, pp 33–37.

8   von Aufschnaiter D: Krankengymnastische Behandlung Zentraler Bewegungsstörungen bei Säuglingen und Kleinkindern. Report of ZVK-Congress Hamburg. München, Pflaum, 1980, pp 159–167.

9   von Aufschnaiter D: Die VOJTA-Methode, eine neurophysiologische Behandlungsform; in Feldkamp M, von Aufschnaiter D, Baumann JU, Danielcik I, Goyke M (Hrsg): Krankengymnastische Behandlung der Infantilen Zerebralparese. München, Pflaum, 1989, pp 127–156.

10 Bauer H, Lint A von der: Aktuelle Neuropädiatrie Bericht über den 15. Jagreskongress der Gesellschaft für Neuropädiatrie; in Weinmann M (Hrsg): EMG – Evaluierung bei Kindern mit Cerebralparesen – Reflexlokomotion nach Vojta. Berlin, Springer, 1990.

11 Schulz P, Vojta V: Zur Effizienz der Physiotherapie bei fixierter Zerebralparese. Kinderarzt 1990;7.

12 von Aufschnaiter D: A new way of treatment for central and peripheral motor disturbances, illustrated by the meningo myelocele. Vortrag, WCPT-Congress, Sydney, 1987.

13 Bauer H, Vojta V: EMG – Correspondence of meuronal activity to the segmental and complex facilitation according to Vojta in plexus paresis. 5th Congress, ISEK – Zdrav Vestn Letrik 51, suppl I, Ljubljana, 1982, pp 21–25.

14 von Aufschnaiter D: VOJTA – eine effektive neurophysiologische Behandlungstechnik oder Qual der Seele; in Born (Hrsg). Stadthagen, BIG, 1991, pp 21–34.

15 Thiessen Hutter M: Psychologie und Neurophysiotherapie Vojtas. Stuttgart, Enke, 1982.

Dorit von Aufschnaiter, PT, Alten Eichen 30, D–W–2800 Bremen 33 (FRG)

Forssberg H, Hirschfeld H (eds): Movement Disorders in Children.
Med Sport Sci. Basel, Karger, 1992, vol 36, pp 16–20

Sensory Integration Theory

Anne G. Fisher, Anita C. Bundy

Department of Occupational Therapy, College of Associated Health Professions,
The University of Illinois at Chicago, Ill., USA

Sensory integration is a theory of brain-behavior relationships. The term *sensory integration*, as it is used here, refers to both a theory, originally developed by Ayres [1–5], and a neurological process that enables the individual to take in, interpret, integrate, and use the spatial-temporal aspects of sensory information from the body and the environment to plan and produce organized motor behavior.

Sensory integration theory is unique among practice models used by occupational and physical therapists for several reasons. First, it is intended to explain mild-to-moderate problems in learning (motor or academic) that are associated with motor incoordination and poor sensory processing that cannot be attributed to frank central nervous system disorders or peripheral sensory loss. Second, the emphasis is placed on normal *central* processing of tactile and vestibular-proprioceptive information and the role of sensory information in motor planning; it does not offer an explanatory model for the neuromotor deficits associated with such problems as cerebral palsy or mental retardation. Third, evaluation and intervention focus on sensory processing and motor planning rather than on the execution of the motor response per se.

Sensory integration theory has three components: the theory itself, associated evaluation methods (i.e. the Sensory Integration and Praxis Tests and related clinical assessments of neuromotor behavior), and specific sensory integration treatment techniques [4, 5]. Associated with each is a major postulate, one that pertains to development and describes normal sensory integrative functioning, one that defines sensory integrative dysfunction, and a third that guides intervention programs that use sensory integration techniques.

The first major postulate is that learning is dependent on the ability of normal children to take in sensory information derived from the environment and from movement of their bodies, to process and integrate these sensory inputs within the central nervous system, and to use this sensory information to plan and produce organized behavior. The second postulate hypothesizes that children who have deficits in processing and integrating sensory inputs are likely to develop deficits in planning and producing behavior, which, in turn, may interfere with conceptual and motor learning. According to the third postulate, the provision of opportunities for enhanced sensory intake, provided within the context of active participation in meaningful activity and the planning and production of an adaptive behavior, will improve the ability of the individual to process and integrate sensory information within the central nervous system, and, in turn, enhance conceptual and motor learning [6].

Ayres conducted eight factor analytic studies designed to identify typologies of sensory integration dysfunction [4, 7–13]. These studies have had an important impact on the revision and evolution of the theory. The identified factors, and their labels, have varied over time, but careful analysis reveals relatively consistent patterns of dysfunction. These are (a) *somatodyspraxia* (somatosensory based dyspraxia associated witah poor tactile discrimination); (b) *poor bilateral integration and sequencing praxis* (BIS) associated with vestibular-proprioceptive dysfunction and a postural-ocular movement disorder (previously referred to as vestibular bilateral integration disorder); (c) *tactile defensiveness* (aversive reaction to being touched) sometimes associated with increased activity level and distractibility; (d) *poor praxis on verbal command* commonly associated with auditory language and motor planning deficits attributable to left hemisphere dysfunction; and (e) a group of interrelated disorders that either may be considered end products of sensory integrative dysfunction or can be attributed to cortical dysfunction: *poor form and space perception, visual construction deficits*, and *poor visuomotor coordination* [6]. See Bundy and Fisher [this vol.] for the specific evaluation signs indicative of each disorder.

Only somatodyspraxia, BIS, and tactile defensiveness are disorders of sensory integration. Tactile defensiveness is one of a group of sensory modulation disorders that also includes *gravitational insecurity, aversive responses to movement*, and *sensory defensiveness*. Sensory modulation disorders, unlike other disorders to sensory integration, are characterized by unusual fear or autonomic nervous system reactions to sensory information.

BIS and somatodyspraxia are hypothesized to represent a continuum of practic disorders associated with poor sensory processing [14]. BIS, the more mild form of dyspraxia, is characterized by deficits in planning and producing bilateral projected action sequences; proprioceptive information, including efference copy (feedforward), has been shown to be critical in the planning of anticipatory and bilateral motor sequences [14, 15]. In contrast, somatodyspraxia is characterized by deficits in planning segmental, responsive motor actions that are more dependent on polymodal (tactile, visual, and vestibular-proprioceptive) sensory information, including that associated with production and outcome feedback. Individuals with somatodyspraxia are thought to be more severely involved because they have impairments of planning feedforward-dependent, projected action sequences as well as feedback-dependent, responsive motor behavior [14–16].

These disorders of sensory integration are not discrete typologies. A child may demonstrate one or more sensory modulation disorders with or without concomitant sensory integrative practic disorders. Moreover, an individual with sensory integrative dysfunction may or may not demonstrate such sequelae as poor form and space perception, visual construction deficits, or poor visuomotor coordination. Finally, while learning disabilities are common, they are not always present.

There are a number of underlying assumptions of sensory integration theory [6]. The first of these is *neural plasticity*. This assumption is central to the theoretical basis of sensory integration intervention programs as acceptance of the concept of plasticity makes it feasible to speculate that it is possible to enhance the function of the nervous system through the provision of controlled tactile, vestibular, and proprioceptive sensory inputs. The second and third assumptions, that the *sensory integrative process occurs in a developmental sequence*, and that *the brain functions as an integrated whole, but is comprised of systems that are hierarchically organized*, are closely related to one another. Such assumptions enable us to conceptualize both the person and the nervous system as open systems that are capable of self-regulation, self-organization, and change along an upwardly spiraling process of sensorimotor and behavioral change that results in self-actualization. In this spiraling process, the action of the system (adaptive behavior and interaction with the environment) becomes the cause (feedback and intake) of system change. Thus, the spiraling process of change is the essence of the fourth assumption: *evincing an adaptive behavior promotes sensory integration, and, in turn, the ability to produce an adaptive behavior reflects sensory integration*.

The final assumption of sensory integration theory is that people have an *inner drive to develop sensory integration through active participation in sensorimotor activities*. Indeed, as reflected in the postulates of sensory integration theory, active participation in meaningful activity, and the planning and production of an adaptive behavior, are critical. Both information processing and action systems models of motor control are compatible with these views [6, 14, 16–18]. Neuronal models of the body and memories of the environment are hypothesized to develop as a result of *active* interaction of the individual with the environment, and then are used to plan *new, more complex* behaviors. New, more complex behaviors are *adaptive*; adaptive implies that change has occurred in order for the individual to meet the demands of new or changing conditions in the environment and now is able to function more effectively within it. *Meaningful* is defined as having significance or purpose, when viewed from the perspective of the client. This volitional component is critical, as volition determines what a person chooses to do. 'For a (person) to move, perception, motivation, plans, physiological status, and affect must all interact with a mechanical system that is composed of muscles, bones, and joints' [18]. Finally, in meaningful activity, it is the goal or anticipated result, rather than the movement, that is the focus of attention. Goal-directed behavior is guided by the sensory information the individual takes in from the environment. Thus, while praxis enables the individual to interact effectively with the environment, the environment also guides praxis. In sensory integration treatment programs, it is the therapist's role is to set up environments that appropriately challenge the individual to evince adaptive behaviors, that, in turn, lead to organized and appropriate occupational behavior, including self-care, play, and school skills through the spiraling process of change.

References

1   Ayres AJ: Sensory Integration and Learning Disorders. Los Angeles, Western Psychological Services, 1972.
2   Ayres AJ: Sensorimotor foundations of academic ability; in Cruickshank WM, Hallahan DP (eds): Perceptual and Learning Disabilities in Children, vol 2. Syracuse, Syracuse University, 1975, pp 301–358.
3   Ayres AJ: Sensory Integration and the Child. Los Angeles, Western Psychological Services, 1979.
4   Ayres AJ: Sensory Integration and Praxis Tests. Los Angeles, Western Psychological Services, 1989.
5   Fisher AG, Murray EA, Bundy AC: Sensory Integration: Theory and Practice. Philadelphia, Davis, 1991.
6   Fisher AG, Murray EA: Introduction to sensory integration theory; in Fisher AG, Murray EA, Bundy AC (eds): Sensory Integration: Theory and Pracatice. Philadelphia, Davis, 1991, pp 3–26.
7   Ayres AJ: Patterns of perceptual-motor dysfunction in children: A factor analytic study. Percept Motor Skills 1965;20:335–368.
8   Ayres AJ: Interrelations among perceptual-motor abilities in a group of normal children. Am J Occup Ther 1966;20:288–292.
9   Ayres AJ: Interrelationships among perceptual-motor functions in children. Am J Occup Ther 1966;20:68–71.

10   Ayres AJ: Deficits in sensory integration in educationally handicapped children. J Learn Disabil 1969;2:160–168.

11   Ayres AJ: Types of sensory integrative dysfunction among disabled learners. Am J Occup Ther 1972;26:13–18.

12   Ayres AJ: Cluster analyses of measures of sensory integration. Am J Occup Ther 1977;31:362–366.

13   Ayres AJ, Mailloux ZK, Wendler CLW: Developmental dyspraxia: Is it a unitary function? Occup Ther J Res 1987;7:93–110.

14   Fisher AG: Vestibular-proprioceptive processing and bilateral integration deficits; in Fisher AG, Murray EA, Bundy AC (eds): Sensory Integration: Theory and Practice. Philadelphia, Davis, 1991, pp 71–107.

15   Goldberg G: Supplementary motor area structure and function: Review and hypotheses. Behav Brain Sci 1988;8:567–616.

16   Cermak SA: Somatodyspraxia; in Fisher AG, Murray EA, Bundy AC (eds): Sensory Integration: Theory and Practice. Phildelphia, Davis, 1991, pp 137–170.

17   Connolly K, Dalgleish M: The emergence of tool-using skill in infancy. Dev Psychol 1989;25:894–912.

18   Thelen E: The (re)discovery of motor development: Learning new things from an old field. Dev Psychol 1989;25:946–949.

Anne G. Fisher, ScD, Department of Occupational Therapy M/C 811,
The University of Illinois at Chicago, 1919 West Taylor Street,
Chicago, IL 60612 (USA)

Forssberg H, Hirschfeld H (eds): Movement Disorders in Children.
Med Sport Sci. Basel, Karger, 1992, vol 36, pp 21–30

Motor Control Models Underlying Neurologic Rehabilitation of Posture in Children

Fay B. Horak

R. S. Dow Neurological Sciences Institute of Good Samaritan Hospital,
Portland, Oreg., USA

Importance of Identifying Motor Control Assumptions

The questions therapists ask when treating postural problems in neurologically impaired children reveal their underlying assumptions about motor control, or how the brain controls movement. It is important that we, as therapists, become aware of our assumptions about motor control, because these assumptions shape and limit our observations and treatments. Our assumptions reflect a theoretical perspective, often held subconsciously, that we use to ask questions regarding the development, assessment, and rehabilitation of neurologic deficits. Therapists who treat children with neurologic deficits often ask questions regarding postural stability in their patients since adequate posture is fundamental to most functional behaviors. Typical questions include: How can I inhibit primitive reflexes and facilitate normal equilibrium responses? How do children learn to orient to a task while maintaining independent equilibrium?

This paper will discuss assumptions of motor control that such neurotherapeutic questions are based upon. The paper presents these assumptions in two models of motor control: the reflex/hierarchical model and the systems/task model.

Reflex/Hierarchical Model

The reflex/hierarchical model of motor control has dominated views of the development and rehabilitation of posture and movement control. As summarized in table 1, the primary assumptions of the reflex/hierarchical model are that (1) sensory inputs determine motor outputs (a reflex assumption), and (2) there is a stage-like development of motor control from low to high nervous system levels (a hierarchical assumption). The

Table 1. Summary of several assumptions and derivative therapeutic aims from the reflex/hierarchical and the systems/task models of motor control

Reflex/hierarchical model	Systems/task model
Assumptions	
Sensory inputs determine motor outputs	Complex systems interact to achieve task goals
Stage-like development from low to high levels	Adaptive, anticipatory behaviors for environment
Therapeutic aims	
Modify CNS through stimulation	Practice the accomplishment of task goals
Facilitate normal patterns	Teach motor problem-solving skills
Inhibit tone and primitive reflexes	Learn efficient, effective strategies
Independent muscle control	Develop appropriate compensations for constraints

first assumption that the brain is an input-output mechanism with which animals react in stereotyped patterns to physical stimuli is based on the work of Sherrington [1] and Magnus [2]. Animals were decerebrated to eliminate spontaneous, functional behaviour which provided a good substrate for studying neural responses to stimuli. These researchers hypothesized that each sensory system is channeled to determine a particular stereotyped pattern of movement called a 'reflex'. The reflex model and derivative therapeutic approaches assume that sensory inputs are necessary for motor outputs and that the nervous system is a passive recipient of sensory stimuli that trigger and coordinate motor patterns that form the basis for normal movement.

The hierarchical assumption was first articulated by Sam Huglings Jackson in 1932 [3] and led to the hypothesis of stage-like development from low to high levels [4]. This assumption is that the most caudal parts of the nervous system control the most primitive, automatic, and stereotyped movements, whereas the most rostral parts control the most mature, flexible and voluntary movements. It also suggests that as a child develops, neural control progresses from the lowest levels by the spinal cord to higher and higher levels of control by the brain stem, midbrain and, finally, cortex (fig. 1, left). Likewise, development of motor control progresses from reflexive to stereotyped reactions, to automatic movements, to voluntary

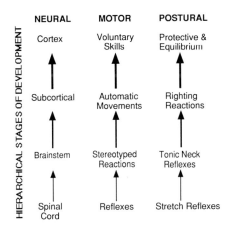

NEURAL   MOTOR   POSTURAL

HIERARCHICAL STAGES OF DEVELOPMENT

Cortex   Voluntary   Protective &
                Skills   Equilibrium

Subcortical   Automatic   Righting
                Movements   Reactions

Brainstem   Stereotyped   Tonic Neck
                Reactions   Reflexes

Spinal   Reflexes   Stretch Reflexes
Cord

Fig. 1. Reflex/hierarchical model of stagewise progression of anatomical, motor, and postural development from low to high levels of control.

skills (fig. 1, middle); and development of postural stability progresses from stretch and supporting reflexes to primitive tonic neck reflexes, to head-in-space and body-on-body righting reactions, to equilibrium and protective responses (fig. 1, right). The reflex/hierarchical model assumes that mature voluntary movements develop through inhibition of lower level reflexes by the cortex or by the reflexes becoming a substrate for voluntary action [5]. It also assumes that postural behaviour progresses in a stage-like fashion of predetermined stages of neural maturation with each stage built upon the previous stage [6]. Thus, postural reflexes must be expressed, and then inhibited or integrated, and the development of equilibrium must progress in chronological order from prone to supine, to sitting, to quadrupedal, to standing [7]. The reflex/hierarchical model assumes that lesions of development arrest of the higher levels result in lack of control, or release, of lower centers and, thus, primitive reflexes dominate motor behaviour [8]. Accordingly, a mature brain is dominated by higher levels, which keep the lower levels under control. The distinction between low and high levels of neural control may have been inherited from the western philosopher Descartes [9], who distinguished human actions as either mechanical, involuntary responses or voluntary commands of the mind [10].

The primary neurotherapeutic aims of therapists using a reflex/hierarchical model of motor control are listed in table 1 [8, 11, 12]. Because the nervous system is passively driven by sensory inputs, therapists provide controlled stimulation to facilitate normal movement patterns and thereby modify, or normalize, the nervous system. Because abnormal movement patterns are assumed to be directly resulting from lack of high-level neural control, therapy is aimed at facilitating high-level, normal patterns, and at inhibiting low-level, abnormal patterns, such as primitive, tonic reflexes and stretch reflexes, which are thought to 'block' normal movements and postural reactions [13]. Numerous reflex identification charts have been developed [4, 14] to help therapists assess a chils's level of motor control. The stepwise levels of control in the hierarchy have been used not only to describe motor development but also to prescribe treatment progressions that begin with stimulating reflexes and progress to facilitating automatic responses and isolating voluntary movements. Therapists help patients move out of low-level, stereotyped patterns to high-level, voluntary control of individual joints and muscles. In fear that abnormal compensatory patterns will become ingrained, they encourage patients not to begin functional activities such as standing and walking too early. Thus, therapeutic questions dealing with identifying or facilitating reflexes and with preventing a child's regression to a lower stage of motor control reflect assumptions of the reflex/hierarchical model.

Many assumptions of the reflex/hierarchical model have not been supported by recent studies in infants and children. For example, far from acting like passive recipients to sensory stimuli, Precht [15] observed spontaneous, functional movements in fetuses even before vestibular reflexes could evoke a response. Unlike reflexive responses to sensory stimuli, babies as young as 60 h use vision to orient the entire head and body to a desired object [16]. Rather than movements being first driven by sensory feedback and then eventually by predictive, central mechanisms, studies have shown that infants only a few weeks old can organize arm movements to moving targets using prediction and only later incorporate sensory feedback [17, 18]. Even early postural behaviors involve not only reflexive responses to vestibular, visual or proprioceptive stimuli, but also anticipatory postural adjustments to displacements that would accompany voluntary reaching [19]. Surprisingly, unlike a stage-like progression from most- to least-stereotyped movement patterns during development, investigators are finding incredible variability of movement in infants and children and quite stereotyped, invariant features of movement patterns in adults [20]. In fact, many aspects of motor development do not progress monotonically but vary through the lifespan [21].

Systems/Task Model

The systems or task model of motor control does not view movements as being prescribed by sensory inputs of by central programs, but rather as

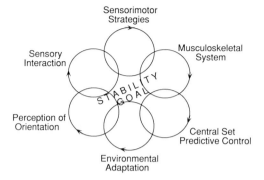

Fig. 2. Systems/task model of interacting systems that contribute to posture control.

a result of an emergent interaction among many systems, each contributing to different aspects of control. The primary assumptions, summarized in table 1, are that: (1) complex systems interact circularly to accomplish functional task goals, and (2) adaptive, anticipatory behaviors allow for effective and efficient solutions for action in a variety of environments. The first assumption is based on the work of Bernstein [22]. It holds that neural control of movement is 'distributed' throughout the nervous and musculoskeletal systems in a flexible interaction. In this view, neural processes are organized around functional, behavioral goals, rather than around predetermined sensorimotor patterns. The second assumption, that animals are active agents adapting to continually changing environments, comes from the work of Gibson [23]. In this view, the function of perception is to identify properties of the environment that have significance to a functional goal, not to trigger reflexes.

Postural control in the systems/task model results from the interaction of systems like those in figure 2 which are organized around the goal of stability. The development of postural stability involves emergence of motor behaviors resulting from finding effective and efficient solutions to the problems underlying postural stability: maintaining optimal equilibrium and orientation for a variety of tasks and in a variety of environments. Equilibrium is control of the body's center of mass over its base of support, and orientation is alignment of body parts in relation to each other and to the environment. Many systems contribute to the goal of postural stability. The *musculoskeletal system* provides dynamic interaction among linked segments and inherent passive elastic stiffness positioned over a variable base of support. *Predictive control*, using central set, allows anticipation of dynamic interactions between the body and environment and between body segments [24]. *Adaptive mechanisms* allow postural movements to be changed or tuned to particular tasks and environments using both sensory feedback and feedforward [25]. *Perception of vertical orientation* using gravity, surface, and visual information helps determine the orientation goal of posture [26]. *Sensory interaction* allows flexible dependence on each sense, given the context, expectation, and prior experience [27]. Innate and learned *sensorimotor strategies* are not prescribed by sensory inputs or central programs but emerge to limit the degrees of freedom of the musculoskeletal system and to optimize obtainment of functional goals.

As summarized in table 1, the neurotherapeutic aims of therapists using a system/task model, are based on helping the nervous system find optimal solutions for motor problems in order to accomplish task goals. Since the same task may be accomplished effectively with a wide variety of movement patterns [28], therapists do not attempt to facilitate an ideal, 'normal' movement pattern but allow patients to learn alternate movement strategies, to coordinate motor behaviors as efficiently as possible, given the constraints of their own systems. Since the nervous system is not a passive recipient of sensory stimuli but actively seeks to control its own perceptions and actions, the child must actively and voluntarily practice motor performance, motivated by the reward of successful accomplishment of task goals. Because the limitations or constraints within a defective neural system may not be amenable to therapeutic intervention, the therapist will help the child develop appropriate compensatory strategies to allow function. Some typical therapeutic questions that emerge from the systems/task model are 'What are the primary constraints limiting a motor behavior?' and 'In which environment is a child most likely to be successful in a particular task?'

According to the systems/task model, the apparently stage-like development of motor behavior does not necessarily depend upon stage-like progression of neural maturation from low, spinal to high, cortical levels [29]. The sudden emergence of a new motor behavior such as independent stance equilibrium results from the summation and interaction among many continuously developing systems that occasionally reach a threshold for emergence of a particular motor milestone. Figure 3 shows a schematic representation of some systems underlying postural stability that are known to change during development [20, 30]. Each system, such as musculoskeletal strength, center of body mass configuration, and dependence on visual or proprioceptive information for orientation, varies in a complex way with age. When these complex, continuous systems summate at any particular age, certain systems provide the primary constraints, or limitations, for the emergence of a postural behavior. The emergence of each behavior (for example, independent stability in standing) may appear

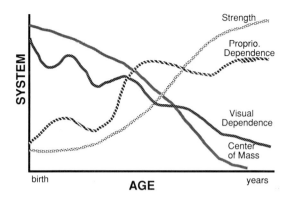

Fig. 3. Schematic representation of summation of changing systems which contribute to developmental constraints for the emergence of postural stability.

abrupt, or stage-like, although independent, underlying neural and musculoskeletal systems are actually changing continuously in a complex manner. One role of the developmental therapist is to identify the primary constraints to motor behavior and to determine whether these constraints can be compensated for or eliminated.

Recent studies have indicated that the constraints imposed upon normal and abnormal postural development are often biomechanical rather than neural. For example, McCollum and Leen [31] predicted that relatively high center of body mass in young children results in body sway too fast to be controllable with a hip strategy for postural correction. Thelen and co-workers [32, 33] has shown that the strength and weight of infants' legs seem to be the most important constraint in the emergence and disappearance of automatic stepping. Berger et al. [34] make a case for changes in muscle fibre mechanical properties that provide an important constraint in spastic gait patterns of children with cerebral palsy. Kugler et al. [35] have proposed that the critical dimensional changes in the body of a young child provide the most important constraints leading to stage-like development. A child moves from stable state to transitional states of instability when previous sensorimotor strategies are no longer optimal for changing body dimensions. In fact, many studies show that normal motor development does not progress monotonically from 'low', immature to 'high', mature levels as predicted by the reflex/hierarchical model but, in may ways, motor control develops unevenly as children improve, regress, and then improve again [36, 37] as predicted by the systems/task model, in which motor behaviors emerge or are constrained by complex, interacting systems.

Conclusions

Models of motor control are only as good as their usefulness. They must help therapists understand the critical questions fundamental to successful assessment and treatment of children with neurologic deficits. Typical questions that reflect our assumptions associated with the reflex/hierarchical model include: Should we try to normalize muscle tone? Will there be carry-over if we facilitate normal movement patterns in the clinic? Will stretching or bracing a spastic leg reinforce abnormal stretch or primitive reflexes and prevent normal movement patterns?

Typical questions that reflect our assumptions associated with the systems/task model include: How do we know when a neural or musculoskeletal constraint can be changed? Is it possible to identify when the most efficient strategy has been found? Which behaviors reflect constraints from the neural lesion and which reflect compensations for those constraints?

By asking helpful questions and by continually questioning our assumptions about motor control, we can contribute to the growth and development of the profession of neurologic rehabilitation.

References

1   Sherrington CS: The Integrative Action of the Nervous System. New York, Cambridge University Press, 1908, p 28.
2   Magnus SR: Body Posture (Körperstellung). New York, Springer, 1924.
3   Jackson JH: In Taylor J (ed): Selected Writings of John B. Huglings. London, Hodda & Stoughten, 1932.
4   Barnes MR, Crutchfield CA, Heriza CB: The Neurophysiological Basis of Patient Treatment. II. Reflexes in Motor Development. Atlanta, Stokesville Publishing Company, 1976, p 241.
5   Twitchell TE: Normal motor development. J Am Phys Ther Assoc 1965;45:419–430.
6   White R: Sensory integrative therapy for the cerebral-palsied child; in Scrutton D (ed): Management of the Motor Disorders of Children with Cerebral Palsy. Philadelphia, Lippincott, 1984, pp 86–95.
7   Schaltenbrand G: The development of human motility and motor disturbances. Arch Neurol Psychiatr 1928;20:720–730.
8   Bobath K, Bobath B: The neuro-developmental treatment; in Scrutton D (ed): Management of the Motor Disorders of Children with Cerebral Palsy. Philadelphia, Lippincott, 1984, pp 6–17.
9   Descartes R: The passions of the soul; reprinted in Cottingham J, Stouthoff R, Murdoch D (eds): Descartes' Philosophical Works. Cambridge, Cambridge University Press, 1986.
10   Reed ES: An outline of a theory of action systems. J Motor Behav 1982;14:98–134.
11   Gordon J: Assumptions underlying physical therapy intervention: Theoretical and historical perspectives; in Carr JH, Shepherd RB, Gordon J, Gentile AM, Held JM

(eds): Movement Science: Foundations for Physical Therapy in Rehabilitation. Rockville, Aspen, 1987, pp 1–30.

12 Keshner EA: Re-evaluating the theoretical model underlying the neurodevelopmental theory. Phys Ther 1981;61:1035–1040.

13 Nelson CA: Cerebral Palsy: Neurological Rehabilitation. St Louis, Mosby, 1985, p 171.

14 Fiorentino MR: Normal and Abnormal Development. Springfield, Thomas, 1972.

15 Precht W: Vestibular mechanisms. Annu Rev Neurosci 1979;2:265–289.

16 Bullinger A, Jouen F: Sensibilité du champ de detection peripherique aux variations posturales chez le bébé. Arch Psychol 1983;51:41–48.

17 Hay L: Spatial-temporal analysis of movements in children: Motor programs versus feedback in the development of reaching. J Motor Behav 1979;11:189–200.

18 von Hofsten C: Predictive reaching for moving objects by human infants. J Exp Child Psychol 1980;30:383–388.

19 von Hofsten C, Woollacott MH: Anticipatory postural adjustments during infant reaching. Soc Neurosci Abstr 1989;15:1199.

20 Woollacott MH, Debu B, Shumway-Cook A: Children's development of posture and balance control: Changes in motor coordination and sensory integration; in Gould D, Weiss M (eds): Advances in Pediatric Sport Sciences: Behavioral Issues. Champaign, Human Kinetics Publishers, 1989, pp 211–233.

21 Woollacott MH, Shumway-Cook A, Williams H: The development of posture and balance control in children; in Woollacott M, Shumway-Cook A (eds): The Development of Posture and Gait Across the Life Span. Columbia, University of South Carolina Press, 1989, pp 77–96.

22 Bernstein N: The Coordination and Regulation of Movement. London, Pergamon Press, 1967.

23 Gibson JJ: The Senses Considered as Perceptual Systems. Boston, Houghton-Mifflin, 1966.

24 Horak FB, Diener HC, Nashner LM: Influence of central set on human postural responses. J Neurophysiol 1989;62:841–853.

25 Horak FB, Nashner LM: Central programming of postural movements: Adaptation to altered support configurations. J Neurophysiol 1986;55:1369–1381.

26 Mittelstaedt H: A new solution to the problem of the subjective vertical. Naturwissenschaften 1983;70:272–281.

27 Nashner LM, Black FO, Wall C III: Adaptation to altered support and visual conditions during stance: Patients with vestibular deficits. J Neurosci 1982;2:536–544.

28 van Sant A: Rising from supine to erect stance: Description of adults' movements and a developmental hypothesis. Phys Ther 1988;68:185–192.

29 Thelen E, Kelso JAS, Fogel A: Self-organizing systems and infant motor development. Dev Rev 1987;7:39–65.

30 Thelen E, Fisher DM, Ridley-Johnson R: The relationship between physical growth and a newborn reflex. Infant Behav Dev 1984;7:79–83.

31 McCollum G, Leen TK: Form and exploration of mechanical stability limits in erect stance. J Motor Behav 1989;21:225–244.

32 Thelen E, Fisher DM: Newborn stepping: An explanation for a 'disappearing' reflex. Dev Psychiatr 1982;18:760–775.

33 Thelen E, Whitley-Cooke D: Relationship between newborn stepping and later walking: A new interpretation. Dev Med Child Neurol 1987;29:380–393.

34 Berger W, Altermueller E, Dietz V: Normal and impaired development of children's gait. Hum Neurobiol 1984;3:163–170.

35 Kugler PN, Kelso JA, Turvey MT: On the control and coordination of naturally developing systems; in Kelso J, Clark J (eds): The Development of Movement Control and Coordination. New York, Wiley, 1982.

36 Shumway-Cook A, Woollacott M: The growth of stability: Postural control from a developmental perspective. J Motor Behav 1985;17:130–147.

37 Butterworth G, Hicks L: Visual proprioceptive and postural stability in infancy: A developmental study. Perception 1977;6:255–262.

Fay B. Horak, PhD, PT, Good Samaritan Hospital and Medical Center, Robert S. Dow Neurological Institute, 1120 Northwest 20th Avenue, Portland, OR 97209 (USA)

Forssberg H, Hirschfeld H (eds): Movement Disorders in Children.
Med Sport Sci. Basel, Karger, 1992, vol 36, pp 31–40

The Nature of Skill Acquisition: Therapeutic Implications for Children with Movement Disorders

A.M. Gentile

Teachers College, Columbia University, New York City, N.Y., USA

The purpose of this paper is to present one model of skill acquisition and, then, to draw implications for therapeutic practice. The model is derived from the movement sciences which, broadly defined, would include research and theory in human ecology, cognitive and developmental psychology, motor learning and control, biomechanics, muscle physiology and neurophysiology. The skill acquisition model to be discussed represents an integration of information that has evolved as a collaborative effort with my colleagues and students at Teachers College, Columbia University [1–6]. The model is still evolving as new information becomes available and as concepts are modified or refined.

In terms of therapeutic practice, there is no 'motor learning model'. There are two reasons for this statement. First, individual perspectives on the same information-base lead to frameworks for describing skill acquisition that differ in detail. Furthermore, deriving therapeutic approaches from any model of skill acquisition represents an artful extension of the available data tempered by clinical experience. Hence, there are (and should be) several attempts to illustrate the application of concepts from the movement sciences to therapeutic practice. For example, Carr and Shepherd [7, 8] and their colleagues [9] have advanced many treatment concepts and have proposed various approaches for physical therapy, while others [10, 11] have described more limited applications for occupational therapy.

Second, the notion of a motor learning model for therapeutic practice sounds too much like a set of techniques and maneuvers which if deployed strictly according to prescribed formulas would produce a desired outcome. One does not do 'motor learning therapy'; it is not a new technique to be put along side others. That is why the phrases 'applications of' or 'implications for' clinical practice are used so frequently. The impact of the movement sciences on therapeutic practice represents a change not in technique but in basic thinking. It reflects a shift in the basic paradigm underlying physical and occupational therapy (similar to the notion of paradigm shifts in science developed by Kuhn [12]). As described so aptly by Gordon [5], the assumptions underlying therapeutic approaches based on the movement sciences are not reconcilable with those underlying traditional, neurotherapies based on a 'facilitative model'. To approach therapy from a movement sciences framework, the therapist must become an active problem solver utilizing a broad knowledge-base to generate ways of helping a particular patient who is attempting to achieve a specific functional goal.

Thus, this paper does not outline a new therapeutic approach. Rather, the intent is to demonstrate how implications for therapy can be drawn from a model of skill acquisition. As the model has been presented in detail elsewhere [1], only a summary is presented here.

A Model of Skill Acquisition

Basic Concepts

The primary focus is on adaptive behaviors through which the individual interacts with the physical environment. These behaviors are directed towards the accomplishment of specific goals, such as maintaining or changing body orientation, maintaining or changing the position of objects, or doing both concurrently.

Goal-directed, adaptive behaviors can be analyzed on three levels: (a) actions; (b) movements, and (c) neuromotor processes. Actions define the relationship between performer and environment. Actions may not always be successful: a change in the performer/environment relationship may occur but not acheive the goal. For example, a therapist may be working with a child on dressing tasks in which the specific goal is to put on a jacket. The therapist is called away for a minute and upon return observes that the jacket is now on the child but backwards. Action is the change in state between child and jacket which, unfortunately, has not been successful. Consistently producing the desired performer/environment relationship is the prime characteristic of skill.

The second level on which adaptive behaviors can be analyzed is in terms of movement strategies and patterns: the means by which actions are realized. Movement emerges from the dynamic interplay of two structured entities: performer and environment. The morphology of the performer and the physical characteristics of the environment shape the topology and metrics of the movement that is observed. In goal-directed behavior, the performer actively attempts to mold movement to relevant features of the environment. These environmental features, critical for performance (i.e. *regulatory* conditions), are specified by the action goal. To be successful in producing a particular outcome, movements must conform to or match these regulatory environmental conditions.

Lastly, goal-directed, adaptive behavior can be analyzed with reference to neuromotor processes. These are the organizational events within the central nervous system (CNS) giving rise to muscular contractions subserving movement. It is assumed that control is distributed across several neural subsystems located at various sites within the CNS. The activity of each subsystem is directed toward the solution of a particular aspect of the overall motor problem (e.g. pattern generation, visuomotor mapping, maintainance of equilibrium). Each subsystem has access to certain information pertaining to the external environment, peripheral events (proprioceptive feedback), or the activity of other subsystems. Within a subsystem, the convergence of input with intrinsic operations yields a consensual determination of network characteristics. Across subsystems, flexible reciprocity prevails. There is no fixed hierarchy. Rather, the locus of control shifts with access to priority information. As so elegantly discussed by Bernstein [13], the localization of coordination within the CNS is in the ongoing interaction among these neural subsystems.

The relationship between these levels of analysis is not one-to-one. There are many movement patterns and strategies that could be used to successfully achieve an action goal (movement equivalence). Similarly, a particular movement pattern is not reducible to one fixed mode of organization within the CNS (motor equivalence). These are flexible means-end relationships. Hence, skill in achieving action goals does not mean that one specific movement pattern is used or that neuromotor processes are organized in one set way. Rather, skill is defined in terms of consistency in achieving a goal, with some economy of effort. Skill involves an individual solution to the problem of specifying these means-end relationships; a solution that produces the desired outcome consistently and efficiently.

Learning

Acquisition of skill can be thought to occur in stages. During the first stage, the task for the performer is to define two means-end relationships: (a) What movement patterns and strategies match the regulatory features of the environment so as to achieve the action goal? and (b) How to organize neuromotor processes so that a specific movement emerges? The learner must engage in active problem solving, generating hypotheses about these relationships to guide a planning process, and evaluating these plans on the basis of performance feedback (about the movement and the outcome actually produced). To do this requires that the learner identify and attend selectively to regulatory features of the environment. There are also demands upon short-term memory processes (STM). For learning to occur, the performer must maintain goal and plans in prospective STM. To evaluate the working hypotheses, the learner must also maintain information feedback about the movement (IF-M) and the outcome produced (IF-O) in retrospective STM. A decision process involving the juxtaposition of goal/IF-O (Did I attain the goal?) and Plans/IF-M (Did I move as planned?) guides the learner's next attempt. Confirmation of both hypotheses results in a general concept of how to proceed to be successful. However, the performer is not skilled.

Skill is acquired during later stages of learning. At this point, learning becomes task-dependent. The structure of the task determines the demands placed upon the performer. Different tasks pose different requirements in terms of information to be analyzed, and constraints on movement and neuromotor processes. To understand these requirements and the processes underlying skill acquisition, we have devised a system for classifying tasks [1–3], a *taxonomy*, based upon two dimensions: (a) the environmental context in which action takes place, and (b) the function of the action.

Tasks are classified in terms of the environmental context by analyzing the regulatory conditions during performance and by examining whether these conditions remain the same or change from one attempt to the next (intertrial variability). During performance, critical features of the environment (objects, other people, the supporting surface) may be either stationary or in motion. Under stationary conditions, movements are controlled only by spatial features of the environment. Timing of the movement is self-paced. In contrast, motion in the environment poses both spatial and temporal constraints upon the movement (externally paced). Now, the performer must pick up cues about these motion characteristics and use predictive processes to compensate for intrinsic time lags in processing information and executing movement. Variability in regulatory conditions across trials affects three important aspects of performance: (a) fixation versus diversification of movement patterns and strategies; (b) attentional processes (monitoring the environment), and (c) reproductive versus generative modes of movement organization.

Summarized in table 1 are the characteristics of four types of tasks classified in terms of environmental context. Clearly, the processes underlyng skill acquisition during later stages of learning differ according to the task demands. For example, in *closed tasks*, practice leads to a fixed and habitual pattern of movement implicating a reproductive mode of organization. As the environment is unchanging, monitoring decreases freeing attentional resources. *Open tasks* involve quite different processes. Move-

Table 1. Environmental context: task characteristics [adapted from ref. 1]

Regulatory conditions during performance	Intertrial variability	
	absent	present
	Closed tasks	Variable motionless tasks
Stationary	Self-paced No predictive demands Movement fixation Reproductive mode Monitoring decreases	Self-paced No predictive demands Movement diversifies Generative mode Monitoring ongoing
	Consistent motion tasks	Open tasks
Motion	Externally paced Predictive demands Movement fixation Reproductive mode Monitoring decreases	Externally paced Predictive demands Movement diversifies Generative mode Monitoring ongoing

ments must be as varied as conditions in the environment, implicating the need to generate new patterns to fit new circumstances. With practice under variable conditions, probability functions develop enhancing predictive capabilities. Monitoring of the environment is ongoing and becomes better attuned to relevant events. Hence, the task, defined according to environmental context, specifies requirements placed upon the performer and determines the nature of skill learning.

Using the second dimension, function of the action, tasks are classified in terms of the body orientation required (stability versus transport) and whether concurrent manipulation is necessary to attain the goal. Presented in table 2 are the characteristics of four types of tasks so classified. Again, demands and underlying processes differ according to task. In *body stability tasks*, upper limbs can become yoked into the postural support system. Furthermore, environmental events fall within fixed boundaries limiting information processing demands. In contrast, *body transport plus manipulation* places dual-task requirements on the performer. Two sources of information must be monitored: the expanding environment and the object to be handled. As these are spatially disparate, attentional resources are taxed. The dual nature of the task also impacts on movement organization. Feed-forward adjustments of body transport mechanisms are mandated to

Table 2. Function of the action: task characteristics [adapted from ref. 1]

Body orientation	Manipulation	
	absent	present
	Body stability	Body stability plus manipulation
Stability	Fixed boundaries Low information processing	Fixed boundaries Modulation of postural system Doing two things at once Moderate information processing
	Body transport	Body transport plus manipulation
Transport	Expanding boundaries Moderate information processing	Expanding boundaries Modulation of postural system Doing two things at once High information processing

preserve balance during independent use of the upper limb/hand. Practice under constraints that differ so markedly leads to those task-specific capabilities mandated by skilled performance.

The complete taxonomy of tasks is derived by combining the four types associated with the environmental context with the four pertaining to the nature of the action to yield a total of 16 different tasks. Each of these 16 categories has unique characteristics, poses different demands upon the performer and involves different processes underlying skill acquisition.

Therapeutic Implications

Responsibility for learning rests with the child. Therapists intervene in this learning process in order to assist the child's development of skill in functionally relevant tasks. Basically, therapists have four tools: (a) verbal instructions; (b) supplementary visual input (highlighting regulatory conditions or using demonstrations); (c) positioning or passive movement of the child, and (d) structuring the environment for practice.

Children with movement disorders attributable to CNS damage display behaviors reflecting such influences as: (a) maturational level; (b) interactions among those neural subsystems that remain intact, and (c) experiential history which may have resulted in compensatory movement behaviors (including learned disuse) or muscular-skeletal changes. Deficiencies in adaptive behavior may reflect a mix of these factors.

The first responsibility of the therapist is to select those functional tasks that are potentially achievable by the child. Understanding task demands and assessing the child's functional capabilities are essential in fulfilling this need. Adapted for the particular patient population, the proposed taxonomy could guide the therapist's approach to assessment and task analysis.

Once a task is selected, the therapist helps the child progress towards skilled behavior. During the first stage of learning, it is important to have the child focus on the action goal (that is, focus is on the outcome to be produced in the environment and not on the movement to be used). The therapist should avoid what we have called 'goal confusion', that is, barely mentioning the goal and emphasizing a specific movement pattern. The child may think the task is to produce a specific movement rather than to produce a specific change in the performer/environment relationship. To ensure a functionally relevant context, the therapist must structure the therapeutic situation so that *all regulatory environmental conditions are present*. Directing the child's attention to these regulatory conditions helps the problem-solving process (especially for children with attentional disorders).

While maintaining a clear focus on the action goal, the therapist can suggest movement strategies and patterns: using demonstrations of various movement possibilities or using verbal cues for children with language capabilities. However, the child has the responsibility for organizing the movement. Only the child can constrain neuromotor process to have a movement emerge. Only through active exploration can the child resolve the problem of matching movement to the environment.

During the child's performance, the therapist observes the movement and its consequences. If the child appears not to retain information, the therapist can serve as an external memory: reaffirming the action goal, re-emphasizing the relevant environmental conditions, or providing augmented IF-O or IF-M. Verbal feedback should be brief and sparing in details in keeping with the child's span of attention. During this initial stage, the therapist should expect movements involving co-contraction of opposing muscle groups as a strategy to safeguard against postural perturbations. The movement will not be smooth and flowing as the child has not learned to account for biomechanical factors impacting on performance (e.g. reactive forces associated with linkage and contact effects, friction, or gravity). It is only later in learning that movement efficiency emerges. At this initial stage, any movement pattern, devised by the child, is acceptable if it attains the goal without leading to immediate or long-term harm (particularly at the muscular-skeletal level). Movement solutions that may limit subsequent actions (e.g. standing with weight bearing on an unaffected leg) can be precluded by altering the task to highlight the solution's inadequacy (e.g. positioning an object to be reached on the impaired side).

Another important role of the therapist is to guide the child's decision processes prior to the next attempt. Encouraging the child to keep on task may be essential if success is not immediately evident. To preclude repetition of ineffectual approaches, the child should be instructed to try alternative movement patterns. Although passively moving or positioning the child may alleviate the therapist's discomfort when confronted with failure, it is the child who must generate the movement for adaptive reorganization of intact neural subsystems to occur.

When the child progresses to later stages of learning, the therapist has two important responsibilities: (a) structuring conditions for practice, and (b) providing augmented feedback. Several concepts related to therapeutic approaches during these later learning stages are described in detail elsewhere [1]; only a few are discussed now. First, the amount of practice is the most important factor in learning. The nature of the task determines how the practice should be structured. When the task involves no intertrial variability, the environmental context for practice can remain the same from one attempt to the next resulting in a fixed and habitual mode of movement organization. However, for tasks involving variable conditions, the therapist must vary the structure of the environment to promote movement diversification. Although practice under constant conditions leads to more immediate success, transfer to variable conditions and retention are poor [14]. Therefore, tasks involving variable contexts have to be practiced under variable conditions. The therapist must structure practice so that the environment changes.

For tasks involving motion of objects, people or the supporting surface, the number and complexity of regulatory conditions should be increased over practice. It is interesting to note that moderately fast moving objects are easier to cope with than slowly moving ones. Also, there may be more transfer from difficult to easier conditions than the reverse. So, practice should be structured towards the limit of the child's present competencies.

Augmented feedback provided by the therapist is also task specific. In *closed* or *consistent motion tasks*, in which movement fixation results, augmented IF-M can be used (verbal, video or demonstration of movement deviations/corrections). However, in *open tasks*, providing feedback about the prior movement is not appropriate as the movement pattern should change on the next attempt when regulatory conditions vary. Thus, the therapist uses IF-O, broadly defined to include information about performer/environment interactions and analysis of the child's movement options under these environmental circumstances. The use of augmented feedback in *open tasks* should support the child's generative processes, facilitating the ongoing problem-solving needed to compose and adapt movement patterns to fit the dynamic context in which action takes place.

Over later stages of learning, augmented feedback can increase in detail but should decrease in frequency. Familiarity with the task allows the child to process more information. However, it is important to decrease reliance on the therapist. Therefore, intermittent feedback, promoting self-evaluation by the child, is better than continuous [15]. Furthermore, providing augmented feedback after a delay rather than immediately seems more beneficial [16] probably because it allows time for the child to analyze the intrinsically available information.

Conclusion

Gordon [5] has described the shift in models underlying therapeutic practice. In contrast to prior 'facilitative' models, in which responsibility for therapy is in the hands of the therapist, the present model anchored in the movement sciences emphasizes the active role of the learner and makes the therapist a partner in the problem-solving process. The proposed model yields no new techniques for handling patients. Rather, it provides a new way of viewing the patient, the learning process and the therapist's role. To derive clinical applications, the therapist is required to become knowledgeable about the current and continuously expanding information-base associated with the movement sciences. Analytic capabilities of the therapist are key. The therapist must decide: (a) What goals/tasks are potentially achievable by this patient? (b) What demands do these tasks place upon the patient? (c) How can the patient be assisted in coping with these task demands? (d) How can the environment be structured to aid learning and make practice realistic and functional? (e) What type, how often and when should feedback be given? and (f) How can transfer of training between tasks be maximized? To evaluate the efficacy of treatment concepts implied by this model, functionally based assessment instruments may have to be developed. Lastly, progress beyond this point will require research at the interface of the basic movement sciences and clinical practice.

References

1   Gentile AM: Skill acquisition: Action, movement and neuromotor processes; in Carr
     JH, Shepherd RB (eds): Movement Sciences: Foundations for Physical Therapy in
     Rehabilitation. Rockville, Aspen, 1987, pp 93–154.
2   Gentile AM, Higgins JR, Miller EA, Rosen, BM: Structure of motor tasks; in Mouve-
     ment, Actes du 7 Symposium en Apprentissage Psycho-motor du Sport. Quebec,
     Professionale de L'Activite Physique du Quebec, 1975, pp 11–28.
3   Higgins JR: Human Movement: An Integrated Approach. St Louis, Mosby, 1977.
4   Higgins S: Motor skill acquisition. Phys Ther 1991;71:123–139.
5   Gordon J: Assumptions underlying physical therapy intervention: Theoretical and
     historical perspective; in Carr JH, Shepherd RB (eds): Movement Sciences: Foundations
     for Physical Therapy in Rehabilitation. Rockville, Aspen, 1987, pp 1–30.
6   Held JM: Recovery of function after brain damage: Theoretical implications for
     therapeutic intervention; in Carr JH, Shepherd RB (eds): Movement Sciences: Founda-
     tions for Physical Therapy in Rehabilitation. Rockville, Aspen, 1987, pp 155–178.
7   Carr JH, Shepherd RB: A Motor Relearning Program for Stroke, ed 2. Rockville,
     Aspen, 1987.
8   Carr JH, Shepherd RB: A motor learning model for rehabilitation; in Carr JH,
     Shepherd RB (eds): Movement Sciences: Foundations for Physical Therapy in Rehabil-
     itation. Rockville, Aspen, 1987, pp 31–92.
9   Ada L, Canning C: Key Issues in Neurological Physiotherapy: Foundations for Practice.
     Boston, Butterworth-Heinemann, 1990.
10   Sabari JS: Motor learning concepts applied to activity-based intervention with adults
     with hemiplegia. Am J Occup Ther 1991;45:523–530.
11   Goodgold-Edwards SA, Cermak SA: Integrating motor control and motor learning
     concepts with neuropsychological perspectives on apraxia and developmental dyspraxia.
     Am J Occup Ther 1989;44:431–439.
12   Kuhn TS: The Structure of Scientific Revolutions, ed 2. Chicago, University of Chicago
     Press, 1970.
13   Bernstein NA: The Coordination and Regulation of Movement. New York, Pergamon,
     1967.
14   Lee TD: Transfer-appropriate processing: A framework for conceptualizing practice
     effects in motor learning; in Meijer OG, Roth K (eds): Complex Movement Behavior:
     The Motor-Action Controversy. Amsterdam, North Holland, Elsevier, 1988, pp 201–
     215.
15   Winstein CJ: Knowledge of results: Implications for physical therapy, Phys Ther
     1991;71:140–149.
16   Swinnen S: Post-performance activities and skill learning; in Meijer OG, Roth K (eds):
     Complex Movement Behavior: The Motor-Action Controversy. Amsterdam, North
     Holland, Elsevier, 1988, pp 315–338.

Prof. A.M. Gentile, Teachers College, Columbia University, 525 West 120 Street,
New York City, NY 10027 (USA)

II. CNS Development after Early Brain Damage (Diagnosis and Treatment)

Forssberg H, Hirschfeld H (eds): Movement Disorders in Children.
Med Sport Sci. Basel, Karger, 1992, vol 36, pp 41–49

What Are the Principles of Motor Development?

Nina S. Bradley

School of Physical and Occupational Therapy, McGill University,
Montreal, Quebec, Canada

Introduction

In *The neuromuscular maturation of the human infant*, McGraw [1] proposed a theoretical framework of eight assumptions for examining the behavior of the infant and young child. These assumptions were based on the view that there is a direct causal relationship between the development of specific neuroanatomical structures and the emergence of motor behavior. For several decades, these assumptions provided a particular point of view for interpretating both behavioral and physiological data. While functional neural substrate is required to initiate behavior, the usefulness of morphologically based 'principles' as a means to understand motor development is now under re-examination, as will be noted by other authors in this volume. Thus, the purpose of this chapter is to examine some of the traditional assumptions and to ask whether they accurately account for the development of motor control, or are there other views that may more effectively advance our understanding.

Revisiting Traditional Views on the Principles of Motor Development

The time-dependent sequence of nerve cell birth, migration, differentiation and maturation was assumed to determine the presence or absence of fundamental movement patterns. Thus, behaviors observed during early periods of development (e.g. infant stepping) were presumed to be under the direct control of subcortical neural structures. Also, because the subcortical structures where considered to be phylogenetically older, the behaviors associated with them were viewed as phylogenetic remnants of primitive behaviors normally exhibited by lower animals. Whereas, behaviors not typically observed until later periods of development (e.g. independent finger movements) were believed to be under the direct control of later developing cortical structures [2]. These cortical structures were also believed to mediate inhibition of primitive behaviors in order for normal development to unfold. Further, based on patterns of morphological maturation, it was assumed that motor development progresses in a cephalocaudal sequence while also progressing in a proximodistal sequence. Additional progressions were subsequently proposed, including: coactive recruitment of antagonist muscles precedes selective recruitment, acquisition of intrasegmental limb control precedes intersegmental control, intralimb control precedes interlimb control and homologous interlimb control precedes homolateral control [3].

Do Traditional Views Accurately Account for Findings in More Recent Studies?

Recently, investigations have begun to question whether the often-cited sequences accurately describe the development of motor control [4, 5]. Even if these sequences do appear to describe behavioral phenomena, should it be assumed that they account for the processes that underly the development of motor control? In a series of studies on neonatal and young kittens, we attempted to identify developmental sequences of skill acquisition for several motor skills in both electromyographic (EMG) and video data [6, 7]. The resulting timeline of skill acquisition in normal kittens (fig. 1A) might be interpreted to support the morphologically-based view of developmental progressions. For example, postnatal onset of forelimb paw shaking 1 week prior to hindlimb paw shaking and initial performance of both paw shaking and scratching in sit prior to performance in stance appear to be consistent with the view that motor development proceeds in a cephalocaudal direction.

However, findings from simultaneous study of these behaviors in littermates after spinal transection challenge a strictly cephalocaudal interpretation. For example, hindlimb paw shaking, a ballistic movement producing high velocities and complex intersegmental dynamics, was evoked in all spinal kittens at 2 weeks postnatally (fig. 1B), 2 weeks earlier than in normal littermates [8]. Onset of hindlimb paw shaking in spinal kittens also preceded forelimb paw shaking in both groups. Thus, the advanced onset of hindlimb paw shaking in spinal kittens indicates that there is sufficient neural substrate to produce elaborate behaviors earlier in the postnatal period than when the onset is typically observed. Further, contrary to the view that inhibitory processes emerge late in development, these data demonstrate that some movements may be initially suppressed and then

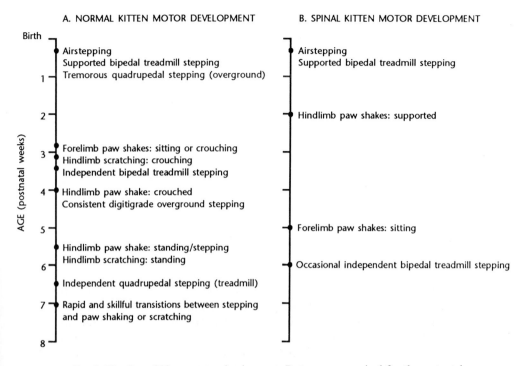

Fig. 1. Timeline of kitten motor development. Data are summarized for the postnatal age at which each behavior was first observed in normal kittens (*A*) and spinal kittens after receiving a low thoracic transection in the neonatal period (*B*).

later released. Similar conclusions were drawn regarding the control of hindlimb movements for stepping [9].

Results of EMG analyses also challenge proposed sequences for the acquisition of organized muscle patterns. A previous EMG study in kittens proposed that hindlimb muscles are not reciprocally active prior to the third postnatal week and that this is due to the immaturity of dendritic branching within caudal spinal motoneuron pools [10]. Thus, it was a surprise to find that the EMG patterns for each of the mature adult behaviors were apparent in recordings from normal kittens during earliest postnatal efforts to step, scratch and paw shake. For example, ankle and knee extensor muscles were co-active while ankle extensor and flexor muscles were reciprocally active during the first recordings of hindlimb stepping and during tremor observed in stance at 3 days of age [6]. Also, EMG patterns for alternating hindlimb steps were observed in spinal kittens during treadmill locomotion within the first postnatal week despite negligible weight support, while in normals, EMG patterns of alternating stepping were seldom observed before acquisition of digitigrade stance at 3–4 weeks of age [6, 9]. From these studies it was concluded that at least some muscle patterns for intralimb and interlimb coordination are established very early in development, but attempts to execute the corresponding behaviors may be delayed until a later age.

Collective review of normal and spinal kitten data across behaviors suggested that the postural requirement to support and adapt a given behavior was the factor that best explained the order of appearance in normal kittens of the various behaviors tested [7]. Further, given the several reversals in onset data for spinal animals, it appeared that more rostral neural inputs inhibited each behavior during initial postnatal development until the corresponding postural requirements could be met. Review of sychronized video data suggested that the order of postnatal onsets for the behaviors was positively related to both the postural context and amplitude of the postural perturbation emergent with execution of each behavior. For example, to initiate hindlimb paw shaking, the last of the behaviors to emerge in normals, the kittens had to maintain a stable tripod stance and abduct the responding limb to execute the shake and, during initial efforts, dramatic postural perturbations were visibly apparent. Whereas, earlier appearing forelimb paw shaking and hindlimb scratching could be initiated while seated, providing a larger base of support for producing stabilizing reaction forces and less dramatic perturbations.

It might be argued that failure to observe the expected developmental progressions in the studies reviewed above only indicates that the progressions occur earlier in development, in the prenatal period. For this reason, studies were initiated to examine motor patterns in the chick embryo during spontaneous motility in ovo. Previous behavioral studies reported that there is a lack of coordination between body parts prior to the onset of prehatching behavior [3]. However, EMG recordings of repetitive limb motions during spontaneous motility revealed that ankle and hip or knee synergist muscles are coactivated and antagonist muscles are reciprocally activated by 9 embryonic days of age, long before chicks initiate coordinated leg movements to hatch and walk [11]. The early presence of coordinated muscle patterns in the leg (distal control) and presumed absence of coordinated body movements (proximal control) also challenge the view that a cephalocaudal progression fully accounts for motor development in the embryonic period. Collectively, the findings from the studies reviewed in this section suggest that the actions of the relatively immature nervous system are complex and dynamic. When constraints, such as postural demands, are too great, the immature nervous system appears to be responsive to those constraints by inhibiting certain actions. This view is contrary to traditional assumptions that imply the immature nervous system is primitive and its responses are stereotypic.

Contemporary Study of the Embryo Challenges Findings of Older Studies

Assumptions of causality, such as those delineated by McGraw [1], were based upon anatomical and behavioral studies of embryos that attempted to control for viability and gestational age, but lacked experimental designs to control for or reveal other possible 'hidden variables' extrinsic to the nervous system that might account for behavioral outcomes. Further, the experimental methods were frequently limited to anecdotal descriptions of behavior and typically lacked quantitative measures now commonly employed to study movement. In general, early studies described embryonic motility as consisting of either synchronous undifferentiated movements of the trunk and limbs, such as mass flexion, or differentiated movements of the trunk and limbs with no apparent coordination between body parts until the final days of incubation [3]. The absence of coordinated movement, however, would appear to be in conflict with the presence of well-ordered recruitment patterns for intralimb control observed in chick embryos [11]. One possible explanation for this discrepancy is that earlier studies did not take into account the contributions of an aqueous medium to the biomechanical dynamics that emerge during movement under bouyant conditions. For example, once movement is initiated, the embryo begins to rock in a rostrocaudal arc and roll side to side about the umbilical vessels that anchor it to the yolk sac [11]. It is possible that emergent biomechanics perturb orderly motor output producing movements too complex for the embryo to accomodate due to the absence of sufficient reaction forces to stabilize the movements in an aqueous medium. It is also possible that these whole body perturbations produce postural variability too complex and unpredictable for the experimenter to visually identify coordinated movement patterns.

The apparent discrepancy between earlier reports of uncoordinated movement and coordinated EMG patterns is currently under investigation. In a recent study of individual kicks during spontaneous motility in chick embryos, kinematic data suggested that leg movements were characterized by a variety of patterns [12]. Given the possible influence of postural perturbations, a study of wing and leg movements at E9 was initiated to examine the kinematic patterns during the portion of motility characterized by continuous movement. Preliminary data suggest that during continuous movement, control of adjacent limb segments is highly organized [13].

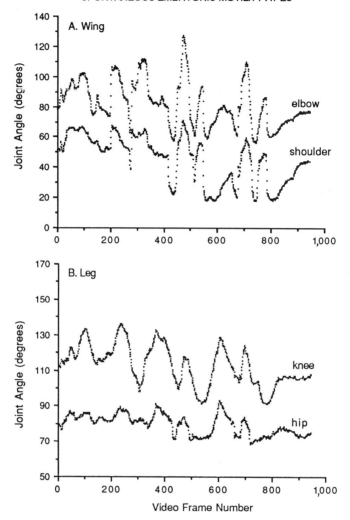

Fig. 2. Joint kinematics for wing and leg movements in chick embryos during spontaneous motility in ovo. Video tape recordings were obtained at embryonic day 9 and computer digitized at a sample rate of 30 frames/s to obtain shoulder and elbow joint angles (*A*) plus hip and knee joint angles (*B*) for a total of 9.7 s of continuous movement.

Alternating flexion and extension motions at the shoulder are accompanied by extension and flexion at the elbow (fig. 2A) while alternating flexion and extension motions at the hip are accompanied by flexion and extension at the knee (fig. 2B). Linear trend analyses for changes in joint angles over time suggest that actions at adjacent limb joints are executed in a reliable pattern for the duration of repetitive flexion/extension motions ($r^2 = 0.74$), with r^2 values approaching 1.0 for several individual cycles per episode of motility. Also, wing and leg movements begin and end coincidently, yet preliminary analyses do not reveal a simple one to one correspondence between wing and leg for repetitive cycles of flexion/extension. One possible explanation for this apparent discrepancy may be that the mechanics of emergent postural perturbations disrupt intrinsic coupling mechanisms. Studies are underway to explore this possibility.

A Call for Multidisciplinary Models of Motor Development

Traditional assumptions regarding motor development, at least in some instances, no longer appear to be sufficient to account for the development of motor control. 'Quantum leaps' in skill acquisition, new skills that suddenly appear, cannot be explained by morphological maturation [14] and proximodistal development of limb control may be too simplistic to be a useful principle [5, 15]. Traditional assumptions may account for the late aquisition of heel strike during gait in normal infants and its loss in victims of cerebral palsy or stroke [16], but proximal control hip abduction and rotation is also lost in these populations. Further, we now know that neonates can initiate visual regard and individuated finger movements [17]. Thus, it is possible that early hand (distal) activity plays a very important role in the development of arm (proximal) control.

Emerging multidisciplinary views of motor control, in contrast, consider the interaction of multiple factors in movement execution, such as the contributions of biomechanics and contextual variables, to the neural control of movement [4, 5, 7, 15, 18]. For example, if we are to identify 'principles of motor development' that account for quantum leaps and other behavioral phenomena, we will need to determine how postural perturbations arising from movement contribute to the ordering or disordering of subsequent movement. If this process is different from what is observed in adults, is it due to differences in morphology, biomechanics, experience, strategy, and/or other contextual variables? In some situations, the ability to estimate postural consequences, the amount of force and/or appropriate timing of actions may be rate-limiting factors that delay execution of a new movement, while in others, movement context may be a critical factor [18]. In conclusion, long-held assumptions regarding causal relationships between morphological development and behavior have provided a particular framework to explain motor development for most of this century. As we approach the end of the century, however, new research developments raise questions that cannot be adequately addressed by older assumptions and provoke us to identify new principles to understand the magnificent achievements of the young and to develop more effective rehabilitation strategies for the physically disabled child.

References

1   McGraw MB: The Neuromuscular Maturation of the Human Infant. New York, Hafner, 1945.
2   Touwen BCL: Primitive reflexes – conceptional or semantic problem? Clin Dev Med 1984;94:115–125.
3   Bekoff A: Development of locomotion in vertebrates: a comparative perspective; in Gollin E (ed): Comparative Development of Adaptive Skills: Evolutionary Implications. New York, Erlbaum, 1985, pp 57–94.
4   Barnes MR, Crutchfield CA, Heriza CB, Herdman SJ: Reflex and Vestibular Aspects of Motor Control, Motor Development and Motor Learning. Atlanta, Stokesville, 1990.
5   Ulrich BD: Development of stepping patterns in human infants: A dynamical systems perspective. J Motor Behav 1989;21:392–408.
6   Bradley NS, Smith JL: Neuromuscular patterns of stereotypic hindlimb behaviors in the first two postnatal months. I. Stepping in normal kittens. Dev Brain Res 1988;38:37–52.
7   Bradley NS, Smith JL: Neuromuscular patterns of stereotypic hindlimb behaviors in the first two postnatal months. III. Scratching and the paw-shake response in kittens. Dev Brain Res 1988;38:69–82.
8   Bradley NS, Smith JL: Early onset of hindlimb paw-shake responses in spinal kittens: a new perspective in motor development. Dev Brain Res 1985;17:301–303.
9   Bradley NS, Smith JL: Neuromuscular patterns of stereotypic hindlimb behaviors in the first two postnatal months. II. Stepping in spinal kittens. Dev Brain Res 1988;38:53–67.
10   Schiebel ME, Schiebel AB: Developmental relationship between spinal motoneuron dendrite bundles and patterned activity in the hindlimb of cats. Exp Neurol 1970;29:328–335.
11   Bradley NS, Bekoff A: Development of coordinated movement in chicks. I. Temporal analysis of hindlimb muscle synergies at embryonic days 9 and 10. Dev Psychobiol 1990;23:763–782.
12   Watson SJ, Bekoff A: A Kinematic Analysis of Hindlimb Motility in 9-Day-Old and 10-Day-Old Chick Embryos. J Neurobiol 1990;21:651–660.
13   Chambers SH, Bradley NS: Intra- and interlimb coordination during motility in chick embryos. Soc Neurosci Abstr 1991;17:937.
14   Connolly K: The nature of motor skill development. J Hum Movement Stud 1977;3:128–143.
15   Schneider K, Zernicke RF, Ulrich BD, Jensen JL, Thelen E: Understanding movement

control in infants through the analysis of limb intersegmental dynamics. J Motor Behav 1990;22:493–520.

16   Leonard CT, Hirschfeld H, Forssberg H: Gait acquisition and reflex abnormalities in normal children and children with cerebral palsy; in Amblard B (ed): Development, Adaptation and Modulation of Posture and Gait. Amsterdam, Elsevier, 1988, pp 33–45.

17   von Hofsten C: The organization of arm and hand movements in the neonate; in von Euler C, Forssberg H, Langercrantz H (eds): Neurobiology of Early Infant Behavior. London, Macmillan, 1989, pp 129–142.

18   van der Weel FR, van der Meer ALH, Lee DH: Effect of task on movement control in cerebral palsy: Implications for assessment and therapy. Dev Med Child Neurol 1991;33:419–426.

Nina S. Bradley, PhD, PT, School of Physical and Occupational Therapy, McGill University, 3654 Drummond Street, Montreal, PQ H3G 1Y5 (Canada)

Forssberg H, Hirschfeld H (eds): Movement Disorders in Children.
Med Sport Sci. Basel, Karger, 1992, vol 36, pp 50–56

Neural and Neurobehavioral Changes Associated with Perinatal Brain Damage

Chuck Leonard

Physical Therapy Department, University of Montana, Missoula, Mont., USA

An observation readily apparent to all medical-care providers involved with neurological rehabilitation is that perinatal brain damage has motor behavioral consequences that are considerably different from those resulting from similar damage occurring in an adult. The differences, although readily apparent, are poorly defined and understood. With the development of new neuroanatomical and neurophysiological techniques, the neural mechanisms subserving behavioral differences have begun to be defined.

Infant Lesion Effect

Generally, scientists have found that perinatal damage to the CNS of neonatal animals has less severe consequences on motor behavior than similar damage occurring in the adult [1–3]. This finding is referred to as the infant lesion effect. Since similar damage results in dissimilar behavioral outcomes, it is probable that different neural mechanisms subserve recovery following perinatal brain damage from that of an adult. The nervous system of a fetus or neonate is considerably different from that of an adult. Maturational processes such as myelinization, cell death, synaptogenesis, dendritic arborization, and the establishment of adult-like neural pathways have not been completed during the perinatal period. Damage to the nervous system prior to or during critical periods of developmemt affects motor behavior differently than damage occurring at other times. The sparing of motor functions following damage to the perinatal nervous system appears to depend on the stage of development not only of damaged neural pathways but also of undamaged pathways at the time the lesion occurs [3, 4]. If brain damage occurs prior to a critical period of development, more plasticity is available to partially damaged pathways and undamaged pathways to help mediate recovery. At different stages of development, comparable behavior may be controlled by different neural circuitry. Certain motor behaviors, therefore, which may be unaffected at the time of a lesion may display deficits during subsequent development. This 'growing into a deficit' seems to be a general behavioral consequence of CNS damage in the infant [2–5].

In summary, several factors contribute to the infant lesion effect: (1) the maturity of the damaged pathway at the time of the lesion; (2) the maturity of undamaged tissue available to mediate compensatory processes, and (3) different neural circuitry appears to control motor behavior at different stages of development and, therefore, depending on the stage of maturation, behavioral consequences of an identical lesion will vary. Two neural maturational processes that are likely affected by these factors are encephalization of function and neonatal neural exuberance.

Encephalization of Function

Encephalization is a term that has been used, somewhat inaccurately, to describe a process whereby, during phylogenetic or ontogenetic development, the control of motor behavior shifts from lower to higher brain centers. It is no longer tenable to regard the development of the nervous system as being based on a hierarchial control model. The development of higher brain centers concerned with motor control does not totally depend on or supercede lower center control. Rather, supraspinal centers become integrated with segmental functioning. This integration, which is greater in humans than in any other species, enhances our movement repertoire, allows fractionation of movement and also appears to decrease the autonomy of spinal cord mediated movement. Encephalization of function, therefore, should more accurately be regarded as the increased integration of higher brain centers in the control of movement. An excellent example of encephalization of a motor behavior is that of placing reactions.

Placing occurs when the dorsum of an animal's paw contacts an object such as the edge of a table. This elicits a reaction which is visually very similar to the human stepping response (i.e. flexion of the paw followed immediately by extension and placement of the limb). Low threshold placing (placing elicited by <980 dyne of force), similar to human infant stepping responses, are present at birth, then become difficult to elicit for a period of time, and then re-emerge during later developmental stages. The sensorimotor (SM) cortex is unnecessary for placing in infant cats but is required in adults [3, 6]. Thus, the cortical mediation of placing develops postnatally. This is an example of encephalization of a postural reflex. Damaging supraspinal centres at a time when placing is mediated solely by segmental spinal circuitry (i.e. during perinatal stages) may leave segmental control in place. Alternatively, sparing of placing following perinatal SM cortex damage may be mediated by plasticity of undamaged supraspinal centers. There appears to be evidence for both and the neural mechanisms involved in the behavioral recovery appear to be dependent upon the location of the damage and which neural pathways are spared. There is evidence that recovered placing reactions following neonatal damage to the SM cortex is the result of compensation from undamaged supraspinal pathways [3, 6]. Placing, however, is spared following neonatal lumbar spinal cord transections [5]. This suggests that placing can develop as a spinal reflex if cortical influences are eliminated prior to the development of cortical mediation of placing. These apparently contradictory findings can theoretically be explained by competitive interactions known to exist between spinal cord and supraspinal projections during development [7] and following CNS damage [8]. Total removal of supraspinal projections by a spinal cord transection removes all possible competition from supraspinal centers and thus may leave the control of placing at the segmental level. Following unilateral SM cortex damage, some supraspinal projections remain intact and may, for an as yet unknown reason, super- cede segmental circuitry in the control of placing. Supraspinal projections undergo dramatic changes perinatally and following damage to the nervous system [3].

Neonatal Neural Exuberance

During various stages of ontogenetic development neural projections exist that are not normally present in the adult [3, 7]. These neonatal 'exuberant' projections appear either to retract or become physiologically latent during development. The extent and time period of this exuberance varies for each neural pathway. For instance, in the cat the corticorubral and corticothalamic but not the corticospinal tracts are exuberent at the day of birth [3]. Neural activity plays a vital role in retraction and segregation within the nervous system [9]. These findings are of importance when considering the potential benefits of early intervention in neurological rehabilitation. The gradual reduction of exuberant projections is related to competition for synaptic sites [8]. There is competition for synaptic sites and early redundancy yields to refinement based upon a proper matching of afferents and efferents. It is of interest to note that the earliest human fetal movements are detected at approximately 8 weeks of gestation [10]. During this time migrating thalamocortical projections interact with SM cortical neurons within the subplate zone near the cerebral ventricle prior to the neuron's migration to the SM cortex [11]. Is this mere coincidence or could early fetal movements be influencing the afferent/efferent connections between the thalamus and SM cortex?

Competitive interactions between projections are modulated by activity. This can be eliminated following damage to brain centers. Removal of competition may result in an abnormal retention of neonatal neural exuberance. Unilateral removal of the SM cortex at birth results in retention of exuberant corticothalamic and corticorubral projections from the contralateral, homotypic, undamaged SM cortex [3]. It appears that this neural retention subserves sparing of some cortically dependent reflex functioning and also subserves some movement dysfunctions seen in neonatally brain-damaged animals [3]. Neonatal neural exuberance and its retention following neonatal brain damage has been found in a number of species and is an important principle underlying the infant lesion effect. Encephalization of function is another principle underlying motor development. What evidence is there, however, that similar neural mechanisms underlie human development and the human infant lesion effect?

Human Infant Lesion Effect

Spastic-type cerebral palsy (CP) is one disorder that may result from perinatal brain damage. Autopsy data and imaging techniques have shown that individuals with CP have damage primarily isolated to the SM cortex, internal capsule and pyramidal tracts [12, 13]. Cerebral vascular accidents (CVAs) in the adult can affect similar cortical areas. Spasticity, abnormal co-contraction during voluntary movement, and alterations in postural reflexes are movement dysfunctions common to individuals with CP or adult-onset CVAs. The movement patterns and postural responses of these two populations, however, are not the same. These observations, together with non-human animal data pertaining to the differing neural consequences for perinatal and adult-onset brain damage suggest that dissimilar neural events subserve the respective movement disorders. Two neural events likely to be affected differently in the human are encephalization of function and neonatal neural exuberance.

Non-human animal data indicate that encephalization of motor function occurs during ontogenetic development and that lesioning the developing brain alters this process. Recent experiments provide indirect evidence of encephalization of human locomotion and an alteration in this process following perinatal brain damage.

All human infants exhibit stepping movements from the day of birth. The response then becomes difficult to elicit until about 8–10 months of age. At this time, the human infant, with its newly refined equilibrium reactions, begins goal-directed bipedal ambulation. Central pattern generators (CPGs) located within the spinal cord mediate locomotion in a variety of vertebrates [14, 15]. The fact that locomotion is apparent even in anencephalic infants at the day of birth [16] supports the existence of CPGs in humans at least early in ontogeny. There is little, if any, evidence of autonomous CPG functioning in adult primates [17] including humans. The autonomy of spinal cord mediated locomotion appears to be lost in humans. What evidence is there that encephalization of function is involved? Electromyographic (EMG) recording from lower extremity muscles during human infant stepping indicate that muscle sequencing is similar during early neonatal stepping and the stepping that re-emerges at 8–10 months of age [18]. After this time, however, the EMG activity and kinematics of walking change quickly and dramatically [19, 20]. Examination of the stepping characteristics of children with known damage to SM cortical projections indicate that their responses are very similar to the initial stepping responses of non-disabled infants [20]. However, at an age and period of development when one would expect gait changes, children with CP do not exhibit typical changes but rather retain characteristics of infant-like stepping [20]. These data suggest that there is encephalization of human locomotion. Initially, stepping responses are mediated at a segmental level but with time, the normal development of gait becomes dependent on supraspinal centers. Alterations in the gait of individuals with CP does not appear to be a totally aberrant development but rather a retention of an earlier developmental stage. Their gait disorders, although of multifarious origin and impacted by musculotendinous changes, represent a lack of integration of higher centers with segmentally mediated movement patterns. This lack of integration of descending systems may also influence subcortical neural development. Alterations in spinal cord neurotransmitter development result from removal of supraspinal input at birth [5].

Another potential change resulting from perinatal brain damage, that is consistent with non-human animal data, is retention of neonatal neural exuberance. Hyperreflexia is a condition common to individuals with CP. Hyperreflexia is usually meant to indicate an exaggerated response to a given reflex-eliciting stimulus. For instance, a tendon tap will cause an increased amplitude in the EMG potentiation of the stimulated muscle. There is evidence that the hyperreflexia associated with CP not only involves an increased amplitude of the deep tendon response but also irradiation of the response onto other muscles [21, 22]. Reflex irradiation is a common feature in non-disabled infants less than 2 years of age [22]. Reflex irradiation is most easily explained by an absence of reflex inhibition from descending systems or by exuberant Ia projections that project to muscles nor normally innervated in the adult. Neonatally exuberant Ia projections may fail to retract following perinatal brain damage. Therefore, a stimulus to a single muscle may spread via exuberant Ia projections to neighboring muscles. It is not yet known whether individuals with adult-onset damage to SM cortical projections exhibit similar patterns of reflex irradiation.

It is an extremely interesting time to be involved in neurological rehabilitation. New methodologies have enhanced our abilities to examine the nervous system and are increasingly providing tools by which we can examine, in humans, the effectiveness of various therapeutic procedures. It is of paramount importance that clinical observations be refined into scientifically testable questions and that the questions result in experiments that elucidate and define the neural mechanisms involved in various neurological disorders. It is probable that apparently similar movement dysfunctions associated with various neurological disorders are subserved by dissimilar neural deficits. Only when this distinction is made, can effective, patient-specific, intervention therapies be established.

References

1 Kennard MA: Cortical reorganization of motor functions (studies of monkeys). Arch Neurol Psychiatr 1942;47:227–240.

2 Hicks SP, D'Amato CJ: Motor-sensory cortex corticospinal system and developing locomotion and placing in rats. Am J Anat 1975;143:1–42.

3 Leonard CT, Goldberger ME: Consequences of damage to the sensorimotor cortex in neonatal and adult cats. II. Maintenance of exuberant projections. Dev Brain Res 1987;32:15–30.

4 Goldman PS, Galkin TW: Prenatal removal of frontal association cortex in the fetal rhesus monkey: Anatomical and functional consequences in postnatal life. Brain Res 1978;152:451–485.

5 Robinson GA, Goldberger ME: The development and recovery of motor function in spinal cats. I. The infant lesion effect. Exp Brain Res 1986;62:373–386.

6 Amassian, VE, Ross, R: Developing role of sensorimotor cortex and pyramidal tract neurons in contact placing in kittens. J Physiol 1978;74:165–184.

7 Stanfield B, O'Leary D, Fricks C: Selective collateral elimination in early postnatal development restricts cortical distribution of rat pyramidal tract neurons. Nature (Lond) 1982;298:371–373.

8 Goldberger ME: Spared-root deafferentation of a cat's hindlimb: hierarchical regulation of pathways mediating recovery of motor behavior. Exp Brain Res 1988;73:329–342.

9 Wiesel TN, Hubel DH: Comparison of the effects of unilateral and bilateral eye closure on cortical unit responses in kittens. J Neurophysiol 1965;28:1029.

10 de Vries JIP, Visser SHA, Prechtl HFR: Fetal motility in the first half of pregnancy; in: Continuity of Neural Functions from Prenatal to Postnatal Life. London, Spastics International Medical Publications, 1983, pp 46–64.

11 Rakic P: Specification of cerebral cortical areas. Science 1988;242:170–176.

12   Kotlarek F, Rosewig R, Brull D: Computed tomographic findings in congenital hemi-
     paresis in childhood and their translation to etiology and prognosis. Neuropediatrics
     1981;12:101–109.
13   Shortland D, Levene MI, Trounce J, Ng Y, Graham M: The evolution and outcome of
     cavitating periventricular leukomalacia in infancy: A study of 46 cases. J Prinatal Med
     1988;16:241–246.
14   Forssberg H: On integrative functions in the cat's spinal cord. Acta Physiol Scand
     1979;474(suppl):1–56.
15   Grillner S, Brodin L, Sigvardt K, Dale N: On the spinal network generating locomotion
     in lamprey: Transmitter, membrane properties and circuitry; in: Grillner S, Stein P,
     Stuart P, Forssberg H, Herman R (eds): Neurobiology of Vertebrate Locomotion.
     Hong Kong, Macmillan Press, 1986, pp 355–352.
16   Thomas A, Autgaerden S: Locomotion from Pre to Post-Natal Life, London, The
     Spastics Society Medical Education Unit/William Heinemann Medical Books, 1966, pp
     1–88.
17   Eidelberg E, Walden JG, Nguyen LH: Locomotor control in macaque monkeys. Brain
     1981;104:647–663.
18   Forssberg H: Ontogeny of human locomotor control. I: Infant stepping, supported
     locomotion and transition to independent locomotion. Exp Brain Res 1985;57:480–493.
19   Okamato T, Goto Y: Human infant pre-independent and independent walking; in:
     Kondo S (ed): Primate Morphophysiology, Locomotion Analyses and Human Bipedal-
     ism. Tokyo, University of Tokyo Press, 1985, pp 25–45.
20   Leonard, CT, Hirschfeld, H, Forssberg, H: The development of independent walking in
     children with cerebral palsy. Dev Med Child Neurol 1991;33:567–577.
21   Myklebust MB, Gottlieb LG, Agarwal CG: Stretch reflexes of the normal infant. Dev
     Med Child Neurol 1986;28:440–449.
22   Leonard CT, Hirschfeld H, Moritani T, Forssberg H: Myotatic reflex development in
     normal children and children with cerebral palsy. Exp Neurol 1991;111:379–382.

Chuck Leonard, PhD, PT, Physical Therapy Department,
University of Montana, Missoula, MT 59812 (USA)

Forssberg H, Hirschfeld H (eds): Movement Disorders in Children.
Med Sport Sci. Basel, Karger, 1992, vol 36, pp 57–64

Morphology of Brain Impairment in Preterm and Term Infants

Olof Flodmark

Department of Neuroradiology, Karolinska Sjukhuset, Stockholm, Sweden

Clinical evaluation of the central nervous system in the neonate is difficult. Cranial imaging has evolved as an important adjunct and has developed in two main directions: computed tomography (CT) and later ultrasonography (US). US has many advantages as the equipment is portable, inexpensive and usually more readily available. The examination can be performed bedside in the incubator. However, the use of US is limited to the first few months of life, and some parts of the brain are poorly visualized. Ultrasonography is operator dependent, thus the quality of the study is intimately related to the skill and experience of the sonologist as well as his/her knowledge of the anatomy and pathology of the neonatal brain. Cranial CT scanning in the premature neonate may provide additional information when US is unsatisfactory and when unusual pathology is encountered. Although ultrasonography may be quite useful, CT, if available, should remain the primary mode of imaging in the term neonate who has suffered hypoxic-ischemic brain damage.

Magnetic resonance imaging (MRI), is now more readily available and has been used to study the pathology and normal development of the neonatal brain. Technical difficulties have so far limited more general use of this technique during the first few weeks of life.

Physiology, Pathophysiology and Pathology

The pattern of cerebral injury in the newborn infant depends on the maturity of the brain at the time of insult. This is due to rapid maturation and changing physiology during the third trimester. Rich vascular supply to the basal ganglia and the germinal matrix characterizes the immature brain. A thin cortex is supplied by numerous small penetrating branches from leptomeningeal vessels with a watershed area between these two vascular territories in the periventricular white matter. Conversely, the vascular anatomy of the brain after 34 weeks of gestation is similar to that of an adult. This evolution of the vascular supply to the maturing brain is the reason why pathology of neonatal hypoxic-ischemic brain injury depends on the maturity of the brain at the time of insult and hence may appear different in term and premature newborns [1]. For the same reason, injury caused by an insult in utero may result in a lesion with characteristics of an injury to the immature brain, i.e. intraventricular hemorrhage or periventricular leukomalacia, despite being seen in a neonate born at term.

Increased cerebral blood flow secondary to damaged cerebral autoregulation is thought to cause *intraventricular hemorrhage* (IVH). Increased blood pressure will lead to increased cerebral perfusion and cause rupture and hemorrhage of the fragile blood vessels in the germinal matrix. The hemorrhage may rupture, usually into the lateral ventricles [1]. The CSF circulation is always compromised as the blood is cleared from the ventricular system, but the development of progressive hydrocephalus requiring permanent shunting is much less common than previously thought [2].

In analogy with the above, hypotension and subsequent hypoperfusion may cause brain damage. Most susceptible to such hypoperfusion is the watershed area in the periventricular white matter, causing *periventricular leukomalacia* (PVL). Lesions occur most commonly close to the trigone and less common adjacent to the frontal horns [3]. In PVL, coagulation necrosis is found initially with subsequent cavitation. These cavities, when small, may collapse and disappear, leading to white matter atrophy and gliosis. Larger cysts may persist and communicate with the lateral ventricles as the ependyma breaks down [4, 5]. PVL is thought to be the pathological substrate of spastic diplegia, a specific form of cerebral palsy most commonly seen in prematurely born children [6]. Episodes of both hypo- and hypertension in the distressed neonate, possibly associated with reperfusion after resuscitation, may cause PVL complicated by secondary hemorrhage and subsequent extensive brain damage. This lesion is usually but not always associated with IVH [7, 8].

As PVL typically is bilateral and more or less symmetrical, a typically unilateral lesion is also seen in the preterm neonate. This lesion is always associated with extensive IVH and is thought to be due to reperfusion following local ischemia in the periventricular white matter caused by the large IVH. Periventricular venous congestion has been suggested. This lesion has been named *hemorrhagic periventricular infarction* and corresponds most closely to the old classification 'grade 4 IVH' [7, 8].

Intracerebral hemorrhage is uncommon in *term neonates* as the germinal matrix is rarely present. If hemorrhage occurs, it is usually due to factors unrelated to asphyxia. Profound and prolonged hypoperfusion with ischemia may lead to cerebral injury in the cortical watershed zones. Diffuse brain injury may occur when the hypoxic-ischemic insult is severe [9]. Cerebral edema is a prominent feature of the pathophysiological process. However, the precise role of cerebral edema in the context of etiology of brain injury is controversial [10].

Permanent damage caused by hypoxic-ischemic brain injury in term neonates is seen as cortical necrosis and large portions of cortex may be replaced by cystic spaces. Central gray matter and cerebellum is usually spared due to redistribution of cerebral blood flow during the gradual onset of hypoxia. Microcephaly associated with severe mental and motor handicap is common in these infants [11]. Other patterns of brain injury can, however, primarily involve the basal ganglia showing gliosis and subsequent severe handicap [2, 12].

Radiology of Neonatal Pathology

The detection of *germinal matrix and intraventricular hemorrhage* is best accomplished by neurosonography [13, 14], which has an excellent sensitivity and specificity for IVH. Although grading systems for IVH exist, there is little reason to use them to grade the amount of intraventricular blood, as there is poor correlation with future outcome [7]. Only posthemorrhagic hydrocephalus can be directly attributed to IVH while future handicap is best related to associated parenchymal damage.

Bilateral, more or less symmetrical parenchymal hemorrhage is presently thought to represent secondary hemorrhage into an area of *periventricular leukomalacia*. This hemorrhage may be a secondary bleed into an ischemic infarction or may represent an extension from the germinal matrix hemorrhage into the ischemic infarction. Such parenchymal hemorrhage is usually combined with IVH, but the lesion can occur in isolation or in the presence of a very small amount of IVH [7].

Extensive IVH may create the necessary scenario for an extensive, usually unilateral hemorrhage (*hemorrhagic periventricular infarction*) into the frontal white matter, the most common location for this form of intraparenchymal bleed but a less common location for PVL [8]. Although many lesions are extensive and carry a poor prognosis, some may be limited in extent or have a more favorable location indicating a better prognosis. Furthermore, US cannot reliably distinguish parenchymal hemorrhage from nonhemorrhagic PVL [15]. Hence, the radiologist must carefully describe the sonographic findings to allow a qualified assessment by the neonatologist in each individual case [16].

Confident diagnosis of *ischemic PVL* is difficult in the newborn. The lesion can readily be found using US when a hemorrhage has complicated the ischemic infarct. This lesion may incorrectly be reported as a grade 4 IVH. PVL without secondary hemorrhage is difficult, unless extensive, to diagnose with US in the neonatal period. Most mild-to-moderate (70 and 45%, respectively) lesions escape detection by any imaging modality during the neonatal period [17, 18], possibly with the exception of MRI. However, the permanent damage caused by PVL can be detected later during infancy by CT or MRI, as both modalities show a typical pattern of atrophy and white matter damage [19–21]. Such damage can be recognized by the characteristic reduction of periventricular white matter with secondary prominence of the deep portions of the Sylvian fissures. Atrophic ventricular dilation and in severe cases large cystic spaces adjacent to the ventricles can occur. These findings have been shown in patients with spastic diplegia, the clinical correlate to PVL. Recent experience with MRI confirms these observations and in addition shows evidence of delayed myelination and gliosis in the remaining periventricular white matter.

It is well documented that CT scanning permits assessment of *hypoxic-ischemic brain injury in term neonates.* Widespread or focal areas of decreased brain tissue attenuation in early CT scans correlate well with adverse neurological outcome [2]. These findings represent cerebral edema developing after hypoxic-ischemic injury with brain tissue attenuation decreasing as the interstitial or intracellular amount of water is increasing. The attenuation of gray matter may approach that of white matter eliminating the distinction between these two tissue types. The brain appears featureless. The edema peaks 72 h following the injury, and this is the ideal time of imaging for prognosis [10]. Even severe edema may have disappeared as early as 5 days after injury. Gradual onset of hypoxia, common in perinatal asphyxia, results in redistribution of regional cerebral blood flow with preferred perfusion of the basal ganglia and cerebellum. Consequently, these structures maintain a more normal attenuation and are clearly visible on the CT image contrasting against the darker background formed by the edematous cerebrum [2, 11].

Focal areas of brain damage and less severe generalized changes may be difficult to evaluate in CT scans during the first few days of life. The findings of prominent but symmetrical areas of low attenuation in the white matter is common and correlates poorly with adverse outcome as long as gray can be distinguished from white matter. Errors in interpretation are common with too much significance attached to findings of prominent white matter. Delayed CT scans at 4–7 weeks of age or later may prove most useful in predicting future handicap in these situations.

Neurosonography can detect cerebral edema secondary to hypoxic brain damage as increased echogenicity. However, this finding is only useful if present as it is very difficult to confidently exclude cerebral edema using sonography.

Severe asphyxia in the term neonate may lead to extensive destruction of brain tissue, i.e. 'multicystic encephalomalacia' in which cystic spaces replace cortical structures. As atrophy progresses, the ventricles dilate [11]. Bright contrast between the relatively normal tissue attenuation in the basal ganglia and low attenuation throughout the rest of the cerebrum may have been mistaken for hemorrhage or even calcifications in the basal ganglia. This very common mistake must be avoided. Confident CT diagnosis of multicystic encephalomalacia depends on careful assessment of brain tissue attenuation. Lesser degrees of atrophy are seen following mild-to-moderate hypoxic-ischemic brain damage. Loss of brain tissue is diffuse and mainly cortical, although axonal degeneration will cause secondary loss of white matter. Associated microcephaly is commonplace, a finding that must be taken into consideration when assessing the degree of atrophy.

Selection of Imaging Modality

Neurosonography and CT scanning remain the primary imaging tools of suspected pathology in the neonatal brain. Both imaging modalities provide similar results but with different sensitivity and limitations depending on the clinical situation. Although the maturity of the neonate and suspected pathology should dictate the choice of imaging modality, other factors come into play and may influence the choice in a sometimes irrelevant way.

Availability of a certain imaging modality is the most important reason to choose a certain mode of investigation. Sonographic equipment of high quality is available in most departments of pediatric radiology. Hence, the radiologists are skilled in the use of this modality. However, accurate interpretation of the study, particularly neurosonography, is possible only if the radiologist has a good understanding of the normal anatomy, pathophysiology and pathology of the neonatal brain. Unless the radiologist is familiar with the limitations of the modality, the results, particularly if negative, are of limited value. The nature of the neurosonographic study is such that a review of the images is of limited value, thus the report of the sonologist is extremely important, but also of limited value if the sonologist is less experienced and skilled. Consequently, positive findings are useful, while the method has limited value in excluding certain types of pathology. This is particularly important in attempting to diagnose cerebral edema in the term newborn. The sensitivity for even severe edema is relatively low and neurosonography should not be relied upon to exclude this pathology [2].

Although CT scanning may not be as readily available as sonography as well as more invasive and cumbersome, the modality has and should maintain an important role in assessing the asphyxiated term newborn. The images are less operator dependent. Accurate interpretation may be as difficult as with neurosonography but the images can be reviewed and reassessed at any time, providing the opportunity for expert evaluation [2]. The role of MRI in the evaluation of the neonatal brain is not yet defined. However, specially designed software and modifications to the magnets and receiver coils may make MRI the preferred imaging modality in some situations [22, 23].

Pathology as an Indicator of Maturity at the Time of Injury

Morphology of a destructive lesion to the brain is more dependent on the stage of maturation at which the injury occurred, than the type of injury. The important difference between the circulatory physiology of the immature brain before and after 34 weeks of gestation has been discussed previously. This difference in the cerebral vascular supply is thought to explain the occurrence of central atrophy (PVL) in the immature brain, as opposed to predominantly peripheral cortical damage with multicystic encephalomalacia in the mature brain, at or near term. It has been shown that assessing the morphology of end-stage cerebral damage and postulating the most likely stage of maturation at the time of injury can be supported by, and complement, clinical assessment [24, 25]. This is not only true for damage between 24 and 34 weeks of gestation as opposed to damage after 34 weeks, but also when cerebral imaging can confirm the presence of a congenital malformation, indicating an injury well before 20 weeks of gestation. Hence, it is possible to state, within limits, at which time in the course of a pregnancy, a cerebral lesion most likely occurred [25].

The implications of this concept are far reaching, particularly in the context of liability suits suggesting that negligence by an obstetrician or perinatologist has caused damage. Radiographic evaluation of the brain, using CT scanning and above all MRI, may provide important evidence, often much more solid and objective, than possible by evaluation of clinical records. Combining the two can often settle a dispute with confidence.

References

1   Pape KE, Wigglesworth JS: Haemorrhage, ischaemia and the perinatal brain. Philadelphia, Lippincott, 1979.
2   Flodmark O: The neonatal brain; in: Syllabus: A Categorical Course in Diagnostic Radiology-Neuroradiology. Oak Brook, The Radiological Society of North America, 1987, pp 43–54.
3   Shuman RM, Selednik LJ: Periventricular leukomalacia: A one-year autopsy study, Arch Neurol 1980;37:231–235.
4   Banker BQ, Larroche JC: Periventricular leukomalacia of infancy. Arch Neurol 1962;7:386–410.
5   DeReuck J, Chatta AS, Richardson EP Jr: Pathogenesis and evolution of periventricular leukomalacia in infancy. Arch Neurol 1972;27:229–236.
6   Volpe JJ: Brain injury in the premature infant: Is it preventable? Pediatr Res 1990;27(suppl):28–33.
7   Volpe JJ: Intraventricular hemorrhage in the premature infant. Current concepts, part I. Ann Neurol 1989;25:3–11.
8   Volpe JJ: Intraventricular hemorrhage in the premature infant. Current concepts, part II. Ann Neurol 1989;25:109–116.
9   Hill A, Volpe JJ: Pathogenesis and management of hypoxic-ischemic encephalopathy in the term newborn. Neurol Clin 1985;3:31–34.
10 Lupton BA, Hill A, Roland EH, Whitfield MF, Flodmark O: Brain swelling in the asphyxiated term newborn: Pathogenesis and outcome. Pediatrics 1988;82:139–146.
11 Naidich TP, Chakera TMH: Multicystic encephalomalacia: CT appearance and pathological correlation. J Comput Assist Tomogr 1984;8:631–636.
12 Roland EH, Hill A, Norman MG, Flodmark O, McNab A: Selective brainstem injury in an asphyxiated newborn. Ann Neurol 1988;23:89–92.
13 Bowerman RA, Donn SM, Silver TM, Jaffe MH: Natural history of neonatal periventricular/intraventricular hemorrhage and its complications: Sonographic observations. AJNR 1984;5:527–538.
14 Kirks DR, Bowie JD: Cranial ultrasonography of neonatal periventricular/intraventricular hemorrhage: Who, how, why and when? Pediatr Radiol 1986;16:114–119.
15 Chow PP, Horgan JG, Taylor KJW: Neonatal periventricular leukomalacia: Real-time sonographic diagnosis with CT correlation. AJNR 1985;6:383–388.
16 Guzzetta F, Shackelford GD, Volpe S, Perlman JM, Volpe JJ: Periventricular intraparenchymal echodensities in the premature newborn: Critical determinant of neurologic outcome. Pediatrics 1986;78:995–1006.
17 Flodmark O, Poskitt KJ, Whitfield MF, Roland EH, Hill A: Inability of neurosonography to diagnose periventricular leukomalacia (PVL). 27th Ann Meet Am Soc Neuroradiology, Orlando, March 19–24, 1989. AJNR 1989;10:891.
18 Hope PL, Gould SJ, Howard S, Hamilton PA, Castello AM de L, Reynolds EOR: Precision of ultrasound diagnosis of pathologically verified lesions in the brains of very preterm infants. Dev Med Child Neurol 1988;30:457–471.
19 Flodmark O, Roland EH, Hill A, Whitfield MF: Periventricular leukomalacia: Radiologic diagnosis. Radiology 1987;162:119–124.
20 Flodmark O, Lupton B, Li D, Stimac GK, Roland EH, Hill A, Whitfield MF, Norman MG: Magnetic resonance imaging of periventricular leukomalacia (PVL) in childhood. AJNR 1989;10:111–118.
21 Wilson DA, Steiner RE: Periventricular leukomalacia: Evaluation with MR imaging. Radiology 1986;160:507–511.

22 McArdle CB, Richardson CJ, Hayden CK, Nicholas DA, Crofford MJ, Amparo EG: Abnormalities of the neonatal brain: MR imaging. I. Intracranial hemorrhage. Radiology 1987;163:387–394.

23 McArdle CB, Richardson CJ, Hayden CK, Nicholas DA, Amparo EG: Abnormalities of the neonatal brain: MR imaging. II. Hypoxic-ischemic brain injury. Radiology 1987;163:395–403.

24 Wiklund L-M, Uvebrant P, Flodmark O: Morphology of cerebral lesions in children with congenital hemiplegia: A study with computed tomography. Neuroradiology 1990;32:179–186.

25 Wiklund L-M, Uvebrant P, Flodmark O: Computed tomography as an adjunct in etiological analysis of hemiplegic cerebral palsy. II. Children born at term. Neuropaediatrics, in press.

Olof Flodmark, MD, PhD, FRCPC, Department of Neuroradiology, Karolinska Sjukhuset, S–104 01 Stockholm (Sweden)

Forssberg H, Hirschfeld H (eds): Movement Disorders in Children.
Med Sport Sci. Basel, Karger, 1992, vol 36, pp 65–71

CNS Morbidity in Preterm Infants[1]

Miriam Katz-Salamon

Department of Pediatrics, Karolinska Hospital, Stockholm, Sweden

The last three decades' development in neonatal intensive care together with the increased knowledge in neonatal physiology have been credited with the significant decline in mortality of very low birth weight infants (birth weight ≤1,500 g). From the early 1950s to the late 1980s the survival rate in these children increased from 28 to 70% (fig. 1). The most substantial improvement of the 1980s over the late 1960s is in the 750–1,000 g birth weight group. Today even those infants have about 70% chance of survival. The survival of infants weighing 500–750 g increased from 21% in 1981–1982 to more than 50% in 1986–1987 [1, 2]. The crucial question is whether the decrease in mortality among very low birth weight infants has been followed by a similar reduction in sequelae. Knobloch et al. [3] found that the incidence of major handicaps among infants with the birth weight of 1,000–1,500 g born in 1952 and 1965–1980 was 48 and 17%, respectively.

The survey comprising developed countries [4] showed a high prevalence of major handicaps among very low birth weight infants until 1960. Since then the prevalence has remained stable and relatively low at 6–8% of livebirths (fig. 2). However, the last decades epidemiological panorama of cerebral palsy (CP) in Sweden [5] has shown a different trend: the decreasing incidence of CP among preterm infants born during the 1950s and 1960s has been replaced by an increase.

Follow-up Studies on Preterm Born Infants

We have a scanty knowledge regarding the neurobiological basis of the development of a very preterm born infant. The need to gain knowledge

[1] The Swedish follow-up study on CNS-morbidity in very preterm infants was supported by the grants from The Bank of Sweden Tercentenary Foundation.

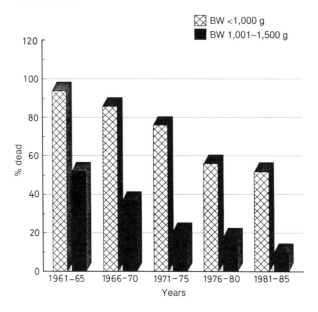

Fig. 1. Morbidity trends in infants with birthweight ≤1,500 g [based on Ehrenhaft et al., 1].

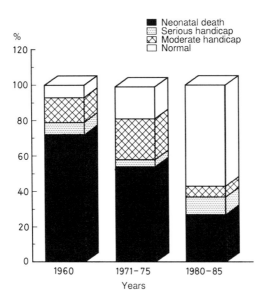

Fig. 2. Changing prognosis of very low birthweight infants [based on Ehrenhaft et al., 1].

about growth and development of very low birth weight infants together with the need for evaluation of the survival rate and morbidity is mirrored in an impressing amount of follow-up studies.

It is agreed that severe sensory-motor handicaps can be recognized before one year of age. However the full extent of less serious impairments cannot be assessed before the age of 6–7 years when learning difficulties become apparent [6, 7]. Thus, the follow-up studies cover the neonatal period, the first 2 years of life (short-term follow-up) and extend until the school age (long-term follow-up).

Neurodevelopmental Disabilities

The pathophysiology of brain impairment in preterm infants is dealt with more in detail in the article above [Flodmark, this issue].

Generally, the most critical determinant of neurological outcome is defined by the *maturity* of the brain at the time of the insult and by the *degree* and *site* of parenchymal injury [8, and Flodmark, this issue]. The adequate development of the preterm brain is jeopardized by a number of factors such as hypoxia/asphyxia, brain hemorrhage, infarctions, infections and hypoglycemia.

The neurological sequelae among very low birth weight infants include: (a) cerebral palsy (spastic diplegia, spastic quadriplegia, spastic hemiplegia, ataxia); (b) epilepsy; (c) visual defects; (d) sensorineural-hearing defect; (e) mental retardation; (f) dysfunction of motor skills, attention and perception; (g) clumsiness; (h) specific learning disorders; (i) attention deficit, and (j) hyperkinesia.

Definition of Handicap

The neurological sequelae of very preterm birth are described as *serious*, *moderate* and *minor* handicaps. In general, a *serious* handicap would prevent a child from attending a normal school, and would include severe cerebral palsy (spastic quadriplegia), visual defect, sensorineural-hearing defect, severe mental retardation and major seizures. A *moderate* handicap is mainly described by an intelligence quotient between 70 and 80 with or without cerebral palsy (diplegia). *Minor* impairment is more difficult to define since it includes many problems which border on normality, such as disturbances in motor skills, perception and attention, clumsiness, specific learning difficulties and hyperkinesia.

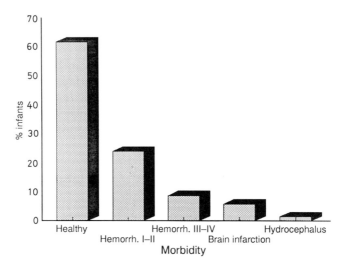

Fig. 3. CNS neonatal morbidity in 138 infants with a birth weight ≤ 1,500 g treated at NICU Karolinska Hospital 1988–1990.

Short-Term Morbidity – Incidence of Brain Impairment

The risk for periventricular and intraventricular hemorrhage is directly correlated to the degree of prematurity [Flodmark, this issue]. Several studies conducted to date have suggested that the neurodevelopmental risk associated with prematurity is concentrated in the subgroup of infants with severe brain hemorrhage. Severe brain hemorrhage range from 100% in infants born at the 24th week of gestation to 7% in those born at the 29th [9]. Other studies have presented a 40% prevalence of peri- and intraventricular hemorrhage in infants with a birth weight below 1,500 g and about 60% in infants born before 28 weeks of gestation [10, 11]. Figure 3 provides the analysis of brain impairment in infants with the birth weight ≤ 1,500 g from the Swedish follow-up study on CNS sequelae in very low birth weight infants [unpubl. data, study in progress]. The majority of these infants (62%) had an uneventful neonatal period, while the prevalence of serious neurological sequelae was 17% (brain hemorrhage grade III–IV, brain infarction, hydrocephalus).

The appearances of cavitating periventricular leukomalacia and subsequent neurodevelopmental and neurological deficits has its highest incidence at and below 27 weeks of gestation and occurs in 15% of these infants [8]. Yet, follow-up studies of preterm infants have indicated repetitively that some preterm children without any evidence of either intraventricular hemorrhage or ventricular enlargement have neurological sequelae while others, with these pathological signs, are free from neurological symptoms [12–14].

Since the survival rate for the smallest premature infants increases, brain hemorrhage will continue to be a major problem in neonatal intensive care.

Long-Term Morbidity

Severe Impairment

The incidence of *severe* handicap increases significantly with decreasing birth weight and gestational age.

The long-term follow-up investigations of the effect of low birth weight on mental and physical development performed before 1965 [15, 16] reported a 20–50% incidence of major neurological handicaps. Studies from North America, Switzerland and Australia showed major handicap rates of 10–30% in very low birth weight infants born between 1970 and 1981. The prevalence of such a handicap in infants under 1,000 g was usually 20–35%. According to Ehrenhaft et al. [1], 41% of infants with birth weight below 800 g had either severe or moderate handicap whereas only 16% of the infants with birth weight between 1,000 and 1,500 g were seriously disabled.

The epidemiological panorama of cerebral palsy over the last 40 years underwent big changes. In Sweden, Hagberg et al. [5] demonstrated an almost 40% fall in the rate of CP, specially spastic and ataxic diplegia, during the years 1954 to 1970. Similar results were published in a British study in 1975 [18]. However, since 1970 there has been an almost constant increase in the prevalence of CP [19]. As a consequence, in the beginning of the 1980s, the rate of CP reached levels observed during the 1950s. The increase in CP is explained by the fourfold increase in survival of very low birth weight infants. However, several other recent studies have shown that the large reduction in mortality is associated with only a small increase in sequelae in quantitative and qualitative terms. Furthermore, these studies provide reassurance that increased survival is accompanied by an increased proportion of survivors considered to be free from neurosensory handicaps.

Mild Impairment

The mild neurological abnormalities encompass motor, sensory, cognitive and emotional spheres. Disabilities in attention, motor control, and perception, so-called *DAMP*, proved to be the most common neurological sequelae among very low birth weight infants at the age of 6.5 years. A follow-up study done in Vancouver [20] revealed the increasing frequency of mild neurological defects at successive age levels among infants born preterm. This was mainly due to the emergence of behavioral and learning difficulties after the age of 2.5 years. The lowest rate of subsequent abnormality was among children without any neonatal abnormal sign. The persistence of abnormal neurological findings through the newborn period indicated the highest probability of abnormality at 1 year of age. Infants with only early or late abnormal neurological signs were in an intermediate position. According to the authors the neurological findings under the neonatal period have a considerable prognostic significance for later neurological and intellectual development.

Follow-up studies performed during the 1950s and 1960s [21] have shown that even preterm children with relatively high birth weight (2,000–2,500 g) were liable to have learning problems in school. Bjerre [22] diagnosed disturbances in attention, motor control and perception in 9.4% of low birth weight children at 5 years of age. Forslund and Bjerre [23] revealed a delayed neurological maturation and mild dysfunction in 18% of preterm infants at 4 years of age as compared with 6.5% in full-term infants. Thus, the described disturbances in perceptual-motor skills and behavioral problems are the most common neurological sequel of low birth weight infants.

Conclusions

One important and challenging issue in pediatrics of today concerns the development of motor skills, perceptive functions, learning capabilities, memory and social behavior in very low birth weight infants. With improved knowledge based on the results from the follow-up studies it has become possible to compensate for some of the effects associated with very preterm birth. To quote from the Lancet [6]: '. . . the leading neonatal units are providing invaluable lessons in the improved care and understanding of preterm babies.'

References

1   Ehrenhaft PM, Wagner JL, Herdman RC: Changing prognosis for very low birth weight infants. Obstet Gynecol 1989;74:528–535.
2   Ferrara TB, Hoekstra RE, Gaziano M, Knox GE, Couser RJ, Fangman JJ: Changing outcome of extremely premature infants (≤26 weeks' gestation and ≤750 gm): Survival and follow-up at a tertiary center. Am J Obstet Gynecol 1989;161:1114–1118.
3   Knobloch H, Malone A, Ellison PH, Stevens F, Zdeb M: Considerations in evaluating

changes in outcome for infants weighing less than 1501 grams. Pediatrics 1982;69:285–295.

4   Stewart AL, Lipscomb AP: Outcome for infants of very low birthweight: survey of world literature. Lancet 1981;i:1038–1041.
5   Hagberg B, Hagberg G, Olow I: The changing panorama of cerebral palsy in Sweden 1954–1970. I. Analysis of the general changes. Acta Paediatr Scand 1975;64:187–192.
6   Anonymous: Editorial article: The fate of the baby under 1501 g at birth. Lancet 1980;i:461–463.
7   Drillen CM: Fresh approaches to prospective studies of high risk infants. Pediatrics 1970;45:7–10.
8   Volpe JJ: Intraventricular hemorrhage in the premature infant–current concepts. Part II. Ann Neurol 1989;25:109–116.
9   Shortland D, Levene MI, Trounce J, Ng Y, Graham M: The evolution and outcome of cavitating periventricular leukomalacia in infancy. A study of 46 cases. J Perinat Med 1988;16:241–247.
10   Wood B, Katz V, Bose C, Goolsby R, Kraybill E: Survival and morbidity of extremely premature infants based on obstetric assessment of gestational age. Obstet Gynecol 1989;74:889–892.
11   Papile LA, Burstein J, Burstein R, Koffler H: Incidence and evolution of subependymal and intraventricular hemorrhage: A study of infants with birth weights less than 1,500 g. J Pediatr 1978;92:529–534.
12   Catto-Smith AG, Yu VYH, Bajuk B, Orgill AA, Astbury J: Effect of neonatal periventricular hemorrhage on neurodevelopmental outcome. Arch Dis Child 1985;60:8–11.
13   Thorburn RJ, Lipsconit AP, Stewart AL: Prediction of death and major handicap in very preterm infants by brain ultrasound. Lancet 1981;i:119.
14   Ment LR, Scott RA, Ehrenkrantz RA: Neonates of ≤1,250 gm birthweight: Prospective neurodevelopmental evaluation during the first year post-term. Pediatrics 1982;70:292–294.
15   Sninnar S, Molteni RA, Gammon K: Intraventricular hemorrhage in the premature infant: A changing outlook. N Engl J Med 1982;306:1464–1467.
16   Benton AL: Mental development of prematurely born children. A critical review of the literature. Am J Orthopsychiatry 1940;10:719–746.
17   Mercer HP, Lancaster PAL, Weiner T, Gupta JM: Very low birthweight infants: a follow-up study. Med J Aust 1978;2:581–584.
18   Davies DP, Tizard JPM. Very low birthweight and subsequent neurological defect (with special reference to spastic diplegia). Dev Med Child Neurol 1975;17:3–17.
19   Hagberg B, Hagberg G, Olow I, IV: The changing panorama of Cerebral Palsy in Sweden. Epidemiological trends 1959–78. Acta Pediatr Scand 1984;73:433–440.
20   Dunn G, Ho HH, Schultzer M: Minimal brain dysfunction; in: Dunn HG (ed): Sequelae of Low Birthweight: A Vancouver Study. 1986, pp 97–114.
21   Drillen CM: Fresh approaches to prospective studies of high risk infants. Pediatrics 1970;45:7.
22   Bjerre I: Neurological investigation of 5-year-old children with low birthweight. Acta Paediatr Scand 1975;64:859–864.
23   Forslund M, Bjerre I: Follow-up of preterm children. I. Neurological assessment at 4 years of age. Early Human Development 1989;20:45–66.

Dr. Miriam Katz-Salamon, Neonatal and Reproduction Laboratory C4 U1,
Department of Pediatrics, Karolinska Hospital, S–104 01 Stockholm (Sweden)

Forssberg H, Hirschfeld H (eds): Movement Disorders in Children.
Med Sport Sci. Basel, Karger, 1992, vol 36, pp 72–79

Early Motor Assessment in Brain-Damaged Preterm Infants

Giovanni Cioni[a], *Fabrizio Ferrari*[b], *Heinz F.R. Prechtl*[c]

[a]Institute of Child Neurology and Psychiatry, University of Pisa and Stella Maris
Foundation, Pisa; [b]Institute of Pediatrics and Neonatal Medicine,
University of Modena, Italy; [c]Department of Developmental Neurology,
University of Groningen, The Netherlands

Preterm infants, born with a very low birth weight, are the neonates at the highest risk for developing a cerebral palsy. Intracranial haemorrhage and especially ischaemic lesions (periventricular leukomacia) are the major cause of motor impairment. These lesions can be identified during the early postnatal period by means of sophisticated and sensitive brain imaging techniques (ultrasounds, CT, MRI). Recent literature on early brain damage [1] has largely documented advantages and limitations of these instruments. On the other hand, few studies have described the early motor behaviour of preterm infants with documented brain lesions.

Neonatal functional assessment is generally carried out by means of classic neurological examination, largely based on muscle tone and elicited responses. This approach has several limitations. The methods of the currently employed examination in newborns and young infants are often strongly influenced by outdated models of brain development and pathology, based on adult neurology and experimental brain lesions. Examples of this can be found in the French neurological examination for the newborn [2], or in Vojta's [3] approach. According to the latter, the infant brain is considered a bulk of 'reflexes', a term which may be appropriate for knee or ankle jerks, but not for the complexity of infant motor repertoire [4].

On a clinical point of view, the most largely applied neurological protocols [5, 6] include items which cannot be used for fragile and preterm infants, who are often intubated and monitored. The assessment is generally carried out only when the infant reaches term age. Longitudinal studies have shown that the diagnostic and especially prognostic value of these methods is limited. At term age preterm infants with brain lesions may show motor abnormalities which gradually normalize in the first months of life. On the contrary, neurological assessment may be transiently falsely negative around term age [7].

New methods of CNS functional assessment, suitable for application even in very immature preterm infants and more reliable for the prognosis, are badly needed. However, to be really useful they have to fulfil a series of basic requirements clearly indicated by Prechtl [8]. They have to include items strictly related to the age-specific repertoire of the CNS, which changes very rapidly during the different pre and early post-natal periods. Moreover, not all the age-specific functions of fetal and neonatal repertoire are suitable for clinical assessment. Diagnostic tools have to be non-invasive, and non-time-consuming. Both conditions are needed to allow repeated observations particularly of newborns in intensive care units. In addition to that, the reliability and prognostic value of these methods have to be carefully tested. Fulfilling the previous conditions, new methods of functional evaluation of the newborns may help in understanding the possible consequences of brain lesions, detected by brain imaging techniques.

Observation of Spontaneous Motility

In several reports, summarized in a recent paper, Prechtl [8] has proposed a new approach to clinical evaluation of fetal and neonatal motility. Endogenously generated motor activity was selected as an observation criterion for the newborn and also for the fetus. The rational for this choice derives from several considerations. In animal embryos autogenetic (spontaneous) activity precedes reflexogenetic activity [9] and it seems to be true also for human fetuses [10]. As from the beginning this activity is very complex, consisting of several movement patterns. Moreover, there are indications that spontaneous activity is more sensitive to adverse conditions than the reactivity to sensory stimuli [8].

By means of on-line observation and replay of long duration video recordings of fetuses and newborns, a comprehensive list of fetal and neonatal spontaneous movement patterns has been provided. It includes more global movements, as general movements, startles or stretches, and isolated arm or leg movements, twitches, etc. The temporal sequence of their emergence during the first months of gestation and their rate of occurence at various gestational ages have been carefully described in healthy fetuses [10], in low-risk preterm infants [11, 12] and in normal full-term infants [13]. These data are a major contribution to the understanding of early motor development and they represent the necessary sound base for the study of abnormal individuals.

Quantification of the movement patterns (i.e. their median rate and quartiles for a given time) were provided for fetuses, preterm and fullterm infants at various ages. The data revealed different trends in the developmental course of the movements, but also a high difference between individual at a particular age, and a low intraindividual consistency from week to week. This held true for fetuses [14], preterm [11, 12] and full-term infants [13] and indicates that quantitative assessment of motility is unlikely to be a good indicator of fetal or neonatal condition.

This has been shown by Prechtl and Nolte [15], who compared the motor behaviour of high- and low-risk preterm infants in their first weeks of life. The quantification of several movement patterns was carried out via 1-min epoch analysis, by direct observation. The differences in the incidence of the movement patterns between the two groups of subjects were minimal.

The limited diagnostic value of quantitative assessment of spontaneous motility in preterm infants was confirmed in a more recent study by Ferrari et al. [16]. Twenty-nine preterm infants with brain lesions documented by imaging techniques, and 14 low-risk infants were video-recorded weekly in the supine position for 1 h from birth to discharge from the hospital, and afterward at longer intervals until the 5th month of corrected age. Incidence and duration of the different movement patterns were assessed during replay of the video recordings. A large interindividual variability and no significant differences between the two groups were confirmed, with the exception of a lower incidence of isolated arm movements and a higher one of tremors in the brain-damaged infants.

Qualitative Assessment of General Movements

In the same study by Ferrari et al. [16] another aspect of spontaneous motility, i.e. the quality of execution of general movements (GMs), was suggested as a better indicator of infant neurological status.

GMs are global and complex movements, involving the whole body, usually lasting from a few seconds to a minute. In normal newborns they are variable in sequence of arm, leg, neck and trunk movements; they wax and wane in intensity, force and speed.

Confirming previous indications by Prechtl and Nolte [15], Ferrari et al. [16] have observed that GMs of the abnormal preterm infants were slow and monotonous, or brisk and chaotic, with a marked reduction of subtle fluctations in amplitude, force and speed. Visual gestalt perception is a powerful instrument to detect these alterations in the complexity of the movement. From the videos of each observation of low-risk and brain-

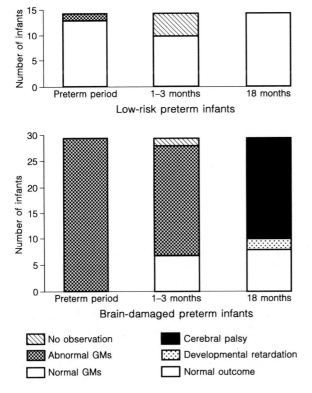

Fig. 1. General movement (GM) quality assessment in the preterm period and 1–3 months of corrected age, and neurological outcome in 14 low-risk and 29 brain-damaged preterm infants. Data from Ferrari et al. [16].

damaged infants, a global impressionist judgement of normal or abnormal motor quality was achieved by the observers, not knowing the history of the infants. The assessment was based on the complexity, fluency, elegance and variability of the GMs. The results of longitudinal observation of the movement quality were compared with the neurological outcome at 18 months.

As reported in figure 1, the movements of low-risk preterms were all judged as normal, with the exception of one infant who showed transient abnormalities in the weeks immediately after birth. In the post-term period they were all normal and so was the neurological outcome. On the contrary, none of the 29 preterm infants with brain lesions (intraventricular haemorrhage and/or periventricular leukomalacia) showed normal movements during the preterm period. In the first weeks after term, 1 infant was not observed, 7 gradually normalized; they had a normal neurological outcome except for one who was judged normal for the GMs at 15 weeks post-term, but later showed a mild monoplegia. Of the 21 infants whose movements were still abnormal at 3 months of corrected age, 19 showed a cerebral palsy (2 monoplegia, 3 hemiplegia, 5 diplegia and 9 tetraplegia), 2 were developmentally retarded and only 1 normalized.

These results indicate a high correlation between early motor assessment, by means of observation of spontaneous motility, and presence of a brain lesion, detected by neuroimaging techniques. When still in the incubator, very consistently during the preterm period, brain-damaged infants show abnormalities in the quality of their movements which are not observable in low-risk infants. These data contrast with the opinion, reported in literature, that after the acute phase newborns with brain lesions be neurologically (silent) and appear normal.

Ferrari et al. [16] have also compared the prognostic value of the quality assessment of motility with the results of a classical neurological examination carried out at term age. In 9 infants with a poor outcome (cerebral palsy), the neurological examination was transiently normal at that age, whereas GMs quality was abnormal. This is probably due to the change of muscle tone from preterm hypotonia to post-term hypertonia. Neural mechanisms of GMs are more complex that those involved in the tonus or in the other responses of the neurological examination. This probably accounts for the different results.

Because of its sensitivity to brain lesions, this technique reveals abnormalities in the movement which not necessarily indicate a severe and permanent motor impairment. In Ferrari's study, about one-third of the infants with abnormal GMs in the first period of life gradually normalized.

If the infants are grouped according to the type of GM abnormality the evaluation increases in specificity. Two main abnormal characters of the movements were described: '*poor repertoire*', when the sequence of successive movement components is monotonous and the movements of the different body parts do not occur in the rich sequence observable in normal GMs; '*cramped-synchronized*', when GMs look rigid, they have not the normal smooth writhing character and all limb muscles contract simultaneously.

The 29 infants with brain lesions were classified according to their movement character; their changes during the preterm and postterm periods were also reported (developmental motor trajectories).

Twenty infants showed cramped-synchronized GMs, often since their first observation in the incubator; 19 of them developed a cerebral palsy and one a developmental retardation. Other 9 infants had a poor repertoire

Case 3

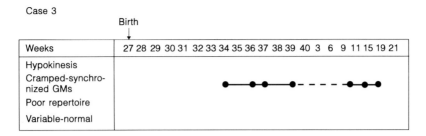

Case 14

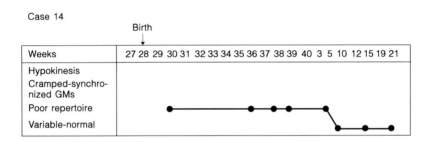

Fig. 2. Developmental trajectories of general movements during preterm and post-term periods in 2 infants from the study by Ferrari et al. [16]: case 3 (spastic tetraplegia) and case 14 (normalized at 10 weeks post-term, normal outcome).

during the preterm period; 8 of them became neurologically normal between 1 and 3 months after term age; one was mentally retarded but without a motor impairment. Two representative cases of these trajectories are reported in figure 2.

Conclusions

A new approach for motor assessment in the newborns is now available, based on the observation of spontaneous motility. This approach takes into account new concepts about the newborn, who is definitively not a bulk of reflexes, but a very complex organism, producing a great deal of movements, both spontaneously generated and elicited by external stimuli.

On a clinical point of view, the assessment of spontaneous movements and of its quality seems to fulfil all the conditions indicated by Prechtl [8]. It is not invasive: even fragile preterm infants still in the incubator can be repetitively evaluated. The results of this assessment correlate very well with the presence of brain lesions, detected by US, CT or MRI, and also with the classical neurological examination, when it can be performed.

The correlation with the outcome is also very high, especially when the results of repeated evaluations and the type of GMs abnormality are taken into account (developmental trajectories).

The observation of infant motility from videotapes is preferable to direct scoring. It is quicker, it permits retesting of the same infant, a full appreciation of the subtle qualities of the movements, data storing and also reliability tests. In fact, this approach based on gestalt perception could be considered as subjective. On the contrary, when the reliability of this evaluation was checked for preterm infants, the interobserver agreement was found to be very high [8]. This technique can be easily learned by persons used to observing newborns and small infants, such as neonatologists, paediatricians and physiotherapists.

Further studies are suitable in order to establish all the potentials of this approach for early diagnosis and prognosis of motor impairment.

References

1 de Vries LS, Dubowitz LMS, Dubowitz V, Pennock FM: Brain Disorders in the Newborn. London, Wolfe, 1990.
2 Saint-Anne Dargassies S: Neurological Development in the Fullterm and Premature infant. Amsterdam, Elsevier, 1977.
3 Vojta V: Die Cerebrale Bewegungsstörungen in Säuglingsalter: Frühdiagnose und Frühtherapie. Enke, Stuttgart, 1974.
4 Touwen BCL: Primitive reflexes: conceptional or semantic problem? In Prechtl HFR (ed): Continuity of Neural Functions from Prenatal to Postnatal Life. Oxford, Blackwell, 1984, CDM No 94, pp 115–125.
5 Dubowitz LMS, Dubowitz V: The Neurological Assessment of the Preterm and Fullterm Newborn Infant. London, Heinemann, 1982, CDM No 79.
6 Prechtl HFR: The Neurological Examination of the Fullterm Newborn Infant, ed 2. London, Heinemann, 1977, CDM No 63.
7 Dubowitz LMS: Clinical assessment of the infant nervous system; in Levene MI, Bennet MJ, Punt J (eds): Fetal and Neonatal Neurology and Neurosurgery. Edinburgh, Churchill Livingstone, 1988, pp 41–58.
8 Prechtl HFR: Qualitative changes of spontaneous movements in preterm infants are a marker of neurological dysfunction. Early Human Dev 1990;23:151–158.
9 Hall WG, Oppenheim RW: Developmental psychobiology: Prenatal, perinatal and early postnatal aspects of behavioural development. Ann Rev Psychol 1987;38:91–128.
10 de Vries JIP, Visser GHA, Prechtl HFR: The emergence of fetal behaviour. 1. Qualitative aspects. Early Hum Dev 1982;7:301–322.
11 Prechtl HFR, Fargel JW, Weinmann HM, Bakker HH: Posture, motility and respiration of low-risk preterm infants. Dev Med Child Neurol 1979;21:3–27.
12 Cioni G, Prechtl HFR: Preterm and early postterm motor behaviour in low risk premature infants. Early Human Dev 1990;23:159–191.

13 Cioni G, Ferrari F, Prechtl HFR: Posture and spontaneous motility in fullterm infants. Early Human Dev 1989;18:247–262.

14 de Vries JIP, Visser GHA, Prechtl HFR: The emergence of fetal behaviour. III: Individual differences and consistences. Early Hum Dev 1988;16:85–103.

15 Prechtl HFR, Nolte R: Motor behaviour in preterm infants; in Prechtl HFR (ed): Continuity of Neural Functions from Prenatal to Postnatal Life. Oxford, Blackwell, 1984, CDM No 94, pp 79–82.

16 Ferrari F, Cioni G, Prechtl HFR: Qualitative changes of general movements in preterm infants with brain lesions. Early Human Dev 1990;23:193–231.

Giovanni Cioni, MD, Institute of Child Neurology and Psychiatry,
University of Pisa and Stella Maris Foundation,
I–56018 Calambrone Pisa (Italy)

Forssberg H, Hirschfeld H (eds): Movement Disorders in Children.
Med Sport Sci. Basel, Karger, 1992, vol 36, pp 80–85

Early Detection of Cerebral Motor Disorders

Elizabeth Köng

Cerebral Palsy Centre, University Children's Hospital, Bern, Switzerland

Patterns in cerebral palsy have changed over the years. The classical pictures of spastics and athetoids have practically disappeared in a considerable part of the western countries. This is due to improved prenatal care, to optimal obstetrics and to intensive neonatal care (primary prevention), also to the teamwork between obstetrics, neonatology and developmental pediatrics, as well as to the advances in early therapy and educational measures (secondary prevention).

Today, a relatively small number of severe multiple handicaps (due to increasing survival of more severely damaged children) remain together with many slight and minimal handicaps.

Severe handicaps are obvious. Early detection of slight cerebral motor disorders is more difficult. It is especially important not to overlook these, because, with early therapy, many of them will have the chance of a practically normal life together with a normal appearance. The abnormal coordination of postures and movements increases only gradually, becomes more dominant and finally obligatory, usually towards the end of the first year of life. Only at this time can we make a definite diagnosis.

Early detection is important due to therapeutic reasons. Therapy is much less effective, when abnormal movement patterns are already habitual. A child may still be able to learn to sit up, to stand up and to walk, but in an abnormal way. Therefore we must start therapy before the diagnosis is definite. We then have a better chance of inhibiting abnormal movement patterns before they have become habitual; this will allow us to facilitate and to build by repetition more normal basic movement patterns (this, if the brain lesion is not too extensive, i.e. causing severe mental retardation and/or severe perceptual problems).

Why Early Diagnosis Is so Difficult?

Slight Brain Lesions May Be Spontaneously Compensated

Many newborns, e.g. after a brain hemorrhage or an asphyxia (so-called risk newborns), show some abnormal neurological symptoms immediately postnatally during the very first months of life. Mostly, these symptoms disappear gradually without any therapeutic measures (transitory symptoms). The central nervous system has a great capability for recovery. The remaining question is therefore, in which cases will the abnormal symptoms disappear spontaneously and in which cases will there be a development towards cerebral palsy. There are not as yet any secure criteria for this.

Dissociated Maturation May Simulate Cerebral Palsy [1, 2]

In these babies, milestones for fine motor development appear at the expected age, while gross motor skills are markedly delayed, especially standing and walking, but without abnormal movement patterns.

There Is a Great Variability of Normal Development

(a) Due to *environmental influences*: (i) Different types of daily handling. Examples: Babies nursed only in the supine position have reduced opportunities for the development of head control, support on elbows and hands, extension and abduction of legs, as developed in the prone position. Babies nursed only in the prone position will develop these functions earlier, but they are often delayed in playing with their feet and may start walking with a Charlie Chaplin gait, especially if they are slightly hypotonic. (ii) Intercurrent illnesses often cause a stand-still in development with transitory hypotonia. These symptoms have disappeared 1–2 weeks after recovery.

(b) Due to *innate genetic differences*, as described by Touwen [3–5] in his study of so-called optimal babies (normal pregnancy, normal delivery, normal neonatal period). He could show that there is a striking variability not only in reaching milestones, but also in the decrease and disappearance of the influence of primitive and tonic reflexes and the development of righting and equilibrium reactions. The beginning and speed of the development of these reactions are variable. Furthermore, there is an inconsistency in the course of development of some reactions, such as placing reaction, Landau reaction, so that we cannot use these for diagnostic purposes. Also, a baby gradually learns a function in different ways, he learns to adapt to different situations. He has several possibilities at his disposal, from which he can choose. Thus, *variabilities and inconsistences are the characteristics of normal sensorimotor development*, whereas stereotyped performances are suspicious for abnormal sensorimotor development.

Stereotyped Movement Patterns in Abnormal Development

In abnormal babies there is a lack of variability and a limited adaptability to different situations (according to Milani-Comparetti [6] a limited freedom of choice of movements and postures). The same stereotyped movement patterns appear with every physical and emotional stress (with pleasure, concentration, crying, hunger, surprise, etc.), i.e. one knows beforehand how the baby will react, e.g. (1) repeatedly with the same asymmetric pattern in the supine position, often combined with opisthotonus, or (2) with an extensor pattern involving the whole body or either more the upper or the lower parts of the body, and/or (3) a flexor pattern in the prone position, together with the impossibility or difficulty of lifting the head against gravity and of bringing the arms forward for support, or (4) a Moro reaction may occur with the slightest noise or other stimulus, or (5) closed fists and clawing of the toes may be seen in any position, evoked by the slightest effort and stress.

To differentiate between normal and abnormal motor development, it is *important to observe the quality of postures and movements* of the baby in different positions (supine, prone, sitting, upright). We see if there is sufficient variability of movements, or if the baby reacts again and again with the same movement patterns. The dominance between normal and abnormal movement patterns is not always clear.

We can get additional information when testing for righting and equilibrium reactions, observing the quality of these reactions, and, furthermore, by testing in suspension positions (ventral, vertical, oblique). Abnormal movement patterns reinforce themselves in suspension positions.

Except in severe cases with obvious dominant abnormal movement patterns, we need to *follow-up* the babies closely. Thus, we are able to observe the development of the variability-stereotypy ratio, i.e. whether there is a development towards normality or towards cerebral palsy. In suspicious cases, the baby should be re-examined after a few weeks, at least after 1 month, e.g. first examination at 3 months, then again at 4 months, and, if the situation is not yet clear, again at 5 and at 6 months.

Indications for Treatment

The increasing dominance of abnormal movement patterns is an indication for treatment, especially from the 4th month onwards.

If *sucking and swallowing difficulties* accompany the motor problem, the treatment should be started immediately, irrespective of the degree of the abnormal motor symptoms. Treatment of feeding difficulties (pre-speech therapy) is the essential basis to obtain understandable speech.

Also, the presence of *strabism* or *epilepsy* is an indication to an earlier start of therapy in questionable cases.

Familial and/or professional situations will sometimes indicate whether to commence treatment earlier or later. When the parents are overanxious and very worried, we might start therapy earlier. If they are farmers or have a hotel business, they will have more time outside their working season. If the parents do not realize their child's problem, one might wait a few weeks, examine the baby again with both parents present, so that they have a better chance of understanding the problem. The positive attitude and cooperation of the parents is essential to give the child a maximal change to get full benefit from the therapy.

The *clinical observation* is *a simple way of assessing the quality of movements*, but, unfortunately, it is *time-consuming* (we usually allow up to one hour per baby). Recently, Prechtl [7] found a way of observing the infant's movements from a replay of videotapes. After an hour of video tape recording (performed by a technician) the videotapes can be reviewed in a few minutes. One can look at them repeatedly in a short time to get a better judgement. The interobserver agreement is high. This method is especially valuable for research purposes, the developmental course of symptoms of cerebral palsy can be fully documented.

Some Specific Diagnostic Difficulties

The *diagnosis of the type of cerebral palsy* is very difficult early on, especially because most cases are mixed forms. The athetoid component is at first obvious by the extreme positions and movements due to the lack of co-contraction; the degree of severity of athetosis is difficult to judge. The spastic component is characterized by lack of mobility, the movements are more slow and smaller, mostly around the mid-positions due to increased co-contraction. The ataxic component shows in most cases only with movements that need more control.

Fortunately, an early diagnosis of the type of cerebral palsy is not important for the physiotherapy, which has to adapt continuously to the individual state and symptoms of a child.

If the abnormal motor symptoms are linked with a *mental handicap* (slight to moderate), the abnormal movement patterns may show later, because the child is less active.

Special attention has to be given to *potential spastic diplegias*. The tendency of the prematures to spastic diplegias does still exist. These babies show often a relatively good development of head control and manipulation, but may still maintain a primitive frog pattern of the legs. The extensor pattern underneath is not striking, one has to look for it. It only becomes evident with extending the legs (slight adduction, slight equinus feet). Increasing of this extensor pattern in the supine and upright positions, together with a remaining flexor pattern of the legs in the prone position points to the development of a spastic diplegia. These symptoms are a clear indication for treatment. It is important to start therapy before the baby uses his hands more intensely, otherwise there will be an associated reaction of the legs with every manual activity, where, in spite of intensive therapy, a diplegic gait can no longer be avoided.

Asymmetry of postures and movements: asymmetry of the whole body or predominantly of the head, of the trunk, hips, legs and feet are evident, they are seldom overlooked. They are the result of a stronger influence of the asymmetrical tonic neck reflex to one side. This can be physiological up to the age of 4–5 months, exceptionally longer. Combined with abnormal tone, they might be transitory symptoms or an early sign of cerebral palsy. Therefore, it is essential to observe and follow these cases closely.

Hypotonias in babies are transitory in most cases. Only when combined with a severe mental handicap, they remain as such. Hypotonias may develop later into athetoids, ataxias, ataxias with athetosis or, less often, into spastic diplegias. Therefore, it is important to look for intermittent spasms, e.g. opisthotonus with feeding, with bathing (signs of an athetoid component), for poor movements, and for fists and clawing of the toes with stress (signs of a spastic component).

Hypotonias are often also the expression of other neurological diseases, such as myopathies, metabolic disorders, and chromosomal and connective tissue anomalies. An exact case history is of great importance.

Conclusions

The majority of babies are neurologically normal. At-risk newborns often show abnormal neurological symptoms during the first months of life. In most cases the nervous system recovers, but a safe prediction is not possible. Therefore, a close follow-up by pediatricians is indispensable for early detection of a cerebral motor disorder. The quality of movements, not a delineated time-schedule of the development of milestones, has to be considered. Variability, inconsistency, adaptability to different situations are expressions of a healthy nervous system. An increasing dominance of stereotyped movement patterns points towards a development of cerebral palsy and is an indication for therapy.

This paper considers only the motor aspects of the baby.

References

1   Hagberg B, Lundberg A: Dissociated motor development simulating cerebral palsy. Neuropädiatrie 1969;1:187–199.
2   Lesigang C: Reifungsdissoziation. Wiener Klin Wochenschr 1977;89:53–58.
3   Touwen BCL: Neurological Development in Infancy. Clin Dev Med, vol 58. London, Heinemann, 1976.
4   Touwen BCL: Variability and stereotypy in normal and deviant development; in Apley J (ed): Care of the Handicapped Child. Clin Dev Med, vol 67. London, Heinemann, 1978, pp 99–110.
5   Touwen BCL: Variability and stereotypy in neurological development; in Köng E (ed): Zerebrale Bewegungsstörungen. Pädiatr Fortbildk Praxis. Basel, Karger, 1982, Bd 53, pp 70–77.
6   Milani-Comparetti A, Gidoni EA: Pattern analysis of motor development and its disorders. Dev Med Child Neurol 1967;9:625–630.
7   Prechtl HFR: Qualitative changes of spontaneous movements in fetus and preterm infant are a marker of neurological dysfunction. Early Hum Dev 1990;23:151–158.

E. Köng, MD, Belpstrasse 3a, CH–3074 Muri/Bern (Schweiz)

Forssberg H, Hirschfeld H (eds): Movement Disorders in Children.
Med Sport Sci. Basel, Karger, 1992, vol 36, pp 86–90

Early Diagnosis of Cerebral Palsy:
Vojta Approach

Ingrid Weinke

Department of Paediatrics, University of Greifswald, FRG

Neurokinesiological diagnosis established by Vojta is based on:
(a) postural ontogenesis; (b) motor ontogenesis, and (c) dynamics of
primitive reflexes.

Postural ontogenesis makes possible the automatic control of posture,
which is inborn and genetically determined in every person [1]. It forms the
background for every motoric behavior and movement of infants from
birth up to the moment of walking independently. Over this period infants
evidence a global motoric pattern appropriate to their age, made up of
partial patterns. Vojta describes the kinesiological content of this global
pattern not as *normal* but as *ideal* (this is not an arbitrary statistical
statement). This can be observed in both postural ontogenesis and motor
activity ontogenesis. Automatic control of posture can be studied according
to Vojta's schedule of 7 provoked postural reactions [1]. Spontaneous
motor activity can be observed in the prone and the supine positions.

The spontaneous motor expressions of the child can be compared with
provoked motor reactions.

Supposing that postural abilities are normal from the prone position,
the ideal motor development proceeds at the age of 4–5 months from the
global pattern of the newborn via the first global posture pattern for visual
orientation to reach the grasping function pattern.

The first global posture pattern for visual orientation is symmetrical
elbow support, which already constitutes part of the genetic programme
in the first 4 months of life and only needs to be brought into function
(fig. 1). When prone, the position of the head in preparation for visual
orientation requires a symmetrical stretching of the neck, a shift in the
center of gravity from the sternum to the pubic symphysis and a forward
movement of the arms. Under these conditions at the age of three months
a support triangle is formed by the medial epicondyls of both humeri and

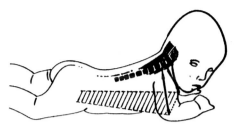

Fig. 1. Symmetrical elbow support.

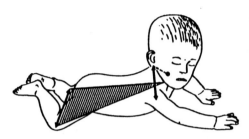

Fig. 2. Single elbow support.

the pubic symphysis. The head – one-third of the child's body weight – is held outside the support line. This is the first expression of balance.

There is a gradual change of posture from the symmetrical elbow support to single elbow support at the age of 4–5 months for the grasping function to be realised (fig. 2). Single elbow support constitutes the first cross motor pattern between the upper and lower extremities, which later forms the basis for crawling and walking [1].

Grasping with one hand in the prone position is possible with triangular support on the contralateral elbow, the ipsilateral advanced knee and the contralateral half of the pelvic girdle. An examination of individual postural reactions thus allows the recognition of spontaneous motor patterns in the prone position.

The motor patterns of postural reactions are described by Vojta as ideal or abnormal. He uses the number of abnormal postural reactions to determine the degree of disturbed central coordination (DCC): very slight (1–3 abnormal postural reactions); slight (4–5 abnormal postural reactions); moderate (6–7 abnormal postural reactions); severe (7 abnormal postural reactions and severe disturbance of muscle tone).

In a normal population 70% of newborns have no DCC. 25% of all newborns have a very slight or slight DCC. 90–75% of these children develop normally without therapy, while approximately 3% may get worse. More than 3% and less than 5% of all newborns have a moderate DCC

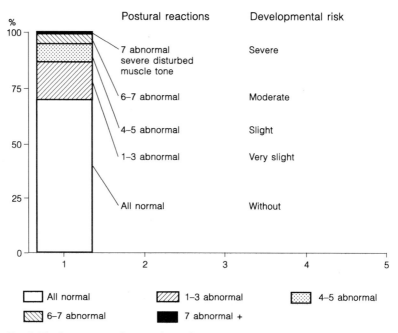

Fig. 3. The importance of postural reactions.

and less than 1% a severe DCC (fig. 3) including severe disturbance of muscle tone (hypertonia or hypotonia) [2]. The group of moderate and severe DCC contains children with mental retardation, severe sensory deficits and cerebral palsy [1, 3, 4]. CP has the following characteristics according to Vojta;

(a) A postural blockade which is already present in the neonatal period.

(b) Abnormal motor patterns.

(c) Pathological primitive reflexes (tonic extensor, Galant reflex, hand grasping and foot grasping reflex, positive supporting reactions of legs) namely blockade in the neonatal period and later or persisting for 3 months or more.

Primitive reflexes are closely tied to postural ontogenesis and when dynamic is taken into account, it is possible to subdivide CP into separate syndromes (table 1). Thus, the spastic and dyskinetic risk can be identified at about 4 months of age [1].

In a longitudinal study, we followed the outcome up to 7 years of 64 high-risk very preterm infants with a gestational age of less than 32 weeks

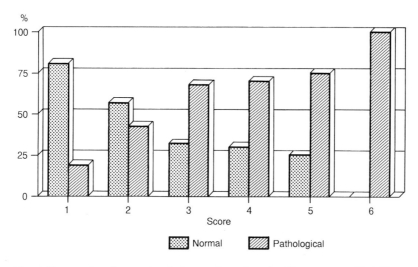

Fig. 4. Frequencies of normal and abnormal reactions by 64 seven-year-old children. 1 = Normal development; 2 = very slight; 3 = slight; 4 = moderate learning disabilities; 5 = severe mental retardation; 6 = severe motor and mental handicaps.

Table 1. Risk for development of spastic or dyskinetic syndrome

	Risk of spastic syndrome	Risk of dyskinetic syndrome
Spontaneous movements	scarcely	dystonic attacks
Muscle tone	without importance	without importance
Clonus	∅	∅
Tonic extensor reflexes	all positive +++	if +/then only crossed in hypertonia
Galant reflex	< - ∅	+++
Positive supportive reactions of legs	+++	+/automatic walking
Lift reaction	+ (abnormal)	+ (abnormal)
Hand grasping	+ + + +	<
Foot grasping	< - ∅	+ + + +

and a birth weight of 1,500 g or less. Each child was categorized into one of six groups depending on their outcome at 7 years of age (fig. 4, see legend). Normal refers to children without or with very slight and slight DCC; pathological means children with moderate or severe DCC when tested at a corrected age of 4 months. All of the infants with moderate and severe DCC received therapy according to Vojta. At the examination at corrected age 4 months, the groups with increased learning disabilities, i.e. groups 3–5, showed a greater frequency of moderate DCC. In the severely handicapped group (group 6) all the children had pathological DCC. This was the only group containing children with spastic CP. The differences between the groups were statistically significant (chi^2, p = 0.1%). The primitive reflexes, especially the tonic extensor and foot-grasping reflexes, indicate that these are related to the severity of later handicap (not shown).

References

1   Vojta V: Die zerebralen Bewegungsstörungen im Säuglingsalter, Aufl 1 1974; Aufl 2 1981; Aufl 3 1984; Aufl 5 1988. Stuttgart, Ferdinand Enke Verlag.

2   Cost GC: Le sette reazioni posturali di Vojta come despitage delle alterazioni neuromotorie del lattante. Esperienza su 2382 soggetti. Pediatr Med Chir 1983;5:59–66.

3   Tomi M: Zur Früherkennung und Frühbehandlung bei Kindern mit cerebralen Bewegungsstörungen in Japan. Deutsch-Japanisches-Symposium, Osaka, 1981. Lübeck, Schmidt-Römhild, 1984.

4   Immamura S, Skuma K, Takahashi T: Follow-up study of children with Cerebral Coordination Disturbance (CCD, Vojta). Brain Dev 1980;5:311–315.

PD Dr. med. Ingrid Weinke, Department of Paediatrics, University of Greifswald, D-O–2200 Greifswald (FRG)

Forssberg H, Hirschfeld H (eds): Movement Disorders in Children.
Med Sport Sci. Basel, Karger, 1992, vol 36, pp 91–97

Effects of Physical Therapy and Infant Stimulation

Frederick B. Palmer

The Johns Hopkins School of Medicine and The Kennedy Institute,
Baltimore, Md., USA

In recent years, strides have been made in providing educational and related therapy services to infants and children with developmental disabilities. In the United States, Federal and State legislation mandates appropriate educational and therapy programs to all handicapped children, including infants and toddlers. The objectives of the legislation related to infants and toddlers are broad and clear-cut:

To enhance the development of infants and toddlers and minimize their potential for developmental delay.

To reduce educational costs by minimizing the need for special education and related services when the children reach school age.

To minimize the likelihood of institutionalization of handi-capped children and maximize their potential for independent living in the community.

To enhance the capacity of families to meet the special needs of their infant or toddler with a handicap [1].

But, this legislation also has the potential effect of contributing to the general acceptance of unproven interventions. If we are to maintain public and governmental support for services to children with handicaps, it is incumbent upon us to critically evaluate effects of traditional treatments and explore new strategies for intervention. Thus, the basic legislative objectives listed above should be framed as broad research hypotheses to be tested in a variety of clinical environments. At this point it is quite clear that our scientific knowledge of the effects of interventions in infants and toddlers lags behind the educational mandate.

Outcome research in the developmental disabilities has not been as extensive or of the quality of that in other branches of medicine. In an article in *Pediatrics* in 1982, Simeonsson et al. [2] evaluated 27 intervention studies in the developmental disabilities according to basic research design criteria. Only about half used defined criteria for subject inclusion; random assignment of subjects to treatment groups was unusual; control or contrast groups were not always used; masked measurements of outcome were used in only three studies (this is especially critical when evaluating traditional therapies where strong opinions about efficacy are held); and outcome measures clearly did not look at the broad range of possible outcomes. In only one case was a family-oriented measure used and usually only single outcome measures were employed. In 1989, Tirosh and Rabino [3] reviewed studies evaluating the effects of motor therapies in cerebral palsy and noted similar problems.

Despite these methodological shortcomings attempts have been made to salvage some meaning from these and similar studies. Shonkoff and Hauser-Cram [4] published a meta analysis combining the results of studies evaluating intervention for disabled infants and their families. Treatment effects were evaluated according to outcome studied, nature of handicap, and characteristics of intervention. The strengths of this statistical approach are that a large sample size can be created to test a single hypothesis by combining similar but not identical studies. The weakness is obvious: the strength of the conclusions depends on the quality of the component studies. By combining studies, the meta analysis noted a marginally positive effect for IQ outcomes but little effect on motor outcomes. A very promising effect was noted for language outcomes. Differences in outcome were noted according to population studied. Children with cerebral palsy or mental retardation showed little or no effect, but children from more loosely defined groups appeared to do somewhat better. Further, highly structured and defined curriculums demonstrated a more positive effect than loosely defined interventions. Extensive parental involvement appeared to have a greater effect than those programs where there was limited or no parental involvement. When the parents and children were programmed together, rather than separately, there appeared to be a greater positive effect. While these findings are encouraging, considerable skepticism is in order because of the limitations of the underlying studies used in the meta analysis. Prospective, well-designed clinical trials will be necessary to confirm or refute them.

In the last 6 years, a few well-controlled clinical trials have been reported. There have been studies addressing both infants at risk and those with diagnosed developmental abnormality. One of each is summarized below as examples of outcome research in developmental medicine.

In 1988, our group at the Kennedy Institute reported the results of a controlled trial contrasting the effects of physical therapy with those of a broad-based infant stimulation curriculum in infants with spastic diplegia

[5]. The objectives of the study were: (1) to evaluate motor and cognitive effects of neurodevelopmental physical therapy, the most commonly used form of physical therapy in the United States, and (2) to determine if earlier physical therapy offered any motor or cognitive advantage. Forty-eight infants with spastic diplegia were enrolled and randomly assigned to either the experimental or contrast group. The experimental group received 12 months of neurodevelopmental physical therapy through biweekly center-based visits and daily home treatment administered by the parents. The contrast group received 6 months of infant stimulation using 'Learningames' [6], a broad-based curriculum developed at the Frank Porter Graham Center at the University of North Carolina, followed by 6 months of neurodevelopmental physical therapy. The only difference between the two treatment groups was the actual treatment content itself. That is, each intervention had identical amounts of professional therapy and home implementation, thereby controlling for treatment intensity and nonspecific professional contact. After 6 months of treatment, the design allowed us to contrast the short-term effects of physical therapy with those of infant stimulation. After 12 months of treatment, the effects of earlier, longer duration physical therapy could be compared with later, shorter duration physical therapy.

We chose outcome measures to sample as wide a range of outcome variables as practical. These included motor, cognitive, neurologic, orthopedic, and psychosocial outcomes. The measures were applied after 6 and 12 months of treatment by observers unaware of treatment group assignment. Because of the lack of universally accepted motor measures, we employed redundant measures of motor function: the Bayley motor quotient, observed functional motor skills, and parental report of functional motor skill attainment. No significant group differences were noted at enrollment in any of the outcome measures.

The results were unexpected. After 6 months of treatment, no advantage favoring physical therapy could be demonstrated in any of the outcome domains. In fact, trends in motor and cognitive development favored infant stimulation. After 12 months, functional motor differences on all measures still favored the contrast group, those who received infant stimulation followed by physical therapy. Thus, no evidence supported the idea that physical therapy started earlier is more effective in infants with cerebral palsy. Using stepwise multiple regression analyses, it was clear that the motor effects of infant stimulation persisted after controlling for any motor, cognitive or demographic differences at enrollment. These findings raise three major points:

(1) Traditionally accepted interventions may not have the effects we anticipate.

(2) In the absence of a no-treatment control group, it is impossible to determine whether group differences were due to beneficial effects of the contrast intervention or deleterious effects of the physical therapy intervention.

(3) Carefully designed clinical trials using accepted methodologies can be applied in evaluating the effects of intervention in the developmentally disabled.

The Infant Health and Development Program (IHDP), under the direction of Gross et al. [7] provides striking further emphasis for this last point. The IHDP is an 8-site multicenter clinical trial in low birth weight premature infants designed to evaluate the efficacy of comprehensive early intervention services in reducing developmental, behavioral and health problems in the first 3 years of life. The study, supported by a number of public and private agencies, used highly rigorous clinical trial methodology. A large sample of premature low birth weight infants ($n = 985$) were randomly assigned to receive either comprehensive services consisting of a center-based developmental curriculum, family support services, and pediatric follow-up (experimental group) or pediatric follow-up alone (contrast group). At 3 years of age the infants were assessed on important developmental, behavioral and health variables. In the experimental group, higher mean IQ scores on the Stanford-Binet were seen: 13.2 IQ points higher in children with birthweight 2,000–2,500 g, but only 6.6 IQ points higher in children below 2,000 g. There was a 2.7 times greater risk of mother-reported behavior problems in the contrast group. Finally, there was a slight increase in reported minor illnesses in the group receiving comprehensive services but this was limited only to the lighter birth weight group and no serious illnesses were noted.

The IHDP clearly indicates that we can have reasonable confidence that prospective clinical trials, even of multicenter design, will be able to effectively test important clinical hypotheses in developmental medicine.

It is important to note that both studies suggest that broad-based developmental curricula with structured parent involvement can have positive developmental benefits, at least in the short term. As you remember, this was also one of the conclusions of the meta analysis. Why such a curriculum should have better motor outcome than neurodevelopmental physical therapy in diplegic infants is unclear. Are there adverse effects of physical therapy? Does the broad-based curriculum offer special advantages? Sparling, one of the authors of the 'Learningames' curriculum, has suggested a number of hypotheses for testing [8]. Does the caretaker regard the individual delivering the broad-based curriculum as more of a colleague than an expert and therefore more readily participate in the intervention? Is the broad-based curriculum more optimistic than the deficit-based approach of motor therapy, again fostering more active caretaker participation? Are the activities of the broad-based curriculum more naturally appealing or more appropriate to the 'relatively undifferentiated' infant? These 'hypotheses' are probably overly simplistic, but they suggest areas for study of the infant-therapy-caretaker interaction and the mechanisms for treatment effect.

Where do we go from here? It is clear that clinical trials, even large multicenter trials, can effectively study the developmental interventions. We can define, enroll, treat, and follow a sufficient number of subjects to test important clinical hypotheses, even in large-scale multicenter trials. We can minimize bias and we can do it with good retention of subjects. Further studies, both small and large, should examine various parameters of treatment in different clinical settings. The following variables characterize an intervention. They are not the only important parameters, but they do indicate areas where research is needed.

Basic content of therapy: Many disciplines are involved in intervention programs; all should be eligible for evaluation. (This includes more traditional or newly popular medical and surgical interventions.) Remember that most interventions are eclectic. Outcomes of an 'infant stimulation' curriculum will not necessarily be duplicated by another 'infant stimulation' regimen where content may be distinctly different. In order to effectively evaluate treatment outcome, the intervention must be well defined and consistently administered. This is difficult to do where individualized treatment plans are used. For research purposes, study treatments need to have a basic consistency yet also meet individual needs. Sequential curricula such as those used in the above-described studies may be helpful.

Treatment intensity: Is there a dose-effect curve for developmental interventions? Or, is there a threshold effect where more adds nothing? Is there a toxic dose?

Duration: This is a similar issue to intensity. How long should therapy be applied?

Age of initiation: When is early intervention early? Is it equally effective to intervene after a period of observation during which an infant's developmental status can be better characterized, or must intervention begin immediately. The desire to study early therapy collides directly with what we know about difficulties with early diagnosis. Most infants 'at risk' will have a good outcome [9] presumably with or without intervention. If we use risk status instead of diagnosis as criteria for enrollment, studies with extremely large sample size and costs will be required. A compromise may be to study therapies at a bit later age than we might ideally desire in order to ensure adequate numbers of abnormal subjects.

Locus of service: Are there different effects for home- vs. center-based interventions?

Parent involvement: This is a very interesting area with major implications for program cost. Can we use parents as surrogate therapists? Most programs do, using the therapist as a coach. Do we gain something extra by improving parents' coping with the handicapped child? The limited data available seem to point in this direction. Could this be a mechanism of treatment effect?

Concurrent treatments: How do we combine therapies? Is there a point where the child's or family's tolerance is exceeded and the treatment becomes detrimental? This is an essential issue in children with multiple handicaps.

In studying these and other aspects of treatment, attention to rigor in design is critical. Special care must be given to eliminating bias whenever traditional therapies are studied. Treatment group assignment must be random and occur after enrollment.

Outcome measures should sample the entire range of pertinent outcomes. Functional measures are essential to assess the true burden of handicap on the individual and family. More basic measures of movement, such as those described by others in this symposium, may be helpful in establishing mechanisms for treatment effect and suggesting additional treatment strategies for study.

Studies using true control groups receiving no treatment should be encouraged in order to explore the possibilities of adverse treatment effect. Outcome measurement must be performed without possible knowledge of treatment group assignment.

We will need to address these issues if we are to provide the quality services handicapped infants and children deserve and preserve the public and governmental support that has resulted in mandates for service. These issues must be part of a research agenda, basic and clinical, aimed at improving the life of children with movement disorders and other developmental disabilities.

References

1   United States Public Law 99-457, Education of the Handicapped Act Amendments of 1986, 1986.
2   Simeonsson R, Cooper D, Scheiner A: A review and analysis of the effectiveness of early intervention programs. Pediatrics 1982;69:635–641.
3   Tirosh E, Rabino S: Physiotherapy in children with cerebral palsy: evidence for its efficacy. Am J Dis Child 1989;143:552–555.

4   Shonkoff JP, Hauser-Cram P: Early intervention for disabled infants and their families: A quantitative analysis. Pediatrics 1987;80:650–658.
5   Palmer FB, Shapiro BK, Wachtel RC, Allen MC, Hiller JE, Harryman SE, Mosher BM, Meinert CL, Capute AJ: The effects of physical therapy on cerebral palsy: A controlled trial in spastic diplegia. N Engl J Med 1988;318:803–808.
6   Sparling JJ, Lewis I: Learningames for the First Three Years of Life. New York, Walker, 1979.
7   IHDP: The Infant Health and Development Program: Enhancing the outcomes of low-birth-weight, premature infants. JAMA 1990;263:3035–3042.
8   Sparling JJ: Narrow- and broad-spectrum curricual: Two necessary parts of the special child's program. Inf Young Children 1989;1:1–8.
9   Nelson K, Ellenberg J: Antecedents of cerebral palsy, multivariate analysis of risk. N Engl J Med 1986;315:81–86.

Frederick B. Palmer, MD, Director of Developmental Pediatrics,
The Kennedy Institute, 707 N. Broadway, Baltimore, MD 21205 (USA)

Forssberg H, Hirschfeld H (eds): Movement Disorders in Children.
Med Sport Sci. Basel, Karger, 1992, vol 36, pp 98–106

Discussion Section II

Carin Allert, Eva Beckung, Christina Erikson, Anette Nylén,
Kristina Persson, Kristina Swanberg

Introduction – Comments to the Lectures

Katz-Salmon presented data concerning the CNS morbidity of preterm infants and showed a significant decrease in mortality during the last decades. Although the majority of infants survive without major sequele there is an increasing incidence of brain damage with decreasing birthweight.

During lectures presented by Seiger and Leonard the development after early brain damage was highlighted. 'Old' knowledge of the CNS development was questioned. Both speakers suggested that early neuronal activity is important for retraction and segregation within the nervous system.

Bradley questioned our traditional view of motor development. The progress of neurological development can no longer be regarded as cephalo-caudal or proximal-distal. Neither is there a strict hierarchical organization. The cortex does not only inhibit spinal reflexes. The activity in supraspinal centers will also be integrated with spinal functions. It seems that many movements are present in the newborn and that the CNS might inhibit several of these waiting for the posture as control system to mature.

According to Horak, the reflex-hierarchical model of assessing motor control and motor development can be questioned as well as the treatments based on it. Two of the treatment models presented in this session (Bobath and Vojta) have been regarded as belonging to this model while the sensory integration theory was not discussed in this respect.

Instead, Horak proposed the system/task model. In this model movements are described as results of an interaction between many systems. The different stages of infant motor development are due to the occasional appearance of posture control contributed by several systems.

The rejection of an hierarchical control was, however, questioned. Forssberg emphasized the well-documented knowledge about the CNS with several motor systems organized in an hierarchical order, such as the locomotor system which has neural networks in the spinal cord controlled by centers in the brain stem.

Three topics were addressed in the discussion:

(I) Early diagnosis – characteristic signs.

(II) The rules of sensory inputs in motor development and treatment.

(III) How to make the bridge between traditional therapy and the motor development.

Early diagnosis

The following questions were put forward:

What are the primary impairments that we can look for in attempting to do early diagnosis? Why should we diagnose early? The discussion was mainly concentrated on early predictors of cerebral palsy. The traditional neurological examination has limited value in this context. Cranial imaging; computed tomography (CT), ultrasonography (US) and magnetic resonance imaging (MRI) can help us to detect infants at risk for later disability but it cannot give us a detailed description of the course and the type of disorder. Floodmark pointed out that the combination of clinical evaluation and a radiographic evaluation of the brain would give better information. Cranial imaging can also add information when the damage occurred.

Following areas of assessment were discussed:

Observation of Spontaneous Mobility

This method was emphasized by Cioni. In his work, led by Prof. Prechtl in Groningen, the observation of spontaneous mobility is used as a tool for early detection of abnormal development [1]. Assessment of the quality of movements, so-called gestalt perception, through videorecording has proven to be a reliable and valid evaluation. This noninvasive method has been performed in preterm low-risk and high-risk infants as well as in full-term infants until the corrected age of 4–6 months.

Giuliani emphasized that it is important to study how the spontaneous movements change over time in development and to define the best parameters to look at.

Thelen pointed out the great need for a prospective study of preterm babies and a control group considering spontaneous movements and that there must be a method to quantify the differences in quality in the movements. There are ongoing studies in Groningen where preliminary results show that quality changes with age in preterm babies.

Köng, a representative of the Bobath concept, stressed the importance of the observation of spontaneous movements and postures. Variability and inconsistency are characteristics of normal motor development.

Analysis of the kinesiology of a child's spontaneous movements in the prone and supine positions is important according to the Vojta concept, as presented by Weinke. This is supposed to measure the deviations from the 'ideal' motor development.

Observation of Postural Reactions

The importance of 7 postural reactions as a compliment to observation of spontaneous or voluntary movements is stressed in the Vojta therapy. Delayed or pathological responses in 6 or 7 of these in conjunction with deficits in spontaneous movements necessitate preventive treatment according to this theory. However, according to Maresova the postural reactions are abnormal in 25% of the whole population and only in 3% of these children is there a risk for motor dysfunction [2, 3]. The value of the postural reactions was questioned by Norén who in a small Swedish study of 25 children found low inter- and intratester reliability [4].

Appearance of Voluntary Goal-Directed Movements

Haley was referring to studies made by Harris using the Motor Assessement Infants test (MAI) [5] as tool for predicting cerebral palsy [6]. In these studies the voluntary movements have been shown to be the most predictable items for abnormal development. He suggested that early diagnosis could be done first at the age of 4–5 months when the infant has started goal-directed movements as reaching.

Tone and Primitive Reflexes

These were referred to by Campbell as perhaps an older approach to evaluate children. Köng meant that there is little use of looking at primitive reflexes and postural reactions while the spontaneous posture and movement are more important.

There seems to be a common view that evaluation of spontaneous movements in the child without too much handling is the best assessment for detecting motor problems and predicting later outcome.

Concerning the question: 'How early can you diagnose cerebral palsy?' there were different opinions. Cioni claimed that the study of qualitative patterns in preterm children by gestalt perception in videorecording was a valid method while Haley proposed the age of 4–5 months. There was another opinion by Leonard that children grow into their pathological pattern and that it might be impossible to see these early because of the ongoing encephalisation of the brain. Campbell claimed that in the USA there is a widespread belief that early diagnosing of motor dysfunction is not reliable before 12 months except for children with severe damage.

We think it is confusing to know what you actually evaluate when searching for the most predictable items for cerebral palsy. For example, when testing postural reactions you evaluate deviant patterns and tone at the same time. In the same way it is difficult to separate and evaluate active tone from spontaneous movements. From the studies of Harris [6], we know that the assessment of tone is considered to be a good predictor for cerebral palsy.

Rules of Sensory Input in Motor Development and Treatment

Neurological Assumptions
From recent studies, we know that fetal movements appear from the 8th gestational week. These movements are generated by neuronal networks and seem to occur without any sensory stimulation. The central part of the spinal cord in which the motoneurons are localized develops first. Movements can be initiated before the sensory nerve fibres enter the dorsal root and establish contact with the motoneuron. However, it is likely that the motor activity and the later coming sensory information from the movements are of importance for development [7].

From the studies of Hubel and Wiesel [8], we know the importance of sensory stimulation. They studied how the organisation of nerve cells in the visual cortex of kittens depended on the influence from visual stimulation. We also know that a newborn brain has redundance of neuron and axonal connections in the CNS while other connections are not established. It is likely that the final connections are partly regulated from activity and are influenced by a rich and stimulating environment. That means that the sensory stimulation can stabilize and fine tailor the neural system. Sensory stimulation can also influence morphological differentiation of the nerve cells and their connections when more dendrites and synapses are developed [9].

Campbell referred to Cioni who had said that early motility takes place without the presence and the need of sensory input and further to clinical researches of postural control (Hirschfeld) and contemporary models of motor control and motor learning (Gentile) which suggest that therapists shall 'take hands off' in therapy as much as possible. She asked: What are the rules of sensory input in motor development, motor control and motor learning? When is it appropriate to use 'hands on' in therapy – positioning that provides passive control? How much can we do by setting the environment to facilitate movements for children who do not produce much movements? Are hands needed?

Feedback

The main question in the discussion was if we can influence the motor pattern by giving sensory stimulation by triggering and guiding movements or shall we, according to the new motor learning methods, take our 'hands off'?

Gentile does not believe that proprioceptive input can alter the organisation in the nervous system or trigger movements that can be comparable with normal movement. 'The important feedback for the child is the feedback from his own movements and no artificial method can replicate that. Passive positioning cannot demonstrate learning.'

Giuliani on the contrary claimed that sensory input is very important and that you have to guide the child when he does not understand the task. The child must initiate movements and teach himself from his own movements. Only by providing some feedback during the movement can you help.

The feedback from the babies' own movements seems to be of great importance to the motor learning process. Cioni pointed out that even during sleep a newborn preterm or full-term baby 'triggers' a certain amount of feedback in the spontaneous movements.

Levitt pointed out that a position is not always passive. The baby becomes active because of the position. For example, it is of great importance for the child in what position he is nursed to get functional movements and to develop the mother-child interaction.

According to the Vojta treatment automatic locomotor programs are provoked by stimulating specific trigger zones of the child's body in specific starting positions. This will give the child an afferent input of body position, and elicit movements regularly shifting the central gravity around the body axis and reciprocally changing the supporting points. This locomotion is supposed to be inborn and can be used immediately after birth and throughout life. The child is doing it actively by himself and gets feedback from his own body.

According to the Bobath concept, the handling and the guiding of the child's movements aim to give a more normal sensation of active movements.

Posture

Cambell asked whether we can provide posture which will allow the child to be more functional? Can we develop postural strategies which will make the child independent without external support?

Hofsten answered the first question with 'yes', demonstrating that newborn babies with supported posture have visually guided arm movements.

Bradley stressed the importance to provide proximal support to give distal activity. That self-generated feedback might provide more proximal actions, e.g. tilting the child forward in a chair gives better functional arm movements. We think this confirms methods already used by physiotherapists.

There were different opinions about postural support. Gordon pointed out that the postural support during reaching has to be separated from proximal-distal sequences in the therapy. You cannot teach the child to stabilize if he has not got a reason for it. The first functional movement is grasping – the ability to do something with your hand makes the use of arm movement useful – then he can learn to stabilize.

Mayston claimed that the difficulty for the child is combining skills, to do both posture and grasping. You can make it easier for the child by choosing an easier condition and train the skills separately and then put them together.

In Vojta treatment posture is not trained separately. He claims that locomotion consists of postural control, rising up against gravity and dynamic movement. The main cue for the child's ability to succeed in voluntary goal-directed movements is how far the child has reached in the postural ontogenes. Can the child in a supine position stabilize well enough on the upper part of the body, shoulder and neck in order to liberate his arms from the body and grasp a toy? This is a question of developing automatic postural reactability according to von Aufschnaiter.

The role of sensory input is still important in both Vojta and Bobath treatment. One difference is that in the Vojta treatment it is important with *hands on* during treatment but after treatment you leave the child to use his spontaneous movements without interfering while in Boboth therapy the caretaker is supposed to give a correcting feedback throughout the whole day. Another difference is that in Vojta treatment you stimulate automatic locomotion but in the Bobath therapy you guide functional goal-directed movements.

According to the model of Gentile, the therapist cannot give sensory feedback by passive movements, only alter the surroundings which gives the child self-generated feedback.

Bridge between Traditional Therapy and Neural Motor Development

Campbell referred to statements from a consensus conference of outcome of physical therapy in the management of cerebral palsy [10]. Evaluating the literature, there was no documentation of a benefit of early treatment. Therefore, she raised the question: Why start early treatment if there is no benefit? There was no evidence for better benefits for one treatment over another or for the ability of physical therapy to decrease muscle tone or abnormal reflexes.

Campbell asked: Do we believe that early treatment may alter and if so what are the outcomes we expect? Is it mainly that we want to diagnose early in order to identify the primary impairment or do we believe that early treatment can reduce primary impairments and make differences in the outcomes? Referring to Palmer, whose study suggested that physical therapy is not more successful than other practical approaches in children with spastic diplegia, she asked if early treatment can do better?

The new concept of motor learning comes from normal development and normal motor control. Do we assume that children with a motor control problem, having difficulties producing voluntary movement, can learn in the same way as healthy children?

Richards continued by stressing the audience: 'It is a shame if people in the audience with experimental evidence and experience in animals and in normal development can't give some indices to physiotherapists to progress in treatment'. She wanted answers to the following questions: How early is early? Matter of intensity? Type of therapy?

One answer was given by Thelen who emphasized the importance of understanding the basic process by which infants learn to control their skills. The general process of development must be the same in normal children and in children with deficits of various severity. She meant that therapy must be given at a time when the system is receptive but that it needs more intensive training. A few minutes a day is not a substitute for the enormous experience normally taking place.

Horak responded to the question of teaching children with motor control problems, by referring to her own studies of teaching monkeys complicated arm movements. They succeded to press a button when they got a reward, which gave them feedback and made them repeat the movements again. It seems as if the brain needs to have a goal to know how to perform the movement and to know how the movement was actually executed. It also needs an error signal to correct the movement. It might be very difficult in a damaged brain.

Mayston replied: What is treatment? For the very young babies treatment should be handling. We ought to find a more sensitive quantitative test to help us evaluate the results in intervention.

Maresova emphasized that treatment must be early (4 months) before the compensatory strategies are obvious. After 9 months it might be very difficult. You have to work preventively. According to Vojta therapy the intensity of the treatment must be high – several times a day – in order to increase the influence of 'ideal' movements.

The implication of early treatment for the mother-child interaction was addressed by Blennow. If treatment should influence the development it must be done when the neural networks are developing. This means early treatment. If we cannot prove that early treatment leads to something positive, it seems unethical to interfere with this very sensitive period between mother and baby.

Another response to the issue of early treatment and the issue of dosage was given by Palmer: Since we know that most children do well without treatment and it is difficult to identify children predictable to cerebral palsy you must decide which children you want to treat. On the issue of dosage, as we do not have an answer we can always say we did not do enough. This has been the response to criticism about efficiency of treatment from certain groups in the USA. In defending a specific treatment some people tend to tell the parents they did not do the treatment well enough. Legislation mandates appropriate educational and therapy programs to all handicapped children in the USA. If they are to maintain public and governmental support for services to children with handicaps, the effects of traditional treatments must be critically evaluated and new strategies for intervention explored.

The symposium questioned the traditional therapies using a motor pattern which is not surely possible to transfer into other situations. Considering early treatment there were suggestions that this might give the best chance to influence an uncoordinated motor pattern within a child because of the plasticity of the brain and the timetable of the developing nervous system. The therapist might have a possibility to intervene and prevent compensatory strategies which lead to secondary impairments. It was also suggested that treatment probably has to be intensive. Concerning the type of treatment there was no answer but the need to evaluate the effect of traditional therapies was strongly stressed also in regard to ethical and economical aspects.

There is still a gap between scientists and clinicians regarding theory and practice in the treatment of children with movement disorders. We have to learn to speak the same language and to take more interest in each others work. Hypothetical questions about treatment must be explored and research results must be brought out and evaluated in the clinical work.

'A theoretical model is not simply right or wrong, it is valid only insofar as it is useful' [Gordon, Movement Science].

References

1   Cioni G, Prechtl HFR: Preterm and early postterm behaviour in low risk premature infants. Early Hum Dev 1990;23:159–191.

2   Costi GC: Le sette reazioni posturali di Vojta come despitage delle alterazioni neuromotorie del lattante. Esperienza su 2382 sogetti. Pediatr Med Chir 1983;5:59–65.

3   Imamura S, Sakuma K, Takahashi T: Follow-up study of children with Cerebral Coordination Disturbance (CCD Vojta). International Congress of Child Neurology. Brain Dev 1983;5:311.

4   Norén L, Franzén G: An evaluation of 7 postural reactions (Lagereflxen) selected by Vojta in 25 healthy infants. Neuropediatrics 1982;12:308–313.

5   Chandler L, Andrews M, Swanson M: in Larsson AH (ed): Movement Assessment of Infants. A manual. Washington, 1980. If interested, write to: Movement Assessment of Infants, P.O. Box 4631, Rolling Bay, Washington, USA.

6   Harris S: Early neuromotor predictors of cerebral palsy in low-birth weight infants. Dev Med Child Neurol 1987;29:508–519.

7   Lagercrantz H, Forssberg H: Hjärnans funktionella utveckling hos fostret och spädbarnet. Läkartidningen 1991;88:1880–1885.

8   Patterson PP, Purves D: Readings in Developmental Neurobiology. Cold Spring Harbor, Cold Spring Harbor, Laboratory, 1982.

9   von Euler C, Forssberg H, Hedner T, Jonsson G, Lagercrantz H, Lundberg P, Olsson L, Seiger Å: Det centrala nervsystemets utveckling-inre och yttre miljöpåverkan. Läkartidningen 1985;38:3177–3190.

10   Campbell S: Consensus conference on efficacy of physical therapy in the management of cerebral palsy. Pediatr Phys Ther 1990.

Christina Erikson, St. Göran Children Hospital, S–112 81 Stockholm (Sweden)

III. Manual Actions: Motor Mechanisms and Perceptual Processes

Forssberg H, Hirschfeld H (eds): Movement Disorders in Children.
Med Sport Sci. Basel, Karger, 1992, vol 36, pp 107–112

Neural Control of Manipulation and Grasping[1]

Roland S. Johansson, Benoni B. Edin
Department of Physiology, Umeå University, Umeå, Sweden

Introduction

Everyone agrees that the human hand is remarkable. It can be used to discriminate between minute differences in textures and yet is capable of handling both a concrete drill and an artist's brush. This exceptional capacity is neither the result of rapid sensory processes, nor of very fast or powerful effector mechanisms. Indeed, some man-made substitutes for both sensors and effectors are vastly superior. Rather, the secret to the functionality of the human hand must be hidden in *how* the manual task is organized and controlled.

During the last decade considerable effort has been spent at the Department of Physiology, Umeå, to elucidate these control mechanisms [1–6]. The task chosen for study was the precision lift: subjects lifted an instrumented object from a support table, held it in the air, and then replaced it on the table. This task is obviously common in daily life and forms part of practically any type of manipulation. The picture that has gradually evolved can shortly be described as follows.

The lifting task is organized in distinct phases linked together, each phase characterized by: (i) a pattern of muscular activity; (ii) specific sensory gating and processing, and (iii) parameters primarily concerned with the magnitude of muscular activity. The passage from one phase to another is triggered by phase-specific patterns of short-lasting sensory inputs. The parameters employed depend on previous experience, visual

[1] These studies were supported by the Swedish Medical Research Council (grant 08667) and the Department of Naval Research, Arlington, Va. (grant N00014–90–J–1838).

and haptic information [7, 8], and sensory information gathered during performance of the task. A detailed account of these interpretations can be found in the cited references. In this paper, however, some points poten-tially pertinent for the understanding and treatment of movement disorders will be outlined.

Sequential Coordination

A fundamental characteristic of the lifting task is that it evolves in a series of phases each delineated by discrete mechanical events and associ-ated responses from sensory organs in the skin of the hand (fig. 1). The contact between the digits and the object marks the beginning of the first phase of the lift. When contact has been established, in a second phase, the *grip force* normal to the contact area and the *load force* start to increase in parallel. This phase in turn is terminated when the load force has overcome the weight of the object and it starts to move. Similarly, at the end of a lifting task, a parallel decrease in grip and load force begins shortly after the object makes contact with the table.

The specific role of sensor organs in the hand in linking the various phases of a lifting task can easily be identified. They inform the nervous mechanisms that particular mechanical events have occurred, for instance, that the digits have made contact with the object, or that the object has started to move. Indeed, the receptors best suited for providing this type of information have been characterized in detail and, in humans, been demonstrated to respond strongly to mechanical events associated with the various phases of the lifting task (fig. 1). Quite predictably, when sensory information is lacking due to nerve damage or an anesthetic block of the digital nerves, the contact force is excessive before the parallel increases in load and grip forces commence, and movement detection may be delayed, resulting in an overshoot of the objects' position.

A sequential organization scheme as the one outlined above display several advantageous features. It allows, e.g., for a considerable *flexibility* when lifting objects of different weights. The extension of the loading phase depends, for example, on the object's weight; with a heavier object, the load force has to reach higher values before the object starts to move. This, in turn, ensures that appropriate grip and load forces are applied during the hold phase; this strategy largely works independently of the the object's weight. Another important advantage is that the system con-trolling the task makes only *limited demands on sensory processing*: rather than relying on continuous sensory processing, specific patterns of short-

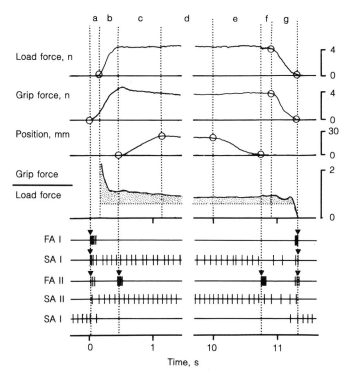

Fig. 1. The phases of a lifting task. The subject establishes the grip in the preload phase *(a)*. During the subsequent loading phase *(b)*, the load and grip forces increase in parallel under isometric conditions until the load force overcomes the object's weight and the object starts to move. The object is lifted to the intended position during the transitional phase *(c)*, which is followed by the hold phase *(d)*. After the replacement *(e)* of the object, there is a short delay *(f)* before the two forces decline in parallel until the object is released during the unloading phase *(g)*. Note the interrupted time scale. The grip:load force ratio has to be larger than the level indicated by a dashed line to avoid slips; the shaded area thus corresponds to the safety margin to avoid slips. *Tactile afferent responses* that are present in every lift are shown schematically below. Note in particular, the burst of impulses in one or several types of afferents early during the preload phase, at object's take-off, when the object is replaced on the table, and when the object is released.

lasting sensory inputs are used to trigger the transition from one operational mode to another. This implies, and indeed has been demonstrated in subjects with digital nerve blocks, that other, less 'specific' sensory inputs may substitute in triggering appropriate phase transitions. Lastly, this scheme is light on memory requirements: it is independent on explicit information on the object's weight.

Parallel Coordination and Choice of Phase Parameters

While the scheme outlined above has a number of innate advantages, it also shows weak sides. It is, for example, incapable of handling objects with different surface characteristics. To ensure a safe grip, the grip:load force ratio has to be above a certain minimal level; if the grip force is too small, slipping will occur. Since it is the ratio of the grip and load forces that is crucial, it is not possible to adapt to objects with different surface characteristics as opposed to different weights by simply changing the duration of one or the other phase. Rather, the relation between grip and load force has to be modified to take different surface characteristics into account. In analogy with computer programs, the *parameters* of various phases have to be changed in order to cope with objects possessing different surface properties.

How are these parameters chosen? The two most important determinants are (i) previous experience, and (ii) afferent information generated during execution of the task. It has been repeatedly demonstrated, for example, that the relation between the grip and load force during the early loading phase matches the relation that was adequate in the preceding lift [1]. Likewise, the first time derivative of the grip and load forces has its maximum when the load force matches about half the weight of the object lifted previously [1, 3], indicating that the generation of the forces was intended to match the object's weight. Furthermore, both frictional and weight information is rapidly transferred from the control mechanisms of one hand to those of the other. Thus, one must hypothesize that *sensorimotor memories* exist that represent both the objects to be manipulated and the appropriate phase parameters.

Again, it has been demonstrated that several types of sensory organs are excited when there is a mismatch between the expected and the actual properties of an object. Receptors in the finger pads (fast adaptive type I, FA I, in particular) differentiate, for example, between surfaces with different frictional characteristics. Pacinian corpuscles (FA II) are extremely sensitive to mechanical transients caused by an object's lift-off, and therefore are capable of detecting that an object has started to move earlier than anticipated if the object is lighter than expected.

In addition to sensorimotor memories and tactile information generated during the performance, both visual and haptic information have been demonstrated to influence a subject's choice of phase parameters [7, 8].

Clinical and Developmental Significance

The large array of factors that necessarily influence the behavior during a lifting task is a challenge to anyone interested in the development of sensorimotor mechanisms or the diagnosis and therapy of movement disorders. Indeed, developmental studies in children show that the adult pattern of control strategies [9], in particular the parallel coordination of muscle activity, develops in a number of definite stages. Furthermore, preliminary studies on patients with somatosensory lesions support some of the predictions from the hypothetized scheme outlined above [10–14]. In patients with peripheral nerve injuries, the sequential coordination of various phases proposed to be delineated by short-lasting sensory events, requiring only limited sensory processing, may appear largely normal, whereas the parallel coordination required for adjustments to frictional conditions is impaired [10]. Conversely, studies on patients with cortical injuries suggest that the automatic tactile control of manipulative coordination may not necessarily involve the use of parietal lobe cortical areas.

It is strongly suggested that the motor behavior displayed by humans is best described as *a discrete event driven control* rather than a continuous closed-loop control. The control mechanisms active when a human lifts an object in a precision grip are basically *anticipatory in nature*, requiring only *intermittent* use of sensory information to update task-phase parameters or to shift from one phase to another. Lastly, the organization of the lifting task involves both sequential and parallel coordination of muscle activity.

Several factors can thus be identified that might appeal to both neuroscientists and clinicians interested in normal and pathological movements. Lifting objects is an integral part of almost any form of manipulation and therefore a task that normally can be carried out with considerable skill even by a child. Despite its apparent simplicity, it may offer insights in not only sensory processing, but also in the parallel and sequential organization of muscle activity. In short, the lifting task may play an important role in elucidating the role of the CNS in sensorimotor integration.

References

1   Johansson RS, Westling G: Roles of glabrous skin receptors and sensorimotor memory in automatic control of precision grip when lifting rougher or more slippery objects. Exp Brain Res 1984;56:550–564.
2   Johansson RS, Westling G: Signals in tactile afferents from the fingers eliciting adaptive motor responses during precision grip. Exp Brain Res 1987;66:141–154.
3   Johansson RS, Westling G: Coordinated isometric muscle commands adequately and erroneously programmed for the weight during lifting tasks with precision grip. Exp Brain Res 1988;71:59–71.
4   Johansson RS, Westling G: Programmed and reflex actions to rapid load changes during precision grip. Exp Brain Res 1988;71:72–86.

5   Westling G, Johansson RS: Factors influencing the force control during precision grip. Exp Brain Res 1984;53:277–284.
6   Westling G, Johansson RS: Responses in glabrous skin mechanoreceptors during precision grip in humans. Exp Brain Res 1987;66:128–140.
7   Gordon AM, Forssberg H, Johansson RS, Westling G: Visual size vues in the programming of manipulative forces during precision grip. Exp Brain Res 1991;83:477–482.
8   Gordon AM, Forssberg H, Johansson RS, Westling G: The integration of haptically acquired size information in the programming of precision group. Exp Brain Res 1991;83:483–488.
9   Forssberg H, Eliasson AC, Kinoshita H, Johansson RS, Westling G: Development of human precision grip. I. Basic coordination of force. Exp Brain Res 1991; in press.
10 Johansson RS, Westling J (eds): Afferent signals during manipulative tasks in humans; in Franzen O, Westman J (eds): Information Processing in the Somatosensory System. London, Macmillan Press, 1991, pp 25–48.
11 Cole KJ, Abbs, JH, Tuner GS: Deficits in the production of grip forces in Down's syndrome. Dev Med Child Neurol 1988;30:752–758.
12 Müller F, Abbs JH: Precision grip in Parkinsonian patients; in Streifler MB, Korczyn AD, Melamed E, Youdim MBH (eds): Advances in Neurology, vol 53: Parkinson's Disease: Anatomy, Pathology, and Therapy. New York, Raven Press, 1990, pp 191–195.
13 Eliasson A-C, Gordon AM, Forssberg H: Basic coordination of manipulative Forces in children with cerebral palsy. Dev Med Child Neurol 1991;in press.
14 Cole KJ: Grasp force control in older adults. J Motor Behav 1991;in press.

Roland S. Johansson, Department of Physiology, Umeå University,
S–901 87 Umeå (Sweden)

Forssberg H, Hirschfeld H (eds): Movement Disorders in Children.
Med Sport Sci. Basel, Karger, 1992, vol 36, pp 113–123

Development of Manual Actions from a Perceptual Perspective

Claes von Hofsten

Department of Psychology, Umeå University, Umeå, Sweden

Introduction

Every coordinated act involves the whole organism and can only be understood as a dynamic interaction between the organism and the external world. Therefore, the development of coordination can never be understood simply in terms of neuromuscular maturation. It is rather a question of acquiring knowledge, tacit knowledge, about one's possibilities and limitations to move, about the external world, and about how to move in the external world. However, above all, it is a question of being able to steer the action on a steady course by extracting the right kind of information at the right time. All of this, requires an acting, perceiving, and thinking child.

The Problems To Be Solved

To get an understanding of what kind of accomplishment a smoothly coordinated action is we need first of all to analyse the problems involved in coordinating an action and how these problems are solved by adult subjects? Several different forces act on the limb or body segment during a movement. There are, of course, torques originating from muscle contractions aimed at moving the segment in question, but because the body is a mechanically linked system, torques are also generated from other moving segments coupled to it. The form of movement is also affected by the pull of gravity which will be different for different orientations of the limb in space. The visco-elastic properties of muscles, joints, and tendons will also affect the final form of movement. To be able to produce an intended movement, the passive forces from other segments and gravity need to be kept under control by the adjustments of active muscular contractions.

Coordination and regulation of purposeful movements are only possible in relation to a stable context – that is, the posture of the body. To be able to act purposefully, we must be able to maintain balance and equilibrium of the body and a stable orientation relative to the environment. The problem is that, because the body is a mechanically linked system, the movements themselves will affect the equilibrium of the body. When a body part is moved, the point of gravity of the whole body is displaced, and if the movement is forceful, it will create a momentum which will push the body out of equilibrium unless it is counterbalanced.

A third set of problems to do with coordinating movements with the external world. As the environment exists independent of ourselves, adaptive coordination is possible only if we can adjust our actions relative to properties of the environment and time them relative to external events. This holds true whether we are walking in a crowded area, catching a baseball, dancing with a partner, or engaging in social communication.

Prospective Control

The role of perception is not so much to evaluate what has been accomplished, but rather to look ahead in time and space and to steer the action on a stable intended course, just like the driver of a car who needs to know how the road is turning ahead, how the paving looks, and what is happening on the road. One reason why we need to know about things ahead of time, whether we drive a car or move a limb, is that there is a lag between the time information enters into the system and the time measures are taken. This lag will introduce an interruption in the flow of action if measures were to be taken after problems arise. However, even if there would be no transmission lag in the system, knowing about a problem when it is already there is too late. The inertia of the system requires changes in the course of movement to be planned. Upcoming events simply have to be dealt with ahead of time. No matter how quickly you get to know that your car has collided with another vehicle no matter how quickly you do something about it, the damage is already done.

If we fail to foresee what is coming up, movements become discontinuous and staccadic. This is what happens, for instance, when posture is suddenly and unexpectedly perturbed as we step on something slippery. The ongoing action has to be interrupted and all attention focused on regaining balance. It is true that we have a rather efficient way of dealing with this problem, the so-called 'stretch reflexes', without which the effects of losing balance would be much worse. However, the 'stretch reflexes' are still *ad hoc* and they cannot prevent the ongoing action from being interrupted. Much better would have been to have perceived the slipperiness ahead of time and been prepared for it. If so, there would have been no interruption of the ongoing activity. On the contrary, we may then even have used the slipperiness to support our locomotion as in a skating movement.

In the same way, if we are prepared for the induced and passive forces that arise during movement we are not only able to control those forces, but we might also use them to our advantage in producing the desired movement as once pointed out by Bernstein [1967].

Development

The child seems well prepared to use perception in a predictive way to steer his or her movements rather than to update them. As soon as infants are able to control purposive movements, they also show clear signs of being able to plan and look ahead. However, the first sign of prospective control may being rather crude and an important aspect of development is the improvement of prospectiveness. In this process, self-produced activity seems to be of crucial importance.

Smoothness of Movements

In a well-functioning perception-action system, perception reaches far into the future, and movements are smooth and continuous. It has long been recognized that such movements are future oriented and characterized by feedforward control. If the movement is quite continuous it is sometimes even called 'ballistic', the term referring to a totally preprogrammed movement. There are probably no such movements. The upcoming reactive forces are never completely predictable. Information has to be taken in and the torques adjusted during the course of the movement [Bernstein, 1967].

In a less-well-functioning system the actor has only a limited knowledge of the task space, and can only perceive the future very shallowly. Problems are not dealt with sufficiently ahead of time to allow smooth and continuous execution of the movement. Such discontinuous movements are traditionally considered as feedback regulated. However, from a functional point of view, the only thing that distinguishes these movements from the more continuous ones is how far ahead the movement is controlled.

Early reaching movements are composed of a number of smaller movements or steps at a base rate of about 4–5 Hz. Each step starts with an acceleration and ends with a deceleration. The trajectory of each step is rather straight with changes in movement direction taking place between steps. Thus, it appears as if movement parameters were reset at those points. This is illustrated in figure 1.

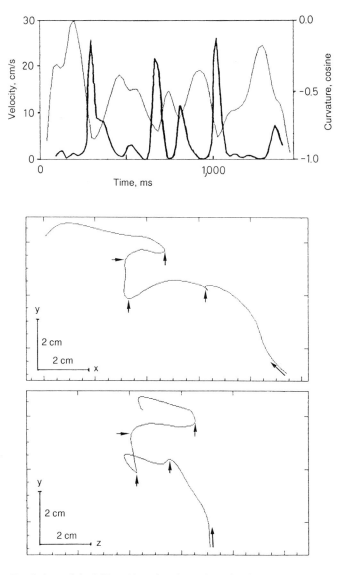

Fig. 1. A reach by LIB at 19 weeks of age. Duration is 1.45 s. The relative straightness, i.e. covered distance divided by shortest distance between the end points, is 1.91. The upper figure shows velocity (thin line) and curvature (thick line) as a function of time. Note the coupling between speed valleys and curvature peaks. The movement consists of 5 action units. Curvature is measured in cosine of the angle. Thus −1.0 equals 180° (i.e. no curvature) and 0.0 equals 90°. The middle figure is a front view of the reach and the bottom figure a side view of the reach. The short arrows indicate the borderlines between action units. The direction of the movement is indicated by the long arrow in each figure [from von Hofsten, 1991].

Thus, in just a few months of active reaching, the structure of the movements changed substantially towards an adult organization [von Hofsten, 1979, 1991]. This can be observed in figure 2. First, the reaching trajectory became straighter. Secondly, the order between the units became more systematic. At the youngest age, von Hofsten [1991] found that the largest unit was positioned at the beginning of the reach in only 50% of the cases, while at the oldest age level, 31 weeks of age, 84% of the reaches started with the largest unit. Thirdly, with age, the duration of the largest unit increased and it covered a larger proportion of the approach compared to the remaining units. Finally, there was a fewer number of units per reach. At 31 weeks of age, more than 50% of the reaches consisted of no more than two units. Reaching trajectories of adults are typically divided up into two functionally different phases, one larger approach phase and one smaller grasp phase [Jeannerod, 1981].

Prospective Postural Control

To be able to act purposefully, we must be able to maintain balance and equilibrium of the body and a stable orientation relative to the environment. Postural control is definitely a limiting factor in action development. Whether newborn infants will perform visually directed arm movements or not seems to depend on the postural support given to the infant. Grenier [1981] found that when the head of the newborn was properly supported, the observed arm movements were more mature. It is also true that in the studies by von Hofsten [1982], the neonates who performed aimed reaches were securely supported. Furthermore, the age when infants start to be successful in their reaching activity at around 4 months of age coincides with the age when they can sit and balance with support.

In order to keep balance during limb movements, the subject has to know about the contingencies between the limb movements, the reactive forces that arise during movement, and the displacement of the point of gravity. Adults seem to counteract such disturbances to the postural system in a precise way. For instance, when adults prepare for pushing or pulling a handle in front of them, they will not only activate the arm that is doing the job, but just before the arm muscles are fired, the appropriate leg muscles that will resist a displacement of the body are activated too [Cordo and Nashner, 1982]. When the handle is pulled, for instance, the gastrocnemius muscles are activated around 50 ms before the pulling starts.

von Hofsten and Woollacott [1990] studied anticipatory adjustments of the trunk in 9-month-old infants reaching for an object in front of them while balancing the trunk. The infants were seated astride on one of the knees of the accompanying parent who was supporting the child by the

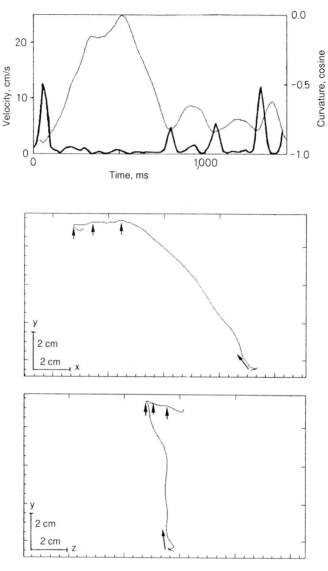

Fig. 2. A reach by LIB at 31 weeks of age. Duration is 1.47 s. The relative straightness, i.e. covered distance divided by shortest distance between the end points, is 1.193. The movement consists of 4 action units. The upper figure shows velocity (thin line) and curvature (thick line) as a function of time. Curvature is measured in cosine of the angle. Thus −1.0 equals 180° (i.e. no curvature) and 0.0 equals 90°. The middle figure is a front view of the reach and the bottom figure a side view of the reach. The arrows indicate the borderlines between action units. The direction of the movement is indicated by the long arrow in each figure [from von Hofsten, 1991].

hips. Muscle responses were recorded from the abdominal and trunk extensor muscles as well as from the deltoid muscle of the reaching arm. The results showed that trunk muscles participated in the reaching actions of 9-month-old infants. It seemed to be the trunk extensors that primarily prepared the reaching. The role of the abdominal muscles in preparing the infant for reaching seems to be less clear cut. The data suggest that the abdominal muscles participate in the reach but less as a preparation for it and more as part of bending the body forward toward the end of the reach (fig. 3).

Postural preparations are not something separate and independent but should be regarded as an integrated part of the action. Reaching for an object does not only involve the upper limb. The whole body is engaged in accomplishing the reaching act and trunk adjustments both before the arm is extended and after it has arrived at its goal are important parts of that process. Figure 3 shows that reaching in 9 month olds is embedded in an envelope of trunk adjustments.

Gearing Action to the Environment

Adaptive coordination is possible only if we can adjust our actions relative to properties of the environment and time them relative to external events. These events exist independent of ourselves and are therefore never totally predictable. Successful coordination is only possible if there is an intimate linkage between perception and action. An important aspect of the development of manual action has to do with establishing such perception-action linkages. The basic ones develop very early.

A smooth reaching action requires that the hand starts to close around the target in anticipation of the encounter with it. The timing needs to be precise if the reach-grasp sequence is going to be smooth and continuous. Such timing is only possible under visual guidance. Tactually controlled grasping is initiated after contact and it will by necessity induce an interruption in the reach-and-grasp act. Thus, the emergence of visually controlled, well-timed grasping is crucial for the development of manual skill. von Hofsten and Rönnqvist [1988] found that at 5 months of age, when the infant has just started to reach and grasp objects successfully, they will also anticipate the encounter with the target and time the grasp appropriately.

The ability to time one's actions relative to external events also develops early. A remarkable timing ability is demonstrated in infant catching behavior. In a series of studies, I have found that infants possess a remarkable capacity to catch objects [von Hofsten, 1980, 1983; von Hofsten and Lindhagen, 1979]. von Hofsten and Lindhagen [1979] found that from the very age an infant starts to master reaching for stationary

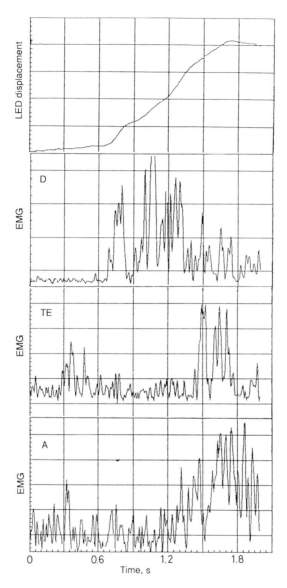

Fig. 3. Example of responses of subject HAW from the deltoid of the reaching arm, the abdominal muscles, and the trunk extensors plus records of the relative displacements of the reaching hand. In this specific example, the reach was performed with the left hand. It can be seen that the trunk extensor muscles (TE) start increasing firing well before the deltoid muscle. The abdominal muscles have some activation before the deltoid muscle too, but the major activation occurs toward the end of the reach [from von Hofsten and Woollacott, 1990].

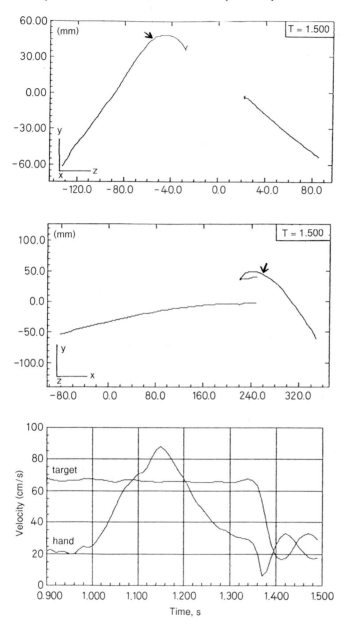

Fig. 4. The catching of an object moving at 65 cm/s by an 8-month-old infant. The upper figure shows a side view of the reach and the middle figure shows a front view of the same event. The lower figure shows the speed profiles of the approaching hand and the moving target. The arrows in the two upper figures indicate the position of the hand at 1.2 s.

objects, he or she will also reach successfully for fast moving ones. Eighteen-week-old infants caught the object as it moved at 30 cm/s. von Hofsten [1983], studying 8-month-old infants, found that they would successfully catch objects moving at 120 cm/s. The initial aiming of these reaches were within a few degrees of the meeting point with the target and the variable timing error was only between 50 and 60 ms. Figure 4 shows the catching of an object moving at 65 cm/s by an 8-month-old infant. Note that the hand decelerates before the encounter with the target. To examine the character of the prospective control in these reaches I have recently started to study catching in infants when the target movement is suddenly stopped.

Development of Skill

One important way in which to get prepared for action is by exploring and acquiring knowledge about the local contingencies between forces during action. This is what happens in development. When the contingencies are known to us, we may prepare ourselves for what is coming up. Motor development in this perspective is a question of getting to know what may be called the 'task space', so that different paths can be taken through it towards the goal and the smoothest and most economical one can be searched for. According to Reed [1990, p. 15]: 'the importance of practice and repetition is not so much to stamp in patterns of movement, but rather to encourage the functional organization of action systems. This principle is constant throughout life: the achievement of an action is not the agent's coming to possess an immutable program, but rather the development of a skill. This means the ability to use perceptual information so as to coordinate movements and postures in a flexible manner that serves to accomplish a desired task.' The task space can never be completely known because it changes a little every time we make a movement. However, we only need to know the task space in an approximate way so perception can be efficient in steering the action through it.

References

Bernstein N: The Coordination and Regulation of Movements. Oxford, Pergamon, 1967.
Cordo PJ, Nashner LM: Properties of postural adjustments associated with rapid arm movements. J Neurophysiol 1982;47:287–302.
Grenier A: 'Motoricité libérée' par fixation manuelle de la nuque au cours des premières semaines de la vie. Arch Fr Pédiatr 1981;38:577–561.

von Hofsten C: Development of visually guided reaching: The approach phase. J Hum
Movement Studies 1979;5:160–178.
von Hofsten C: Predictive reaching for moving objects by human infants. J Exp Child Psychol
1980;30:369–382.
von Hofsten C: Eye-hand coordination in newborns. Dev Psychol 1982;18:450–461.
von Hofsten C: Catching skills in infancy. J Exp Psychol 1983;9:75–85.
von Hofsten C: Structuring of early reaching movements: A longitudinal study. J Mot Behav
1991;in press.
von Hofsten C, Lindhagen K: Observations on the development of reaching for moving
objects. J Exp Child Psychol 1979;28:158–173.
von Hofsten C, Rönnqvist L: Preparation for grasping an object: A developmental study. J
Exp Psychol 1988;14:610–621.
von Hofsten C, Woollacott M: Postural preparations for reaching in 9-month-old infants.
1990; in preparation.
Jeannerod M: Intersegmental coordination during reaching at natural visual objects; in Long
J, Baddeley A (eds): Attention and Performance IX. Hillsdale, Earlbaum, 1981, pp
153–168.
Reed ES: Changing theories of postural development; in Woollacott M, Shumway-Cook A
(eds): Development of Posture and Gait Across the Life Span. Columbia, University of
South Carolina Press, 1990.

Claes von Hofsten, Department of Psychology, Umeå University,
S–901 87 Umeå (Sweden)

Forssberg H, Hirschfeld H (eds): Movement Disorders in Children.
Med Sport Sci. Basel, Karger, 1992, vol 36, pp 124–129

Roles of Proprioceptive Input in Control of Reaching Movements

James Gordon[a,b], *Claude Ghez*[a,1]

[a]Center for Neurobiology and Behavior, New York State Psychiatric Institute,
and [b]Program in Physical Therapy, College of Physicians and Surgeons,
Columbia University, New York, N.Y., USA

Almost 100 years ago Mott and Sherrington [1] established what has become a critical paradigm in the study of motor control: the deafferentation experiment. In order to determine the 'influence of the sensory nerves on the movements of the limbs', they cut off sensory input from an upper or lower limb in rhesus monkeys by surgical transection of the dorsal roots of the spinal cord. This procedure left the motor nerves intact, since they exit from the spinal cord through the ventral roots. The results were dramatic. Although some crude automatic movements remained, virtually all volitional movements in the deafferented limb were permanently abolished, especially those involving distal segments. The monkeys simply did not use the limbs for any purposeful activities. Thus, Mott and Sherrington concluded that sensory input from the limbs was essential for the production of purposeful movements.

Why should sensory input from the limbs be essential for movement? A simple answer was that all movement involves simple spinal reflexes, or chains of such reflexes, an idea that was current throughout the first half of the twentieth century. Later, Merton [2] developed a more sophisticated formulation, the follow-up servo model, in which gamma motor neurons activated muscles indirectly by way of muscle spindles. In any case, the assumption that sensory input is a prerequisite of voluntary movement became the cornerstone of the neurophysiological approaches to rehabilitation of brain-injured patients that developed in the middle part of this century and are still in use today [3]. In general, each of these 'facilitation' approaches attempted to restore normal movement by providing some form of enhanced proprioceptive input, usually to elicit simple reflexes.

[1] We thank Dr. Maria Felice Ghilardi for invaluable assistance with some of the experiments described. Supported by NIH grant NS-22715.

Beginning in the 1960s, however, the tide of scientific opinion began to change, as increasing evidence developed that sensory input was not essential for generation of voluntary movement. In particular, Taub and Berman and colleagues [4–6], in a series of studies, provided definitive evidence that monkeys with deafferented limbs are indeed capable of making skilled voluntary movements, if they are provided with training and sufficient incentive to relearn the use of the deafferented limb.

These and other experiments led to increasing acceptance of a 'motor program' theory of movement [7] which held that complex patterns of movement can be generated by the central nervous system without specific sensory input from the limbs. This idea, although overly simplistic in its initial formulations, became the basis for increasingly sophisticated analyses of the nature of central representations of movement. An example was the demonstration by Polit and Bizzi [8] that a deafferented monkey could produce reasonably accurate arm movements even when the limb was transiently perturbed before or during the movement. They concluded that the monkey could program a desired elbow angle by setting the appropriate ratio between agonist and antagonist muscle forces and allowing the spring-like properties of the muscle to bring the arm to a new equilibrium position [9].

By the early 1980s, the pendulum had swung to the other extreme and the dominant view in motor physiology was that sensory input was not essential for control of movement, but was useful merely for assuring its 'normal elegance' [10]. Then in 1982, Rothwell et al., [11] described a series of studies of a 'deafferented man', a human patient with generalized large-fiber sensory neuropathy. This rare condition leads to loss of all proprioceptive input and tactile sense from the limbs, but leaves intact the motor nerves. They described an individual profoundly impaired in activities of daily living, especially those requiring fine movements of the hands, but surprisingly normal in most standard laboratory tasks. They attributed many of the functional difficulties to a loss of sensory feedback, that is, an inability to correct small errors based on proprioceptive information, and they discovered a laboratory task that demonstrated this deficit convincingly. When asked to maintain a target isometric force or position with the thumb, the patient could do so very well when allowed to view at the same time an oscilloscope trace of his motor output. But, if this visual feedback was removed, the force or position began to fluctuate in a random fashion, without the subject being aware that this was happening. Normal subjects, in contrast, could easily maintain a steady force or position without visual feedback. This inability of deafferented patients to maintain a constant level of muscle contraction can be demonstrated clinically by asking them to hold their hands steady in front of the body and then to close the eyes.

They then exhibit slow drifts in hand and finger position, a symptom referred to as 'pseudoathetosis,' because of the similarity to the slow writhing movements of athetosis.

Thus, sensory input from the limbs acts as *feedback* in certain types of sustained activities, such as holding a cup of water, allowing the nervous system to maintain a desired force output by signalling when errors occur [11–14]. Presumably, such feedback is necessary because the state of the muscles and joints is not stable over time, so that a steady neural output has varying effects, as factors such as fatigue and subtle changes in load change the response of the muscles. In the absence of sensory input from the limbs, visual feedback can at least partially substitute, and thus these patients are highly visually dependent. However, since visual reactions are known to be slower than kinesthetic reactions [15], these patients must slow their movements, so they will have time to make visually determined corrections.

In our laboratory, we have had the opportunity in the past few years to study patients with large-fiber sensory neuropathy [16–19]. These patients, although able to initiate and carry out complex movement sequences, were severely impaired in most functional activities. For example, none could successfully reach for and drink from a cup of water without spilling it. Since other investigators had found clear evidence of a disturbance in feedback control of movement, we addressed a different question: whether these patients have deficits in *feedforward* control of movement. In other words, is there an impairment in their ability to program in advance the appropriate set of commands to make accurate goal-directed movements?

We examined the ability of 3 patients to make accurate reaching movements *without visual feedback* to different targets on a horizontal surface. In comparison to normal subjects, the patients made large errors in their movements, both in direction and extent, and these errors were present from the very beginning of the movement. Some of these errors could be attributed to an incorrect estimate of the inertial loads opposing movement, which differ for movements in different directions [19, 20]. Thus, sensory input from the limb is important not just for providing input about errors after they have developed (feedback control), but also for planning the movement (feedforward control). We also found that, if the patients were allowed to look at their arm prior to movement, their accuracy was substantially improved, although never to normal levels. This prior visual input about the state of the arm was particularly effective if the patients could see their arm in motion, thereby gaining information about the dynamic properties of the limb, that is, how it responds to motor commands. Therefore, we hypothesize that deafferented patients use visual information about their limb to update internal representations, or models, of the current position and mechanical state of their limbs, and that such models are necessary for accurate control of limb movement.

Thus, proprioceptive input from the limb is critical, not just for feedback corrections, but also for feedforward control of voluntary movement. Why has this role of sensory input received so little attention? One reason may be that other investigators who saw relatively little effect of deafferentation on programming mechanisms examined single-joint movements [8, 11]. Reaching movements, on the other hand, require movement at more than one joint, introducing complexities, such as inertial differences with different directions of movement, that are not present in single-joint movements. Reaching movements are also notable because they require a complex sensorimotor transformation, from the extrinsic coordinates in which a target is first represented in the visual system, to intrinsic body-centered coordinates in which the joint movements to get the hand to that target are represented [21, 22]. Apparently, the dynamic stage of this transformation, the specification of the muscle forces needed, requires up-to-date information regarding inertial and other loads acting on the limb. The muscle receptors, especially spindles and tendon organs, are of course especially well adapted for this purpose.

Another reason that the effects of deafferentation are not always evident in laboratory situations is that these often involve discrete tasks in which the patient is able to focus on controlling a single variable. Real life tasks, on the other hand, typically require control of many variables simultaneously. Vision is not well suited to monitoring and controlling several different components of a task at the same time. We saw an example of this problem when one of our patients tried to learn to use a walker to compensate for her poor balance. She could grip the walker using visual feedback, but, as soon as she tried to pick up the walker and move it forward, her grip would falter or the walker would tilt to one side or the other. She could use the vision to monitor only one aspect of her performance at a time. This emphasizes an important advantage of using proprioceptive and tactile inputs to control specific components of a task. In contrast to visual feedback, the nervous system can apparently set up several somatosensory feedback operations to operate in parallel. Once these feedback loops are enabled, they can presumably operate automatically, without requiring conscious intervention.

Finally, our results emphasize the importance for motor control of internal neural models of the mechanical properties of the peripheral musculoskeletal system. We might think of these in sum as the *body image*. However, these models must include, besides a static representation of limb positions, information about the dynamic behavior of the muscles and joints – how they respond to specific motor commands. It is possible, even likely, that interference with the acquisition and updating of these internal models is one of the consequences of damage to the brain.Thus, one of the goals of rehabilitation in many cases should probably be to restore working models of the body's mechanical properties. In other words, the patient learns improved motor control by learning about the properties of his or her peripheral system. This kind of learning is unlikely to be facilitated by eliciting stereotyped reflexes. Rather, treatment approaches that allow the patient to use the available sensory inputs to explore the mechanical properties of their neuromuscular system, ideally while attempting to carry out meaningful tasks, are most likely to be successful.

References

1   Mott FW, Sherrington CS: Experiments upon the influence of sensory nerves upon movement and nutrition of the limbs. Proc R Soc Lond [Biol] 1895;57:481–488.
2   Merton PA: Speculations on the servo-control of movement; in Wolstenholme GEW (ed): The Spinal Cord. London, Churchill Livingstone, 1953, pp 247–255.
3   Gordon J: Assumptions underlying physical therapy intervention: Theoretical and historical perspectives; in Carr JH, Shepherd RB (eds): Movement Science: Foundations for Physical Therapy in Rehabilitation. Rockville, Aspen, 1987, pp 1–30.
4   Knappp HD, Taub E, Berman AJ: Movements made in monkeys with deafferented forelimbs. Exp Neurol 1963;7:305–313.
5   Taub E, Berman AJ: Avoidance conditioning in the absence of relevant proprioceptive and exteroceptive feedback. J Comp Physiol Psychol 1963;56:1012–1016.
6   Taub E: Somatosensory deafferentation research with monkeys: Implications for rehabilitation medicine; in Ince LP (ed): Behavioral Psychology in Rehabilitation Medicine: Clinical Implications. Baltimore, Williams & Wilkins, 1980, pp 371–401.
7   Keele SW: Movement control in skilled motor performance. Psychol Bull 1968;70:387–403.
8   Polit A, Bizzi E: Characteristics of motor programs underlying arm movements in monkey. J Neurophysiol 1979;42:183–194.
9   Feldman AG: Functional tuning of the nervous system with control of movement or maintenance of a steady posture. III. Mechanographic analysis of the execution by man of the simplest motor tasks. Biophysics 1966;11:766–775.
10 Bossom J: Movement without proprioception. Brain Res 1974;71:285–296.
11 Rothwell JL, Traub MM, Day BL, Obeso JA, Thomas PK, Marsden CD: Manual motor performance in a deafferented man. Brain 1982;105:515–542.
12 Marsden CD, Rothwell JC, Day BL: The use of peripheral feedback in the control of movement; in Evarts EV, Wise SP, Bousfield D (ed): The Motor System in Neurobiology. Amsterdam, Elsevier, 1985, pp 215–222.
13 Sanes JN, Mauritz K-H, Dalakas MC, Evarts EV: Motor control in humans with large-fiber sensory neuropathy. Hum Neurobiol 1985;4:101–114.
14 Forget R, Lamarre Y: Rapid elbow flexion in the absence of proprioceptive and cutaneous feedback. Hum Neurobiol 1987;6:27–37.

15   Poulton EC: Human manual control; in Brooks VB (ed): Handbook of Physiology, sec
      1. The Nervous System, vol 2. Motor Control, part 2. Bethesda, American Physiological
      Society, 1981, pp 1337–1389.

16   Ghez C, Bermejo R, Gordon J: Impairment in programming of response direction and
      amplitude in deafferented patients. Soc Neurosci Abstr 1988;14:953.

17   Gordon J, Iyer M, Ghez C: Impairment of motor programming and trajectory control
      in a deafferented patient. Soc Neurosci Abstr 1987;13:352.

18   Gordon J, Ghilardi MF, Ghez C: Deafferented subjects fail to compensate for
      workspace anisotropies in 2-dimensional arm movements. Soc Neurosci Abstr
      1990;16:1089.

19   Ghez C, Gordon J, Ghilardi MF, Christakos CN, Cooper SE: Roles of proprioceptive
      input in the programming of arm trajectories. Cold Spring Harbor Symp Quant Biol
      1990;55:837–847.

20   Hogan N: The mechanics of multi-joint posture and movement control. Biol Cybern
      1985;52:315–331.

21   Soechting JF: Elements of coordinated arm movements in three-dimensional space; in
      Wallace SA (ed): Perspectives on the Coordination of Movement. New York, North-
      Holland, 1989, pp 47–83.

22   Soechting JF, Terzuolo CA; Sensorimotor transformations and the kinematics of arm
      movements in three-dimensional space; in Jeannerod M (ed): Attention and Perfor-
      mance. XIII. Motor Representation and Control. Hillsdale, Lawrence Erlbaum, 1990,
      pp 479–494.

James Gordon, EdD, PT, Center for Neurobiology and Behavior,
New York State Psychiatric Institute, and Program in Physical Therapy,
Columbia University, 722 W. 168th Street, New York, NY 10032 (USA)

Forssberg H, Hirschfeld H (eds): Movement Disorders in Children.
Med Sport Sci. Basel, Karger, 1992, vol 36, pp 130–136

Development of Anticipatory Control Mechanisms for Manipulation

Andrew M. Gordon

Nobel Institute for Neurophysiology and Department of Pediatrics,
Karolinska Institute, Stockholm, Sweden

During active manipulation of objects, anticipatory control of the motor output is required to produce well-coordinated transitions between the various movement phases due to the long delay between the motor command and feedback. If the termination of the force increase during a simple lift of a small object using the thumb and forefinger (precision grip) was based only upon signals from tactile afferents at lift-off, the delay would result in a large vertical acceleration of the object and an overshoot in the grip force. Therefore, adults normally base the programming of the isometric force output before lift-off upon an internal neural representation (e.g. a sensorimotor memory) of the object's size [1–3], weight [4] and friction [5]. This anticipatory control is characterized by bell-shaped force rate profiles [6] which are appropriately decreased prior to lift-off to harmonize with the physical properties of the object. Figure 1 illustrates a schematic diagram of the processes underlying the anticipatory control of a grip/lift movement. Anticipatory control of manipulation involves a nervous system which can efficiently monitor sensory information. The sensory information must be properly integrated and stored in an internal neural representation of the object to be manipulated. The representation must be translated into motor programs, which are appropriate for the specific task, controlling the gain of both the grip and load force (vertical lifting force) generating circuits. Finally, the motor program must issue motor commands stabilizing the trunk and executing the grip/lift movement, and information regarding the outcome of the movement must be used to update the internal representation.

Precision grip is controlled by the motor cortex via the corticospinal tract [7, 8]. It normally develops during the later part of the first year and is dependent on the maturation of the corticospinal tract [9]. During a grasp with the precision grip, adults typically generate the grip force and

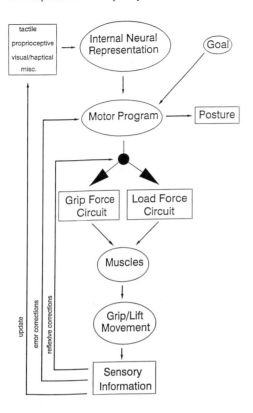

Fig. 1. Schematic diagram of mechanisms underlying the anticipatory control of grip/lift movements.

load force in parallel after the initial contact with the grip surface [Johansson and Edin, this vol.]. This reflects a functional synergy coupling grip and loads force generators, which serves to simplify the movement. When the precision grip first emerges, children do not generate the forces in parallel [10]. They initiate the grip force in conjunction with a negative load force, pushing the object against its support. By the onset of positive load force, there is already a substantial grip force, and subsequent increases in the isometric grip and load force during the loading phase are not in parallel [10]. The sequential activation of the forces and an excessive grip force likely allow children to obtain additional information regarding the surface friction and to stabilize the grasp, as well as to provide a strategy less dependent on anticipatory control. There is a large intra-subject variability in the force amplitudes and temporal parameters, which

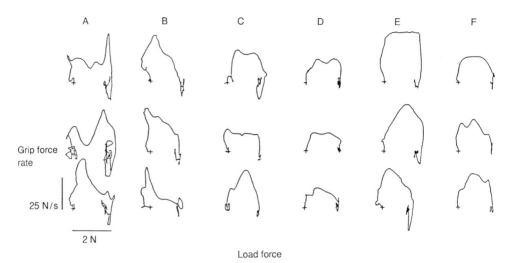

Fig. 2. Grip force rate as a function of load force for *(A)* a 10-month-old child; *(B)* a 2-year-old child; *(C)* a 4-year-old child; *(D)* an 8-year-old child; *(E)* a 12-year-old child, and *(F)* an adult. Grip force rate is shown using a ±10 point numerical differentiation. Modified from Forssberg et al. [10].

may allow the CNS to explore and evaluate different response patterns [11].

Likewise, young children do not exhibit the bell shaped force rate profiles seen in adults [10] (fig. 2). In contrast, these children have multi-peaked force rate profiles which resemble those seen during a 'probing strategy' [2] in which small increments in force occur until terminated by sensory feedback at lift-off (i.e. from FAII afferents) [Johansson and Edin, this vol.]. During the later part of the second year the grip force and load force start to be generated in parallel and the force rate profiles become increasingly bell shaped with small irregularities. Subsequent development is gradual and approximates adult-like coordination by the time children reach 8–10 years of age, and subtle improvements occur until adolescence.

When the weight of the object is varied while the visual appearance of the object remains constant, adults use an anticipatory strategy in which the amplitude of the isometric grip and load forces during the loading phases are scaled towards the object's weight [4]. This anticipatory control results in force rates which are critically damped at lift-off, providing similar vertical accelerations independent of the object's weight [3] (fig. 3). In contrast, the force development for young children is not influenced by

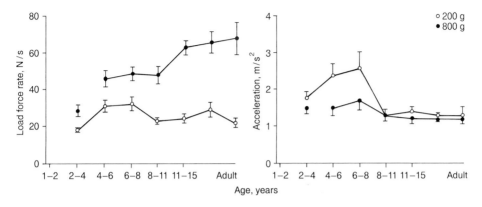

Fig. 3. The influence of 200 and 800 g weight (400 g for the 1- to 2-year-old children) on the peak load force rate and the peak vertical acceleration. Modified from Forssberg et al. [in press].

the object's weight [12] (fig. 3). These children obtain higher forces mainly by prolonging the duration of isometric force increase. Yet, they are capable of adapting the forces to the object's weight during the static phase, when the object is held in the air, indicating that somatosensory weight information can be used to adjust the force output. Concomitant to the emergence of the mainly single peaked force rate profiles, children begin to scale the amplitude of the forces according to the object's weight during the second year [12]. The influence of the object's weight in the previous trial increases gradually until 6–8 years, when the vertical acceleration of the object following lift-off becomes similar for various weights (fig. 3). Interestingly, anticipatory control of the precision grip may develop later than anticipatory control underlying other grasping movements [see von Hofsten, this vol.] and children with cerebral palsy never develop anticipatory control of the precision grip [13; see Eliasson, this vol.].

Weight information may also be gained from visual [1, 3] and haptical [2] size cues when an additional transformation is made based on a predicted relationship between the object's size and weight. When both the size and weight of an object attached to an instrumented grip handle are covaried (i.e. the weight is kept proportional to the volume), the forces are appropriately scaled toward the expected weight relative to the volume. Interestingly, when only the size of the object attached to the grip handle is changed while the weight is kept the same [1, 2], a size weight illusion occurs, in which adults perceive the smaller object to be heavier [14]. Yet these subjects still employ higher forces for the larger objects, indicating a

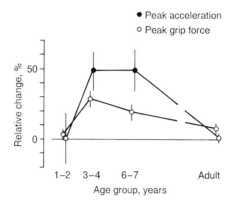

• Peak acceleration
○ Peak grip force

Fig. 4. Relative change in peak grip force and vertical acceleration, between a small and large box (both 500 g) for children of various ages and adults. Modified from Gordon et al. [in press].

dichotomy between perceptual and motor systems [1]. In the latter case, the size influences on the force output are relatively small compared to the size weight covariation [3] and the influence of the previous weight [4]. Therefore, adults are capable of attenuating the influences of size cues when they are not purposeful.

The force output for children under the age of $2\frac{1}{2}$–3 years is not influenced by the object's size, regardless of whether the weight is kept the same or covaried [15] (fig. 4). This suggests that an additional year of development is necessary before children can make an associative transformation between the object's size and weight. This likely involves additional demands on cortical processes, requiring further cognitive development. When this ability emerges, these children exhibit much larger visual size influences than adults when only the size is varied, suggesting that they are incapable of attenuating size information when it is not purposeful [15] (fig. 4). One possible interpretation of these findings is that children rely more on vision [16]. However, others have found that children are less likely to integrate sensory information from various modalities than adults [17]. The maintained large but inappropriate size influences may correspond to a later development of mechanisms integrating visual size information and somatosensory weight information gained during earlier manipulative experience.

In conclusion, anticipatory control of precision grip is not innate; rather it gradually develops. Although the youngest children can regulate their grip force during the static phase, they appear to have difficulties in forming an internal representation or translating the representation into motor commands. The lack of anticipatory control in young children may explain their excessive force generation, prolonged movement phases and large intra-subject variability. When anticipatory control emerges, it appears that children are not capable of appropriately integrating sensory information into the internal representation of the object. The ability to deduce one physical property from another probably requires additional cognitive development. It appears that the continued development of anticipatory control, the ability to proper integrate sensory information and the ability to transform size information (fig. 1) may reflect an important maturation of mechanisms controlling grasping. Objectives for clinicians treating children with motor disorders involving manipulative functions should perhaps include (1) helping to facilitate the relationship between physical properties of objects and movement parameters; (2) teaching these children to compensate for their disabilities by relying on alternative strategies when necessary (e.g. feedback control), and (3) when possible, allowing vision to compensate for other sensory deficits by using it to extract physical properties of objects prior to manipulation.

Acknowledgements

The author was supported by a grant from the Fulbright Commission and Stiftelsen Wenner-Gren Center. These studies were supported by Stiftelsen Sven Jerrings Fond, The Swedish Medical Research Council (projects 5925, 8885 and 08667), The First of Mayflower Annual Campaign for Children's Health, Stiftelsen Solstickan, Sunnerdahls Handikappfond, and the University of Umeå. Appreciation is extended to Hans Forssberg for reviewing an earlier version of this manuscript.

References

1   Gordon AM, Forssberg H, Johansson RS, Westling G: Visual size cues in the programming of manipulative forces during precision grip. Exp Brain Res 1991;83:477–482.
2   Gordon AM, Forssberg H, Johansson RS, Westling G: The integration of haptically acquired size information in the programming of precision grip. Exp Brain Res 1991;83:483–488.
3   Gordon AM, Forssberg H, Johansson RS, Westling G: Integration of sensory information during the programming of precision grip: Comments on the contributions of size cues. Exp Brain Res 1991;85:226–229.
4   Johansson RS, Westling G: Coordinated isometric muscle commands adequately and erroneously programmed for the weight during lifting task with precision grip. Exp Brain Res 1988;71:59–71.
5   Johansson RS, Westling G: Signals in tactile afferents from the fingers eliciting adaptive motor responses during precision grip. Exp Brain Res 1987;66:141–154.

6   Brooks VB: How are 'move' and 'hold' programs matched? in Bloedel et al (eds): Cerebellar Functions. Berlin, Springer, 1984, pp 1–23.

7   Lawrence DG, Kuypers HGJM: The functional organization of the motor system in the monkey. I. The effects of bilateral pyramidal lesions. Brain 1968;91:1–14.

8   Muir RB, Lemon RN: Corticospinal neurons with a special role in precision grip. Brain Res 1983;261:312–316.

9   Conel JL: The Postnatal Development of the Human Cerebral Cortex, vol 1. The Cortex of the Newborn. Cambridge, Harvard University Press, 1939.

10   Forssberg H, Eliasson AC, Kinoshita H, Johansson RS, Westling G: Development of human precision grip. I. Basic coordination of force. Exp Brain Res 1991;85:451–457.

11   Touwen B: Variability and stereotypy in normal and deviant development; in Touwen B (ed): Neurological Development in Infancy. London, SIMP and Heinemann Medical Books, 1978, pp 99–110.

12   Forssberg H, Kinoshita H, Eliasson AC, Johansson RS, Westling G, Gordon A: Development of human precision grip II. Anticipatory control of isometric forces targeted for object's weight. Exp Brain Res, in press.

13   Eliasson AC, Gordon AM, Forssberg H: Impaired anticipatory control of isometric forces during grasping in children with cerebral palsy. Dev Med Child Neurol 1992;34:216–225.

14   Charpentier A: Analyse expérimentale de quelques élements de la sensation de poids. Arch Physiol Norm Pathol 1891;3:122–135.

15   Gordon AM, Forssberg H, Johansson RS, Eliasson AC, Westling G: Development of human precision grip. III. Integration of visual size cues during the programming of isometric forces. Exp Brain Res, in press.

16   Lee DN, Aronson E: Visual proprioceptive control of standing in human infants. Percept Psychophys 1974;15:529–532.

17   Forssberg H, Nashner LM: Ontogenetic development of postural control in man: Adaptation to altered support and visual conditions during stance. Neuroscience 1982;2:545–552.

Andrew M. Gordon, Nobel Institute for Neurophysiology and Department of Pediatrics, Karolinska Institute, S–104 01 Stockholm (Sweden)

Forssberg H, Hirschfeld H (eds): Movement Disorders in Children.
Med Sport Sci. Basel, Karger, 1992, vol 36, pp 137–143

Perceptual Determinants of Precise Manual Pointing in Children with Motor Impairments

Birgit Rösblad

Department of Psychology, Umeå University, Umeå, Sweden

Most movements are goal directed and purposeful. We see, feel, hear, smell and taste our own body and the objects and events with which we are surrounded. The information provided to our senses will invite us to act and enables us to plan and guide our movements. The ability to utilize sensory information for movement control appears very early in infancy. Crude examples of sensorimotor integration are already seen at birth. A newborn will reach for a seen object [1]. When hearing a sound the newborn will turn towards it [2] and is also capable of following a moving object with eyes and head [3]. During infancy and childhood the ability to utilize information for controlling movements improve considerably. However, not all children seem to develop these capabilities equally well. This paper is concerned with impaired perceptual control of goal-directed arm movements in children with motor impairments.

Perceptual Control of Arm Movements

When performing goal-directed arm movements we need information about the layout of the environment, our own body, as well as the relation between the hand and the environment [4]. Vision and proprioception are the two major sources of information used to supply these varieties of information. Vision specifies the form of the object and its position in space and is also used to specify the position of the hand towards the end of the approach. In fact, seeing the hand as well as the object is necessary for pointing with precision and for fine grasping movements, e.g. picking up small objects [5, 7].

Proprioception is used here to define the information provided by receptors in muscles, tendons, joints and skin about one's own movements and positions of limbs and body parts. The role of proprioception for goal-directed movements is more complicated to study than the role of vision. One can easily prevent the subject from seeing the hand but not from feeling it. From deafferentation experiments in monkeys and from studies of patients with reduced or absent afferent feedback from the moving limb, one can draw the conclusion that coordinated movements can to some extent be performed without proprioceptive information [8, 9]. However, coordination of movements involving several joints as well as maintaining stable postures [10, 11] are impossible.

von Hofsten and Rösblad [12] studied how children develop their ability to utilize vision and proprioception for manual control. 270 children aged between 14 and 12 years participated in the study. The task was to place pins underneath a tabletop at positions seen or felt on the tabletop. When a position was felt, the child was asked to place the index finger of the other hand on the tabletop at the position to be pointed at and then close the eyes and point. Normally, when performing a precise pointing task visual feedback of the pointing hand is required. It is likely to assume that when unable to see the hand the child will substitute visual feedback with proprioception. One main finding was that performance was superior when visual information about the position of the target was provided. This was true for all age groups. In the condition where the child closed the eyes and pointed at the felt or remembered position of the target, the youngest children had marked problems. However, between 4 and 8 years of age, random error was substantially reduced in those conditions.

Movement Control in Children with Motor Impairments

Little is known about the degree to which motor impairments in children are determined hy poor perception. Some attempts have been made to study this problem in 'clumsy children'.

Hoare and Larkin [21] tested a large sample of clumsy children on a variety of perceptual judgement items, trying to clarify the relationship between proprioception and clumsiness. They demonstrated that the clumsy children, as a group, were deficit in 3 of 7 proprioceptive tasks, including both passive and active movements.

Laszlo and Bairstow [13] also tested the proprioceptive sensitivity in clumsy children. They reported a marked inability to process propriocep- tive information in a group of clumsy children and stated that propriocep- tive sensibility deficits is one of the causes of clumsiness in children. They carried out a proprioceptive training intervention with children performing poorly on their test and concluded that training of the proprioceptive sensibility improved motor abilities dramatically [14]. The findings reported by Laszlo and Bairstow have been questioned from several standpoints; failures to replicate the studies [15, 16] as well as methodological problems [17].

Hulme and his associates [18–20] argue that deficits in visual perception is a crucial factor causing clumsiness in children. They studied a variety of tasks, with and without visual information, and found indications of an association between visual perceptual deficits and impaired motor performance.

Vision and proprioception do not only have to function in an optimal way by themselves in making well-coordinated movements but the two systems also have to be coordinated and calibrated to each other. According to Lee [4], the proprioceptors are subject to drift and need to be continuously calibrated with vision. In a hand alignment task, Lee et al. [22] found cross-modal functioning to be impaired in cerebral-palsied children. When aligning the unseen hand to a seen target they performed less accurately than when the target as well as the hand were unseen.

In order to study the role of visual and proprioceptive perception in goal-directed arm movements in children with motor impairments the pointing task used by von Hofsten and Rösblad [12] was administered to a group of 29 children with motor impairments, including spina bifida, cerebral palsy and developmental coordination disorder, with a mean age of 10 years. The essential feature of developmental coordination disorder is marked impairment in the development of motor coordination which is not a function of mental retardation and is not due to a known physical disorder, [23]. This group of children would be similar to what is often called 'clumsy children'.

In figures 1–3, the performance of these groups are plotted relative to a group of 7-year-old normal children. The mean age in the three clinical groups was 10 years so the comparison with the normal 7-year-old children is reasonably conservative.

It is clear from figures 1–3 that the children with motor impairments exhibited large variability in pointing accuracy compared to the normal children. A main finding in von Hofsten and Rösblad [12] was the superior pointing performance with visually defined targets. This effect was found to be even larger in the study of motor-impaired children. If the child cannot see the target during the pointing action, the impairment is more obvious. This is well in agreement with Henderson [unpubl. manuscript] who, in collaboration with the present authors, administered a similar test to a group of children with developmental coordination disorders and compared them with a control group.

These results suggest that many motor-impaired children are dependent on having a visual frame of reference when planning and guiding

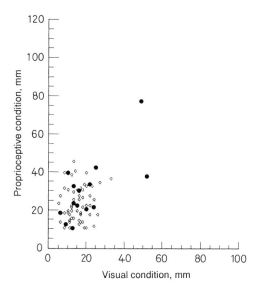

Fig. 1. Absolute error for visual and proprioceptive condition in children with cerebral palsy (●) and a group of 7-year-old normal children (◇).

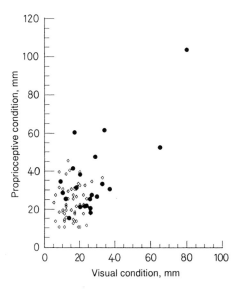

Fig. 2. Absolute error for visual and proprioceptive condition in children with developmental coordination disorder (●) and a group of 7-year-old normal children (◇).

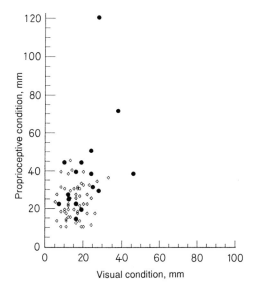

Fig. 3. Absolute error for visual and proprioceptive condition in children with spina bifida (●) and a group of 7-year-old children (◇).

movements. Although the common feature is a dependency of visual control this is not true for all children tested. Instead, some had problems matching the unseen pointing hand to the seen target. This could indicate that the visual space and proprioceptive space of their bodies were uncoordinated. Some children had large errors both when the target was seen and felt which could indicate an impaired proprioceptive sensitivity. However, other children performed very well despite their motor difficulties.

Conclusion

The variability in results from different studies and the large variability within studies indicates that we cannot expect just one perceptual factor to cause all the movement problems in a specific diagnosis group. Both visual and proprioceptive deficits may contribute to movement disorders in children. To be able to understand the specific problems of each child and to develop treatment programs adapted to these problems, it is of crucial importance to develop instruments for testing the perceptual abilities underlying coordinated movements.

Perception and action are tightly coupled. We have to take perception into account when we try to understand disturbed or delayed motor behavior. It is important both when it comes to assessing and planning treatment for children with motor impairments as well as when stimulating the delayed child. Vision is very powerful for stimulating the motor system and for controlling movements and perhaps especially so in young children and children with motor impairments. Is the role of vision for movement control and motor learning fully recognized among therapists? To give the child proprioceptive input in order to facilitate motor output is a technique common to several therapeutic methods. Have we been giving enough consideration to how the child itself is using proprioceptive information for perception of its own body and how this 'body image' can be disturbed and affect motor performance.

References

1   von Hofsten C: Eye-hand coordination in the newborn. Dev Psychol 1982;18: 450–467.
2   Mendelson MJ, Haith MH: The relation between audition and vision in the human newborn. Monogr Soc Res Child Dev 1976;41:
3   Aslin RN: Development of smooth pursuit in human infants; in Fisher DF, Monty RA, Senders JW (eds): Eye Movements: Cognition and Visual Perception. Hillsdale, Lawrence Erlbaum, 1981.
4   Lee DN: The function of vision; in Pick HL, Salzman E (eds): Modes of Perceiving and Processing Information. Hillsdale, Lawrence Erlbaum, 1978, pp 159–169.
5   Buyakas TM, Vardanyan G, Gippenreiter Yu B: On the mechanism of precise hand movements (in Russian). Psicholigitsheskij J 1980;1:93–103.
6   Helms Tillery SI, Flanders M, Soechting JF: A coordinate system for the synthesis of visual and kinesthetic information. J Neurosci 1991;11:770–778.
7   Jeannerod M: The Neural and Behavioural Organization of Goal-Directed Movements. Oxford, Clarendon Press, 1988, pp 173–178.
8   Taub E, Berman AJ: Movement and learning in the absence of sensory feedback; in Freedman SJ (ed): The Neurophysiology of Spatially Oriented Behavior. Homewood, Dorsey Press, 1968, pp 173–192.
9   Polit A, Bizzi E: Characteristics of motor programs underlying arm movements in monkeys. J Neurophysiol 1979;42:183–194.
10 Rothwell JC, Traub MM, Day BL, Obeso JA, Thomas PK, Marsden CD: Manual performance in a deaferrented man. Brain 1982;105:515–542.
11 Sanes JN, Mauritz KH, Dalakas MC, Evarts EV: Motor control in humans with large-fiber sensory neuropathy. Hum Neurobiol 1985;4:101–114.
12 von Hofsten C, Rösblad B: The integration of sensory information in the development of precise manual pointing. Neuropsychologia 1988;20:461–471.
13 Laszlo JI, Bairstow PI: The measurement of kinesthetic sensitivity in children and adults. Dev Med Child Neurol 1980;22:454–464.
14 Laszlo JI, Bairstow PI: Kinesthesia: Its measurement, training and relationship to motor control. Q J Exp Psychol 1983;35:411–421.

15   Lord R, Hulme C: Kinaesthetic sensitivity of normal and clumsy children. Dev Med Child Neurol 1987;29:270–275.
16   Sugden D, Wann C: The assessment of motor impairment in children with moderate learning difficulties. Br J Educ Psychol 1987;57:225–236.
17   Doyle AJR, Elliott JM, Connolly KJ: Measurement of kinaesthetic sensitivity. Dev Med Child Neurol 1986;28:188–193.
18   Hulme C, Biggerstaff A, Moran G, McKinley I: Visual, kinaesthetic and cross-modal judgements of length by normal and clumsy children. Dev Med Child Neurol 1982;24:461–471.
19   Hulme C, Smart A, Moran G: Visual perceptual deficits in clumsy children. Neuropsychologia 1982b;20:475–481.
20   Lord R, Hulme C: Visual perception and drawing in clumsy and normal children. Br J Dev Psychol 1988;6:1–9.
21   Hoare D, Larkin D: Kinaesthetic abilities of clumsy children. Dev Med Child Neurol 1991;33:671–678.
22   Lee DN, Daniel BM, Turnball J, Cook ML: Basic perceptuo-motor dysfunction in cerebral palsy; in Jeannerod M (ed): Attention and Performance. XIII. Motor Representation and Control. New York, Lawrence Erlbaum, 1990, pp 586–603.
23   DSM III R: Diagnostic and Statistical Manual of Mental Disorders, ed 3. Washington, American Psychiatric Association, 1987.

Birgit Rösblad, Department of Psychology, Umeå University, S–901 87 Umeå (Sweden)

Forssberg H, Hirschfeld H (eds): Movement Disorders in Children.
Med Sport Sci. Basel, Karger, 1992, vol 36, pp 144–150

Manipulative Forces in Grasping of Children with Cerebral Palsy

Ann-Christin Eliasson

Nobel Institute for Neurophysiology and Department of Pediatrics,
Karolinska Institute, Karolinska Hospital, Stockholm, Sweden

Children with cerebral palsy (CP) usually have a disturbed hand function. The character of the impairment varies according to age, localization and size of the cerebral damage [1–3]. Major lesions involve the sensorimotor cortex and the corticospinal tracts, which has great implication for hand motor control since the precision grip and independent finger movements are controlled by this system [4, 5]. Children with CP are known to have deficits in motor control with impaired temporal and spatial coordination during locomotion, posture and isometric muscle contractions [6–9]. Sensory mechanisms, such as two-point discrimination, stereognosis and kinesthetic sensitivity are also known to be disturbed [10–12]. The handling of various objects's requires an intricate control of manipulatory forces. In this paper, I summarize studies on children with CP (diplegia and hemiplegia) during a simple lifting task [13, 14]. For details about the methods see Gordon and Johansson and Edin [this vol.].

Coordination of Grip and Load Force

During a lift, 6- to 8-year-old children with CP and a control group grasped and lifted the instrumented grip handle with a precision grip and held it in the air. The children in the control group grasped an object with a short delay between finger contacts. The grip force only increased slightly prior to the increase of load force. Thereafter, during the loading phase, there was a parallel increase of grip and load forces followed by a static phase when the object was held stationary in the air (fig. 1).

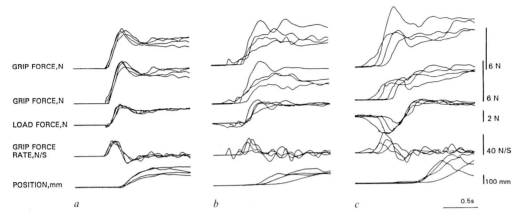

GRIP FORCE,N

GRIP FORCE,N

LOAD FORCE,N

GRIP FORCE
RATE,N/S

POSITION,mm

6 N

6 N

2 N

40 N/S

100 mm

a   *b*   *c*   0.5s

Fig. 1. Grip force for thumb and index finger, load force, grip force rate (dGF/dt) and vertical position as function of time for four superimposed lifts for one child in the control group (*a*), one child with diplegia (*b*), and one child with hemiplegia (*c*). The weight of the instrument was 200 g. Grip force rate is presented using ±20-point numerical differentiation.

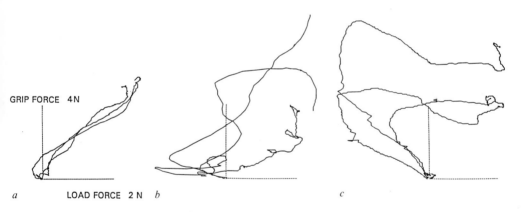

GRIP FORCE 4N

a   LOAD FORCE 2 N *b*   *c*

Fig. 2. Grip force in the preload and loading phases, plotted against load force. Three trials superimposed for one child in the control group (*a*), one child with diplegia (*b*), and one child with hemiplegia (*c*).

The coupling of grip and load force generators providing the parallel force output can be thought of as a lifting synergy simplifying the control of the grip-lift movement [15]. The forces were scaled in a bell-shaped force rate profiles target to the weight of the object, indicating that the force output was programmed in advance (fig. 3).

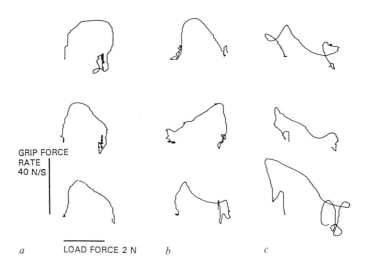

GRIP FORCE
RATE
40 N/S

a   LOAD FORCE 2 N   *b*   *c*

Fig. 3. Grip force as a function of load force in three consecutive trials for one child in the control group (*a*), one child with diplegia (*b*), and one child with hemiplegia (*c*).

The principal evidence for the programming is the bell-shaped force rate profile [16].

In children with CP the formation of finger contact was prolonged. They increased the grip force prior to the load force in a sequential order resulting in a long preload phase. The instrument was often pressed down against the table, resulting in a negative load force before onset of a positive load force (fig. 1, 2). Instead of bell-shaped force rate profiles the grip and load force rates increased in a stepwise and irregular fashion, until the object started to move (fig. 3). The temporal parameters were disrupted. In addition to a long delay between first and second finger contact children with CP increased the grip force rate early, the peak occurred sometimes during the preload phase instead of the loading phase. There was also a prolonged delay between lift-off and the grip force peak (fig. 1). The grip force was excessive compared to the control group. The children with CP used 50% sometimes up to 70–80% of their maximum grip strength in the grip force peak to lift an object of 200 g, compared to less than 14% in the control group. The control group performed this task consistently while there was large intra- and intersubject variation in the group of children with CP (fig. 1–3). To the same extent, these children exhibit a similar immature pattern as children below 2 years, although it was exaggerated [17; Gordon, this vol.].

Anticipatory Control of Isometric Forces

Anticipatory control, i.e. programming of the forces prior to the movement, is crucial to achieve smooth movements. The long delay between the arrival of sensory signals and the release of muscle commands makes the use of sensory feedback less purposeful in this context. Already during the preceding reaching phase the hand forms according to the size of the object and starts closing before hand contact [18]. Anticipatory hand closure seems to emerge at 9 months [19]. However, patients with hemiplegia cannot shape the hand properly and do not initiate closure during the reaching phase [18]. During the lift with the precision grip, a prolonged duration between first and second finger contact also indicated an impaired anticipatory hand closure.

Adults and children above 8–9 years of age program the isometric grip and load force increase prior to the movement indicated by a bell-shaped force rate profile targeted to the weight of the object (fig. 3) [20, 21]. To program the forces adequately, the sensory information of the object's physical properties achieved during earlier manipulation has to be stored into an internal representation and later transformed into appropriate motor programs [22, 23]. In the control group there was a mature programming resulting in a low load force rate at lift-off leading to constant acceleration independent of objects weight. Almost none of the children with CP could produce bell-shaped force rate profiles and the amplitudes were not scaled to the previous weight of the object (fig. 3) except in a few children. Differences in the peak grip force were achieved by a stepwise force increase of the isometric force until lift-off, resulting in much longer duration of the loading phase. Yet, the peak of grip and load force rates occurred later for the heavier object than for the lighter object indicating that also children with CP can to some extent scale the temporal aspect of force generation. The acceleration at lift-off was also influenced by the previous weight, i.e. there was a higher acceleration following a heavy than a light weight (fig. 4).

The impairment of the anticipatory scaling in children with CP may occur at different levels. The adaptation of grip force to different weights during the static phase indicates that the sensory system is efficient in modifying the ongoing motor output via feedback mechanisms. On the other hand, the sequential initiation of grip and load forces and the disturbed temporal pattern with prolonged durations of the various phases indicate a disturbed sensorimotor performance. The formation of an internal representation of the object's physical properties is of fundamental importance for the anticipatory control. At the moment it is impossible to judge whether children with CP cannot form such an internal representation or whether they cannot transform it into adequate motor commands.

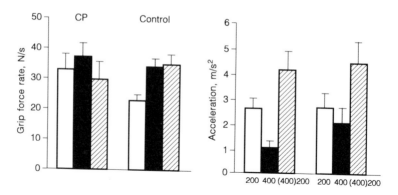

Fig. 4. Mean and SE for (*a*) the first peak of grip force rate, and (*b*) the maximum vertical acceleration for the 200 and the 400 g weights in constant series, and 200 g weight preceding a lift with 400 g weight (brackets) in both children with CP and the control group.

Conclusion

All children with CP have to the same extent a disturbed control of the force generation during lifting even if they have a mild diplegia with minor functional deficit in the hand or a spastic hemiplegic hand. However, the children with hemiplegia are more disturbed than children with diplegia in coordination of the isometric force generation and the temporal patterns (fig. 1, 2). There is no difference in anticipatory control between the different types of CP, although the results indicate that smoothness and efficiency in manipulation are disturbed in both groups. The sequential initiation of grip and load forces, the prolonged phases and inability to scale the forces in advance partly explain the jerky and slow movements typically seen in children with CP. However, there may be functional reasons to maintain the sequential initiation of forces to compensate for the impaired motor and sensory functions. The large grip force and the negative load force during the prolonged preload phase may help the children to establish a grasp and to prevent the object from slipping during the lift. Since these control mechanisms are impaired, the treatment has to focus on compensatory mechanisms. The control mechanism functions at an unconscious level, although motor learning strategies can be used to different extents. Vision is crucial for sensory information during fine prehension. It is used to focus the object, yet it also speeds up the movements and is essential when somatosensory information is impaired.

Acknowledgements

This study was supported by the Swedish Medical Research Council (projects 4X-5925, 4P-8885), Stiftelsen Sven Jerrings Fond, The First of Mayflower Annual Campaign for Children's Health, Stiftelsen Solstickan, Sunnerdahls Handikappfond, Josef and Linnea Karlssons Minnesfond, The Bank of Sweden Tercentenary Foundation.

References

1 Koeda T, Suganuma I, Kohno Y, Takamatsu T, Takeshita K: Comparative study between preterm and term infants. Neuroradiology 1990;32:187–190.
2 Wiklund LM, Uvebrant P: Hemiplegic cerebral palsy: Correlation between CT morphology and clinical findings. Dev Med Child Neurol 1991;33:512–523.
3 Shortland D, Levene MI, Trounce J, NG Y, Graham M: The evolution and outcome of cavitating periventricular leukomalacia in infancy. A study of 46 cases. J Perinat Med 1988;16:241–247.
4 Lawrence DG, Kuypers HGJM: The functional organization of the motor system in the monkey. I. The effects of bilateral pyramidal lesions. Brain 1968;91:1–14.
5 Muir RB, Lemon RN: Corticospinal neurons with a special role in precision grip. Brain Res 1983;261:312–316.
6 Forssberg H: Ontogeny of human locomotor control. I. Infant stepping, supported locomotion and transition to independent locomotion. Exp Brain Res 1985;57:480–493.
7 Berger W, Quintern J, Dietz V: Pathophysiology of gait in children with cerebral palsy. Electroencephalogr Clin Neurophysiol 1982;53:538–548.
8 Nashner LM, Shumway-Cook A, Marin O: Stance posture control in select groups of children with cerebral palsy: Deficits in sensory organization and muscular coordination. Exp Brain Res 1983;49:393–409.
9 Neilson PD, O'Dwyer NJ, Nash J: Control of isometric muscle activity in cerebral palsy. Dev Med Child Neurol 1990;32:778–788.
10 Lesny I: Disturbance of two-point discrimination sensitivity in different forms of cerebral palsy. Dev Med Child Neurol 1971;13:330–334.
11 Uvebrant P: Hemiplegic cerebral palsy aetiology and outcome. Acta Paediatr Scand (Suppl) 1988;345.
12 Opila-Lehman J, Short MA, Trombly CA: Kinesthetic recall of children with athetoid and spastic cerebral palsy and of non-handicapped children. Dev Med Child Neurol 1985;27:223–230.
13 Eliasson AC, Gordon AM, Forssberg H: Basic coordination of manipulative forces in children with cerebral palsy. Dev Med Child Neurol 1991;33:659–668.
14 Eliasson AC, Gordon AM, Forssberg H: Impaired anticipatory control of forces during grasping in children with cerebral palsy. Dev Med Child Neurol, in press.
15 Bernstein N: The Coordination and Regulation of Movements. Pergamon Press, Oxford, 1967.
16 Brooks VB: How are 'move' and 'hold' programs matched; in Bloedel, et al (eds): Cerebellar Functions. Springer, Berlin, 1984, pp 1–23.
17 Forssberg H, Eliasson AC, Kinoshita H, Johansson RS, Westling G: Development of human precision grip. I. Basic coordination. Exp Brain Res 1991;85:451–457.
18 Jeannerod M: The formation of finger grip during prehension. A cortically mediated visuomotor pattern. Behav Brain Res 1986;19:305–319.

19   von Hofsten C, Rönnqvist L: Preparation for grasping an object: A developmental study. J Exp Psychol 1988;4:610–621.

20   Johansson RS, Westling G: Coordinated isometric muscle commands adequately and erroneously programmed for the weight during lifting task with precision grip. Exp Brain Res 1988;71:59–71.

21   Forssberg H, Kinoshita H, Eliasson AC, Johansson RS, Westling G, Gordon A: Development of human precision grip. II. Anticipatory control of isometric forces targeted for object's weight. 1991;submitted.

22   Johansson RS: How is grasping modified by somatosensory input? In Humphrey DR, Freud H-J (eds): Motor Control: Concepts and Issues. Chichester, Wiley, 1991, pp 331–355.

23   Gordon AM, Forssberg H, Johansson RS, Westling G: Integration of sensory information during the programming of precision grip: Comments on the contributions of size cues. Exp Brain Res 1991;85:226–229.

Ann-Christin Eliasson, Nobel Institute for Neurophysiology and
Department of Pediatrics, Karolinska Institute, Karolinska Hospital,
S–104 01 Stockholm (Sweden)

Forssberg H, Hirschfeld H (eds): Movement Disorders in Children.
Med Sport Sci. Basel, Karger, 1992, vol 36, pp 151–158

Discussion Section III

*Ann-Christin Eliasson, Charlotte Häger, Lena Krumlinde, Karin Melén,
Marion Mähler, Birgit Rösblad*

Manual Actions – Based on the Capacity to Use Sensory Information

This discussion dealt with principles for sensorimotor control in
general and not only with hand and arm function. There was an emphasis
on how the sensorimotor systems are utilized for fine control of reaching
and grasping movements. Perception and action are intimately linked
together, e.g. when performing a movement there is already an ongoing
preparation for the next action on the bases of perception [von Hofsten,
this vol.]. Preparation of movement occurs in the whole body before
reaching. In the normal child, the various sensory systems provide information about the state of the limb which is preparing to move or is moving.
There is an integration of sensory signals at several levels at the central
nervous system. However, specific sensory information may be essential in
certain conditions.

Anticipatory Control

The debate initially focused on 'anticipatory control'. R. Johansson,
J. Gordon, C. von Hofsten and A. Gordon demonstrated that movement
depends on sensory mechanisms and are programmed in advance. What
does this concept mean to us as clinicians and therapists and how can we
incorporate it into our clinical analysis and treatment? It seems that the
significance of 'anticipatory' or 'prospective' control is somewhat unclear to
therapist in general. An attempt will be made here to summarize a few
points. The majority of voluntary movements are believed to depend on
programmed patterns based on internal representation or 'sensorimotor
memories' [Johansson et al., this vol.]. These neural internal representations are mainly acquired during early practice in childhood and are used
to scale the motor activity. We select among the internal representations
when we plan and perform an action. When needed, the programmed

patterns are updated through sensory information concerning the properties of handled objects, our body and its relation to the environment. Vision, for instance, has a strong sensory influence on movement control, especially when somatosensory input is not available. Deafferented patients who received visual information of the hand and arm prior to movement onset in a reaching task and not only during the movements, improved in accuracy. This indicates that their anticipatory control was enhanced by the visual input [J. Gordon, this vol.]. Thus, anticipatory control implies actions based on predictions that the role of perception is one requirement for coordinated manual action. Another requirement is to understand the dynamics of the body in matching the features of the task. Somehow these two demands must be integrated to successfully accomplish a task as pointed out by Shumway-Cook.

Cutaneous information from receptors in contact with the object is critical for adjusting the forces when restraining an object that moves in an unpredictable way [1]. Moreover, if the optimal sensory input for movement control is not available, other sources of information may compensate. Häger reported that subjects with anesthetized fingertips show a better grip force control of the moving object when the arm is not supported compared to situations with arm support. Thus, the flexibility of the nervous system enables several possibilities of using various sensory information to grade motor behavior. A child with motor disabilities may not have the neural prerequisites to develop in a normal way. However, it was suggested that one might consider the child's performance as a compensatory strategy to cope with his deficits; the child may choose one out of a several sets of solutions which enables him to realize the goal. The anticipatory control is a general feature for all normal movements and Campbell suggested that a deficit in this function may be one of the primary impairments in children with cerebral palsy. If the cerebral palsy child moves very slowly, it may be due to his basic problems with anticipatory control. His inability to modulate the grip force may make him compensate and grip almost at his limits in order to not risk dropping a lifted object. What we observe might be his best solution according to his sensorimotor capability [Eliasson, this vol.].

Assumptions Underlying Treatment

Passive versus Active Movements. Active movement is crucial to produce proper sensory feedback during ongoing movement, stated by Johansson. There is a completely different sensorimotor process when a person *actively* explores the environment compared to *passive* movements, i.e. when a therapist is moving or guiding the limb. It is essential for normal motor development to actively explore the possibilities of the body in the environment in order to organize multiple solutions for activity. Yet for the child with sensorimotor impairments, there is most likely a limited set of solutions. In agreement with earlier concepts for treatment, children often have been taught to react to proprioceptive input rather than to use proprioceptive information to improve their movement patterns. This emphasizes the role of sensory information from the environment to improve function. Horak referred to results from haptic research that subjects moved their hands differently if asked to identify the shape of an object than when asked to describe the surface of the object. Likewise, it is known from studies on monkeys that they receive different sensory input if the surface is drawn over their hand versus if they explore the surface with an active movement. However, passive sensory stimulation might cause adaptive changes in the somatosensory primary fields of the brain, but whether this has any functional consequence is not known. There was a general agreement among therapists that the passive movement approach has been left behind in favor of active movements.

Transfer of Function. An issue that was brought up several times throughout the conference was the ability to transfer a learned coordinated movement pattern to various functional situations. This belief in transfer of function has been a general assumption in treatment and it may be one of the reasons why there has been so little attention on training of arm hand function. A. Gordon presented one argument against such a transfer; a learned isometric force contraction cannot automatically be used when the position is changed. The learned movement has to be relearned during different constraints. Training in a real context is therefore probably important to improve function. For example, it was found that children with CP could perform a wider range of movement in a pronation-supination task when they had to hit a drum instead of simply performing pronation-supination of the arm, referred by Bradley. The attention was directed to a specific goal of the task in a real situation, and performance improved. Maybe one of the therapist's goals should be to provide various solutions to specific actions, instead of expecting generalization of a learned pattern.

Another question was whether a hemiplegic child could transfer somatosensory information from the nonhemiplegic hand to the affected side. Normal children can transfer sensory information from one hand to the other in a lifting task, reported by A. Gordon. We still don't know if this is also the case in hemiplegic children, but it is certainly an interesting question for therapists.

Proximal versus Distal Control. The often debated issue of motor development in a proximodistal sequence was clarified in the talk given by

Bradley in a previous session. The theory of proximodistal direction of development is based on morphological studies which show progress in cephalocaudal sequences. However, this theory might not account for development of motor control. Distal movements already occur in the fetus before the control of forces against gravity, stated by Cioni. Some patterns of intra- and inter-limb coordination are established very early, i.e. infant grasping occurs before the infant can control posture against gravity [von Hofsten, this vol.]. It was pointed out in the discussion that there is no evidence for a development in proximal to distal direction in normal infants, or that manipulatory actions should be dependent on proximal control. Anatomical and neurophysiological studies have shown that shoulder movements and fine finger movements are controlled by different pathways in the CNS [2, 3]. Reaching and manipulation of objects are two different functions which probably have quite different control mechanisms underlying the movements. In children with motor disorders there is no evidence that the distal control is more impaired than proximal according to Bradley. She even suggested that early manual activity might play an important role for the normal development of proximal control.

Traditionally, treatment of manipulatory actions has focused on preparation for function by inhibition of postural reflexes, often by the adjustment of the sitting position. The question of trunk stability in relation to perception and arm movements was raised, but never really answered. It seems difficult to find any evidence in the literature that the sitting position is crucial for arm and hand function. Some studies compare the performance of manipulatory tasks during various sitting positions, while others compare movement trajectories in reaching in order to understand the arm hand function in relation to posture. However, biomechanical differences in posture seem not to influence the control of movements [4]. Reaching also involves trunk movement since the body can be used to prolong the arm. Moreover, Giuliani reported that fixation of the body suppresses arm movements in normal children. Whether fixation of a child with bad postural control restrains or improves arm and hand movements needs to be further examined.

It is important to sort out which assumptions treatment is actually based on and possibly reevaluate the assumptions which modern neuroscience question [5]. However, assumptions do not necessarily have to be right or wrong, but they can be more or less useful, as stated by Horak [this vol.].

Therapeutic Considerations and Speculations

In the traditional methods for treatment of children with motor impairments, few ideas are offered on how to deal with arm and hand function. However, the assumption of a proximodistal sequence of development has been fundamental. Thus, the training has focused on proximal stability and postural control. If it is assumed that a 'correct' sitting position of a child with motor impairments will support hand function, what actually is intended: will a good sitting position provide symmetry; or normalized muscle tone; or an opportunity for visual control of the hands? What are the key features that we believe are important? During the session Campbell pointed out that from clinical experience we feel by setting the posture the child improves in function. Nevertheless, until we know the underlying causes we cannot sophisticate the treatment.

However, since a child with cerebral palsy seldom or never develops normal postural control or proximal stability, treatment rarely arrives at more specific training of arm and hand function. On the other hand, in activities of daily living (ADL) training of arm hand function becomes both necessary and natural. It is goal directed and the motivation of the child is essential. In order to obtain the primary goals, i.e. get clothes on and off, eat and so forth, compensatory strategies must be allowed. It seems that such a goal-directed training offers a valid platform from which we can further develop treatment strategies.

Enhancement of Function through Compensatory Mechanisms

A child with cerebral palsy does not have the neural requirement to perform a task in a way that children normally do. Children with cerebral palsy have to, as pointed out earlier, choose a compensatory strategy. Then we should ask ourselves as therapists: do we allow and accept these compensatory strategies or do we try to modify them? The gait of impaired children is a good example of a chosen strategy; they probably walk in the way which is least energy consuming and tiring. However, how can we as therapists know that a child's compensatory strategy is the best solution? For example, a child who has problems in stabilizing his gaze when performing a fine manipulatory task may prefer not to look at what he is doing since this would only deteriorate function. Should we accept the child's solution to the problem and try to enhance the ability to use proprioceptive information as we train the skills? Or maybe a better way is to train the child to stabilize the gaze and use visual information for movement control? Important questions are: Are supports or constraints provided in therapy? Could we as therapists change some environmental constraints to make the task easier for the child? Hence, compensatory strategies might not always be the most effective way of solving a motor function. During the discussion, Maystone suggested that it can be of value to provide a cerebral palsy child with an experience of normal movement by facilitation, an experience the child otherwise would not have had. We still do not have the answers to whether a present compensatory strategy is the best available solution or when we should try to find other solutions for the child. Nevertheless, we should always pay attention to the child's own solution, as pointed out from the audience during the discussion.

The control of movements is often automatic and does not require conscious intervention. Yet, in a patient with sensorimotor problems, would a more direct control by volition and increased attention during training influence the motor behavior beyond the training situation? Lee reported while biofeedback is used to improve movement, most studies indicate that the feedback does not have a long term effect. However, movement can be learned, monkeys with one forelimb deafferented only use the normal forelimb, but if prevented from doing so the deafferented limb will recover function to a higher degree [6].

The Application of Knowledge of Normal Development

Children normally have an innate drive to learn. We have all seen their eagerness to practice a skill over and over again. When stimulating the delayed or retarded child, maybe we can apply the knowledge we have from normal sensorimotor development. Often movements in a baby are due to a perceptual process. The baby turns its head towards a sound and in a dialogue with the mother or father, the infant will perform a whole variety of arm and hand movements. A moving object will invite the child to reach for it. Likewise, a child in prone position will try to lift its head in order to better view the environment. It is also known that as a baby quickly habituates to an object, it will soon lose interest if the stimulus does not change over time. In treatment of impaired children there might be better ways of utilizing the stimuli which invite normal babies to move. Traditionally, movements in therapy have often been triggered by different facilitation techniques like tilting, pushing or pulling the child.

Assessment of Function

Most evaluation scales for arm hand function in children are descriptions in relation to normal development, i.e. looking at 'milestones' such as when different grips emerge. By tradition we have compared the grasps of the impaired child with those of the normally developed child and tried to determine which stage of development this particular child has reached. The grasps developed by a child with cerebral palsy probably do not follow the normal development. This comparison might lead us to the conclusion that the goal of treatment is to obtain a movement as normal looking as possible. However, this may not be the best solution for the child. To consider the child's ability to perform a task is probably more revealing than a comparison with normal development.

In both by von Hofsten and Rösblad's presentations and the discussion it was stressed that the perception of the child is very important to consider when trying to assess his motor activity. A true understanding of the problems a child has when moving cannot be achieved unless there is an estimation of the child's sensorimotor capacities. There is a need to analyze the sensory processes underlying coordinated movements and not only look at the capacity of isolated movements. Observations of the actions of the child in more functional situations are requested. Clinicians must attempt to get an idea of how the child perceives his own body in the environment and if he can use this information for movement control. When treating a child with movement disorders, therapists can ask themselves questions which to some extent will help them analyze the perceptive abilities of the child. Some examples of questions are: How is his sense of position? Is the child capable of using the proprioceptive information, i.e. does the child know where the parts of the body are even if not looking at them? Can the child perform a manual task only when able to control the movements of the hand visually and not only when somatosensory information from the hands is provided? It is known that cutaneous information is disturbed in some children. Some examples to examine those questions are: When buttoning the button on a shirt, could the button under the chin be buttoned when visual information is not available? Another question: Is it possible for the child to maintain a stable hand position in a task like holding a glass of water, only when watching the hand? Or will the water spill when he looks in another direction?

Can the child use visual information in a sufficient way for movement control? Does the child look at his hands when using them? If not, why doesn't he? Lee et al. [7] reported that children with CP often do not know where their eyes are looking. However, development of vision is highly important for the progress of many motor skills. To see is a complicated task per se. There is a need of linking information from mechanoreceptor in the body with visual information in order to know where the gaze is directed. Moreover, vision must be controlled in relation to the environment, for instance, stabilization of gaze on an object. These fundamental abilities might be impaired in children with cerebral palsy.

New Perspectives on Treatment – A Problem-Solving Approach?

Fisher appropriately concluded the discussion by stating that a real task in a real situation is crucial for motor learning: In a recent study adults showed bell-shaped velocity curves when eating real food from a real bowl. This was not the case during imaginary conditions, even when subjects used the proper tools. This indicates that when training reaching (for a glass), the child should actually reach for a real glass of water and probably most important, he should want to have a drink!

Gentile proposed that treatment should focus on solving manipulatory actions in different contexts to find functional strategies. Therapists might try to use more functional goal-oriented tasks (making sure that the child knows what the goal is), provide enough, but not too much, information and consider the motivation of the child. However, even if focusing on task-specific training and compensatory strategies to a higher extent, we must not forget the more biomechanical aspects of movements.

In conclusion, the debate has identified a series of issues that need to be studied further. However, a good way to proceed in treatment might be to question our way of working in relation to what is said by the authors of this book. J. Gordon [5] has adequately stated that basic science will never provide us with new techniques – therapists have to be innovators and deal with the clinical implications themselves.

References

1   Johansson RS, Häger C, Bäckström L: Somatosensory control of precision grip during unpredictable pulling loads III. Impairments during digital anesthesia. Exp Brain Res 1992; in press.

2   Lawrence DG, Kuypers HGJM: The functional organization of the motor system in the monkey. I. The effects of bilateral pyramidal lesions. Brain 1968;91:1–14.

3   Muir RB, Lemon RN: Corticospinal neurons with a special role in precision grip. Brain 1983;261:312–316.

4   McPherson JJ, Schild R, Spaulding SJ, Barsamian P, Trason C, White SC: Analysis of upper extremity in four sitting positions: A comparison of persons with and without cerebral palsy. Am J Occup Ther 1991;45:2:123–129.

5   Gordon J: Assumptions underlying physical therapy intervention: Theoretical and historical perspectives; in Carr JH, Shepherd RB, Gordon J, Gentile AM, Held JM (eds): Movement Science: Foundations for Physical Therapy in Rehabilitation. Rockville, Aspen Publishers, 1987, pp 1–30.

6   Taub E, Berman AJ: Movement and learning in the absence of sensory feedback; in Freedman SJ (ed): The Neurophysiology of Spatially Oriented Behavior. Homewood, Dorsey Press, 1968, pp 173–192.

7   Lee DN, Daniel BM, Turnball J, Cook ML: Basic perceptuo-motor dysfunction in cerebral palsy; in Jeannerod M (ed): Attention and Performance. XIII. Motor Representation and Control. New York, Lawrence Erlbaum, 1990, pp 586–603.

Birgit Rösblad, Department of Psychology, University of Umeå,
S–901 87 Umeå (Sweden)

IV. Control of Locomotion, Posture and Spasticity

Forssberg H, Hirschfeld H (eds): Movement Disorders in Children.
Med Sport Sci. Basel, Karger, 1992, vol 36, pp 159–168

Neural Control of Innate Behavior[1]

Judith Schotland

The Nobel Institute for Neurophysiology, Karolinska Institute, Stockholm, Sweden

Introduction

The control of many complex motor behaviors is greatly simplified by instantiating much of the organization within the anatomical connections of the neural circuitry directly generating that behavior. For example, the neural control of walking and other locomotor behaviors involves control signals to initiate the rhythmic, alternating movements of the limbs, and, in turn, is closely regulated by signals relaying the current state of the limbs. However, the control of the rhythmic, alternating limb movements themselves are largely coordinated by specialized networks of neurons located in the spinal cord. Because these neuronal networks are capable of *generating* complex *patterns* of motor activity and because of their localization within the *central* nervous system, they have been referred to as *central pattern generators* (CPGs). Perhaps most widely studied has been the network controlling the rhythmic, reciprocally coupled movements involved in locomotion – be those movements of wings (birds, insects), body musculature (lampreys), or limbs (cats, humans). Therefore, the rest of this discussion will largely focus on the neural network coordinating locomotion.

We will begin by a closer examination of these central networks – both the behavior of these circuits and the neuronal connections of which they are composed. Next we will examine how these circuits are controlled, both by descending inputs from higher levels of the nervous system and by proprioceptive feedback.

[1] A lecture on neural control of innate motor behavior was presented by Prof. S. Grillner, The Nobel Institute for Neurophysiology, Karolinska Institute, Stockholm, Sweden. We appreciate Dr. J. Schotland, working at Prof. Grillner's laboratory, for contributing this paper.

Central Pattern Generating Networks

A CPG is defined as a 'network of neurons . . . able to produce a repetitive, rhythmic output . . . that is automatic and independent of necessary sensory feedback' [1]. These neuronal networks have been postulated to control many rhythmic motor behaviors such as locomotion in cat [2, 3], lamprey [4], and locust [5], scratch reflexes in cat and dog [6, 7] and turtle [8, 9], mastication [reviewed in 10], and respiration [reviewed in 11]. Key elements in this definition include: 'network of neurons' emphasizing the anatomical and/or physiological integrity of the neurons participating in the generation of the behavior; 'repetitive, rhythmic output' indicating the rhythmical nature of the behaviors coordinated by CPGs; 'automatic' referring to the generation of these behavioral patterns in the absence of descending and/or conscious control; 'independent of necessary sensory feedback' pointing to the capacity for generation of the basic pattern in the absence of any sensory feedback regarding the current state of the system.

Because the pattern can be generated in the absence of afferent input, and because motor neurons are the output channels [12], the 'network of neurons' constituting the locomotor CPG of the lumbar spinal cord comprises the interneurons interposed between afferent and efferent systems. In describing the interneurons that constitute the locomotor pattern generating network, however, it is instructive to include the distribution and organization of afferent input to these interneuronal circuits and the organization of the motor pools to which they project.

Most cutaneous, muscle, and joint afferents are very sensitive to mechanical stimulation and are normally phasically active during locomotion [13]. In addition, their distribution tends to be local, rather than widespread, e.g., the monosynaptic projection of spindle afferents is limited to motoneurons of the homonymous muscle and its close functional synergists [14].

Motor neurons directly control muscles producing movements of the joints and are localized into motor pools subserving single muscles or muscle groups of similar function. The motor pools of axial muscles are located medial to those controlling limb muscles. There is a further division of flexors dorsal to extensors.

Corresponding to the distribution of motoneurons, interneurons with long axons that span several segments are distributed bilaterally to medial parts of the spinal gray matter, thereby being in a good position to influence axial muscles involved in postural stability, whereas those with short axons that have a fairly localized action are distributed ipsilaterally in the lateral parts of the spinal gray matter, near motor pools controlling limb muscles. The dendritic arrays of these lateral interneurons span a maximum of 2–3 segments in the spinal cord and thus may be involved in coordinating motor nuclei of functionally similar muscles [15]. In addition they are known to receive convergent input from both primary afferents and supraspinal centers. There is a good 'match' between afferents, interneurons, and motoneurons and the muscles coordinating trunk and limb movements, and as we shall see, this anatomical specificity extends beyond local spinal circuits.

The second part of the definition of CPGs is that they have a 'repetitive, rhythmic output', i.e. movements such as mastication, respiration, and locomotion (whether it be flying, swimming, walking, or running) may be considered to be coordinated by the CPG. How is this rhythmic activity generated? This question is addressed by a second definition of the CPG as '... an assembly of neurons which, by virtue of their *intrinsic properties and synaptic interactions*, is capable of generating and controlling the spatial and temporal activity of motor neurons' (emphasis added) [16]. Unfortunately, the complexity of the mammalian nervous system has made efforts to unravel the detailed cellular properties and synaptic interactions of the interneurons comprising the locomotor CPG very difficult [4, 17]. However, simple vertebrate preparations such as the lamprey share most of the systems level characteristics of higher vertebrates, yet have relatively fewer kinds and numbers of neurons, making them a tractable model system for elucidating CPG function [18, 19].

Synaptic connectivities consist of the actual contacts made between various cells in the CPG. Particular patterns of synaptic connections can generate rhythmic activity. As long ago as 1911, Brown [2] hypothesized that in the locomotor CPG the left and right sides of the spinal cord ('half centers') had inhibitory connections with each other, such that when one side was active, it inhibited the other and vice versa. This general pattern of organization is termed reciprocal inhibition, and has been found to play a role in behaviors ranging from swimming in *Tritonia* [20] to flying in flies [21], to the concurrent inhibition of antagonist motor neurons during excitation of agonists in cats [22].

These patterns of synaptic connectivities are, however, not immutable. For example, in the lobster stomatogastric and pyloric ganglia, the output of a CPG defined by synaptic connectivities can be restructured by neuromodulators that 'can "tune" the output of the synaptically and anatomically "hard-wired" circuit in a different way, thus evoking a different output' [23, 24].

The efficacy of synaptic connectivities is further influenced by properties inherent in the cells they contact. Cells in many different species exhibit unique time and voltage dependent ionic conductances that lead to oscillations or plateaus in membrane potential. For example, in the presence of the neurotransmitter NMDA, many of the neurons of the lamprey locomotor CPG exhibit regular depolarizations and hyperpolarizations in membrane potential, even when all synaptic activity has been pharmacologically blocked [25]. Synaptic input will have a different effect depending upon whether it reaches those cells when they are depolarized and close to threshold for firing action potentials or whether they are hyperpolarized [26]. Somewhat closer to humans, is the demonstration that cat motoneurons exhibit prolonged depolarized plateaus after a barrage of excitatory input, thus changing their responsiveness to incoming signals for a prolonged period of time [27].

Pattern generators are also 'automatic', i.e. behaviors coordinated by CPGs can function independent of descending command signals. One of the earliest demonstrations of the independence of CPG output from descending command signals was provided by Brown [2] who showed that cats generate walking movements following transection of the spinal cord. Later on, spinal cats injected with *L*-DOPA were shown to exhibit hindlimb walking on a treadmill [28]. In the lamprey, excitatory amino acid neurotransmitters applied to the solution bathing the isolated spinal cord are sufficient to elicit the pattern of reciprocally organized bursts of activity in segmental oscillators (CPGs) that generates swimming in the intact animal [29, 30].

Finally, a central pattern generator is defined by its capacity to continue to generate a rhythmic output 'independent of necessary sensory feedback'. In the intact animal, of course, feedback plays an important role in modulating motor output. But it is nevertheless clear that sensory feedback is not *necessary* in order for the spinal network to generate the complex pattern of muscle activity underlying the coordination of locomotion [3]. Again, one of the earliest demonstrations goes back to Brown [2] who showed that cats that had their spinal cords transected after having the dorsal roots cut, nevertheless generated walking movements. A clear contemporary demonstration of the independence of CPG circuitry from sensory information again comes from fictive locomotion induced in the isolated lamprey spinal cord, which has no afferent input [29].

Descending Control

Although the rhythmic alternating movements constituting locomotion can be generated solely by spinal networks, these networks are normally activated by signals descending from higher levels of the nervous system. Tonic stimulation of a specialized region of the brain stem known as the mesencephalic locomotor region leads to normal walking on a treadmill in decerebrate cats [31]. Likewise, stimulation of brain stem reticulospinal neurons in the isolated brain stem-spinal cord preparation of the lamprey leads to generation of the locomotor rhythm [32]. In the intact animal, all types of sensory information – visual, auditory, somatosensory, vestibular – have access to spinal locomotor networks through descending inputs. In mammals, these signals are transmitted to spinal networks via three major descending motor systems, the ventromedial, dorsolateral, and corticospinal pathways [33].

There are three major components of the ventromedial pathway; vestibulospinal fibers originating in the vestibular nuclei carrying input important for the regulation of equilibrium, tectospinal fibers carrying input from the tectum important for coordinating eye and head movements toward targets, and reticulospinal fibers carrying input from the medullary and pontine reticular formation important for the maintenance of postural tone. Medullary reticulospinal fibers are inhibitory and pontine reticulospinals are excitatory to extensor tone. These fibers descend in the ventral funiculus of the spinal cord where their terminals are distributed widely, and often bilaterally, to the ventromedial gray matter where they influence both axial muscles and the medial and long propriospinal interneurons that project in turn to axial muscles. This system, with its strong inputs related to postural adjustments, is in good anatomical relation to the location of motoneurons and interneurons coordinating axial musculature that would be required for those postural adjustments.

The dorsolateral pathway originates primarily from the red nucleus in the midbrain and descends in the dorsolateral portion of the spinal cord to terminate in the dorsolateral part of the spinal gray matter where it influences the motoneurons and short, lateral interneurons involved in the coordination of girdle and limb muscles.

The corticospinal tract is most highly developed in humans and only partially or not at all developed in lower vertebrates. It is specialized for the fine motor control required for independent movements of the digits [34]. Neurons of this pathway originate in the cortex and make direct connections to motoneurons and premotor interneurons. Some of the interneurons that are targets of corticospinal neurons are also involved in the coordination of spinal reflexes, and perhaps also, of the locomotor CPG. For example, a single corticospinal neuron can monosynaptically excite a motor neuron and at the same time excite an interneuron that inhibits the antagonist muscle [35]. Corticospinal neurons also project to the brain stem where they have the opportunity to influence ventromedial and dorsolateral descending pathways.

In addition to these three major descending pathways, the output of spinal CPG circuitry is also influenced by the cerebellum and basal ganglia, and by secondary motor cortical areas. Like the cerebral cortex, the cerebellum has a topographic organization. It receives ascending input from the periphery as well as descending signals from the cortex and brain stem. In this way the cerebellum is able to compare the descending motor command with feedback related to movement to provide on-line correction of movements. The output of the cerebellum is directed via specialized cerebellar output nuclei to the ventromedial, dorsolateral, and corticospinal systems, as well as back to the cortex. Cerebellar lesions result in a distinctive set of symptoms related to movement execution, including difficulty initiating and terminating movements, dysmetric movements, and difficulty performing rhythmic, alternating movements [36].

The basal ganglia [37] receive input from all areas of cortex and project primarily to prefrontal, supplementary motor, and premotor cortices via the thalamus. These secondary motor areas also receive input directly from posterior parietal cortical areas that in turn receive input from somatosensory and visual cortices. The substantial input of preprocessed sensory information is important to the function of these areas in the planning and execution of movements. Supplementary motor cortex [38, 39] plays a role in planning movement sequences. In addition to cortical inputs, it receives a dominant input from the basal ganglia via the thalamus. The activity of neurons in this area is not tightly coupled to individual muscles or movements; it can be activated merely by thinking about a movement sequence [40]. Premotor cortex is largely concerned with orientation of the body for sensory guided movements [41, 42]. In addition to direct input from posterior parietal cortex, the cerebellum provides a major input via the thalamus. Premotor cortex projects to the reticulospinal system and to ventromedial gray areas of the spinal cord coordinating axial and proximal musculature that would be important in correctly orienting the body for movements.

Afferent Modulation

The output of the neural network coordinating locomotion in the cat, rather than merely consisting of alternating flexor and extensor activity, consists of complex and detailed patterns of muscle activation. Although this detailed pattern of motor output is preserved quite well under deafferentation, the timing of muscle activity and joint motion is less precise and movements are weaker and not as well coordinated or adapted [3, 13, 43]. Normally, CPG output is subject to modulation by sensory feedback – directly, through primary afferent connections to spinal interneurons and motoneurons – and, indirectly, via sensory input through the thalamus to the cortical and subcortical pathways outlined above and via spinocerebellar pathways conveying information about muscle activity [44] and spinal interneuronal processing [45] to the cerebellum and once again to the descending pathways.

Identical sensory input does not always have the same affect on motor output. The efficacy of sensory input from skin, muscle, and joints directly to the CPG circuitry varies as a function of the phase of the CPG. Afferent input may effectively modulate the CPG during specific phases of the flight rhythm in locust [46] and the same sensory signal may prolong extension during one phase of the locomotor cycle and flexion during another [47, 48]. These kinds of observations point to the delicate interplay normally present between afferent, descending, and CPG circuitry.

Conclusion

The neural control of innate behaviors such as locomotion is greatly simplified by building much of that control into neural circuitry that is capable of generating a complex motor pattern. The anatomy of spinal locomotor circuitry is tailored both to the particular muscles coordinating different categories of movements, such as orienting movements or grasping movements, and to the descending inputs that require access to those muscle groups. Local afferent feedback modulates and adapts movements, both directly at the level of the spinal cord and at higher levels of the nervous system, such that descending commands can be adjusted to current conditions.

References

1   Delcomyn F: Neural basis of rhythmic behavior in animals. Science 1980;210:492–498.
2   Brown TG: The intrinsic factors in the act of progression in the mammal. Proc R Soc Lond [Biol] 1911;84:308–319.
3   Grillner S, Zangger P: How detailed is the central pattern generation for locomotion? Brain Res 1975;88:367–371.
4   Grillner S: Neurobiological bases of rhythmic motor acts in vertebrates. Science 1985;228:143–149.
5   Wilson DM: The central nervous control of flight in a locust. J Exp Biol 1961;38:471–490.
6   Berkinblit MB, Deliagina TG, Feldman AG, Gelfand IM, Orlovsky GN: Generation of scratching. I. Activity of spinal interneurons during scratching. J Neurophysiol 1978;41:1040–1057.

7   Sherrington CS: The Integrative Action of the Nervous System. New Haven, Yale University Press, 1906.

8   Mortin LI, Keifer J, Stein, PSG: Three forms of the scratch reflex in the spinal turtle: Movement analyses. J Neurophysiol 1985;53:1501–1516.

9   Robertson GA, Mortin LI, Keifer J, Stein PSG: Three forms of the scratch reflex in the spinal turtle: Central generation of patterns. J Neurophysiol 1985;53:1517–1534.

10 Lund JP, Enomoto S: The generation of mastication by the mammalian central nervous system; in Cohen AH, Rossignol S, Grillner S (eds): Neural Control of Rhythmic Movements in Vertebrates. Wiley Series in Neurobiology. New York, Wiley, 1988, pp 41–72.

11 Feldman JL, Smith JC, McCrimmon DR, Ellenberger HH, Speck DF: Generation of respiratory pattern in mammals; in Cohen AH, Rossignol S, Grillner S (eds): Neural Control of Rhythmic Movements in Vertebrates. Wiley Series in Neurobiology. New York, Wiley, 1988, pp 73–100.

12 Grillner S, Buchanan JT, Wallen P, Brodin L: Neural control of locomotion in lower vertebrates: From behavior to ionic mechanisms; in Cohen AH, Rossignol S, Grillner S (eds): Neural Control of Rhythmic Movements in Vertebrates. New York, Wiley, 1988, pp 1–40.

13 Rossignol S, Lund JP, Drew T: The role of sensory inputs in regulating patterns of rhythmical movements in higher vertebrates. A comparison between locomotion, respiration, and mastication; in Cohen AH, Rossignol S, Grillner S (eds): Neural Control of Rhythmic Movements in Vertebrates. New York, Wiley, 1988, pp 201–284.

14 Eccles JC, Eccles RM, Lundberg A: The convergence of monosynaptic excitatory afferents on to many different species of alpha motoneurons. J Physiol 1957;137:22–50.

15 Jankowska E, Lundberg A: Interneurons in the spinal cord. TINS 1981;4:230–233.

16 Getting PA: Comparative analysis of invertebrate central pattern generators; in Cohen AH, Rossignol S, Grillner S (eds): Neural Control of Rhythmic Movements in Vertebrates. New York, Wiley, 1988, pp 101–128.

17 Selverston AI: Are central pattern generators understandable? Behav Brain Sci 1980;3:535–571.

18 Grillner S, Wallen P, Dale N, Brodin L, Buchanan J, Hill R: Transmitters, membrane properties and network circuitry in the control of locomotion in lamprey. TINS 1987;10:34–41.

19 Grillner S, Wallen P, Brodin L, Lansner A: Neuronal network generating locomotor behavior in lamprey: Circuitry, transmitters, membrane properties, and simulation. Ann Rev Neurosci 1991;14:169–199.

20 Getting PA: Mechanisms of pattern generation underlying swimming in Tritonia. II. Network reconstruction. J Neurophysiol 1983;49:1017–1035.

21 Wilson DM: Central nervous mechanisms for the generation of rhythmic behavior in arthropods. Symp Soc Exp Biol 1966;20:100–228.

22 Jankowska E, Roberts WJ: An electrophysiological demonstration of the axonal projections of single spinal interneurons in the cat. J Physiol 1972;222:597–622.

23 Marder E: Mechanisms underlying modulation of small networks; in Stein PSG (ed): Motor Control: From Movement Trajectories to Neural Mechanisms. Washington, Soc Neurosci, 1985, pp 81–94.

24 Dickenson PS, Mecsas C, Marder E: Neuropeptide fusion of two motor-pattern generator circuits. Nature 1990;344:155–158.

25 Sigvardt KA, Grillner S, Wallen P, van Dongen PAM: Activation of NMDA receptors

elicits fictive locomotion and bistable membrane properties in the lamprey spinal cord. Brain Res 1985;336:390–395.

26   Wallen P, Grillner S: The effects of current passage on NMDA induced TTX resistant membrane potential oscillations in lamprey neurons active during locomotion. Neurosci Lett 1985;56:87–93.

27   Hounsgaard J, Hultborn H, Jespersen B, Kiehn O: Intrinsic membrane properties causing bistable behavior of alpha-motoneurons. Exp Brain Res 1984;55:391–394.

28   Jankowska E, Jukes MGM, Lund S, Lundberg A: The effect of DOPA on the spinal cord. 5. Reciprocal organization of pathways transmitting excitatory action to alpha motoneurons of flexors and extensors. Acta Physiol Scand 1967;70:369–388.

29   Cohen AH, Wallen P: The neuronal correlate of locomotion in fish. 'Fictive swimming' induced in an in vitro preparation of the lamprey spinal cord. Exp Brain Res 1980;41:11–18.

30   Wallen P, Williams TL: Fictive locomotion in the lamprey spinal cord in vitro compared with swimming in the intact and spinal animal. J Physiol 1984;347:225–239.

31   Shik ML, Severin FV, Orlovsky GN: Control of walking and running by means of electrical stimulation of the mid-brain. Biophysics 1966;11:756–765.

32   McClellan AD, Grillner S: Activation of 'fictive swimming' by electrical microstimulation of brainstem locomotor regions in an in vitro preparation of the lamprey central nervous system. Brain Res 1984;300:357–361.

33   Lawrence DG, Kuypers HGJM: The functional organization of the motor system in the monkey. II. The effects of lesions of the descending brainstem pathways. Brain 1968;91:15–36.

34   Lawrence DG, Kuypers HGJM: The functional organization of the motor system in the monkey. I. The effects of bilateral pyramidal lesions. Brain 1968;91:1–14.

35   Jankowska E, Padel Y, Tanaka R: Disynaptic inhibition of spinal motoneurons from the motor cortex in the monkey. J Physiol (Lond) 1976;258:467–487.

36   Holmes G: The cerebellum of man (the Hughlings Jackson memorial lecture). Brain 1939;62:1–30.

37   Carpenter MB: Anatomy of the corpus striatum and brain stem integrating systems; in Brooks VB (ed): Handbook of Physiology, sect I. The Nervous System, vol II: Motor Control. Bethesda, American Physiological Society, 1981, pp 947–995.

38   Penfield W, Welch K: The supplementary motor area, in the cerebral cortex of man. Trans Am Neurol Assoc 1949;74:179–184.

39   Penfield W, Welch K: The supplementary motor area of the cerebral cortex. Arch Neurol Psychiatry 1951;66:289–317.

40   Roland PE, Larsen B, Lassen NA, Skinhoj E: Supplementary motor area and other cortical areas in organization of voluntary movements in man. J Neurophysiol 1980;43:118–136.

41   Fulton JF: A note on the definition of the 'motor' and 'premotor' areas. Brain 1935;58:311–316.

42   Moll L, Kuypers HGJM: Premotor cortical ablations in monkeys: Contralateral changes in visually guided reaching behavior. Science 1977;198:317–319.

43   Grillner S, Zangger P: The effect of dorsal root transection on the efferent motor pattern in the cat's hindlimb during locomotion. Acta Physiol Scand 1984;120:393–405.

44   Arshavsky YI, Berkinblit MB, Fukson OI, Gelfand IM, Orlovsky GN: Recordings of neurons of the dorsal spinocerebellar tract during evoked locomotion. Brain Res 1972;43:272–275.

45   Arshavsky YI, Berkinblit MB, Gelfand IM, Orlovsky GN, Fukson OI: Activity of the

neurones of the ventral spino-cerebellar tract during locomotion. Biophysics 1972;17:926–935.

46   Pearson KG, Reye DN, Robertson RM: Phase dependent influences of wing stretch receptors on flight rhythm in the locust. J Neurophysiol 1983;49:1168–1181.

47   Forrsberg H, Grillner S, Rossignol S: Phase dependent reflex reversal during walking in chronic spinal cats. Brain Res 1975;85:103–107.

48   Forssberg H: Phasic gating of cutaneous reflexes during locomotion; in Taylor A, Prochazka A (eds): Muscle Receptors and Movement. London, Macmillan, 1981, pp 403–412.

Judith Schotland, PhD, The Nobel Institute for Neurophysiology,
Karolinska Institute, S–104 01 Stockholm (Sweden)

Forssberg H, Hirschfeld H (eds): Movement Disorders in Children.
Med Sport Sci. Basel, Karger, 1992, vol 36, pp 169–173

Development of Locomotion from a Dynamic Systems Approach

Esther Thelen

Department of Psychology, Indiana University, Bloomington, Ind., USA

Less than 20 years ago, the accepted account of the development of locomotion was rather a simple one. Infants are born with reflex mechanisms for producing stepping movements, probably mediated by the spinal cord or brainstem. These reflexes become inhibited as higher brain centers mature, and walking develops as the motor cortex assumes control of the lower nervous system mechanisms [1]. The process driving this developmental sequence was believed to be neural maturation, although *what* matures, or most importantly, *why* it matures was not specified.

In the last decade or so, we have learned more about the mechanisms of early infant motor activity and have found that the process of learning to walk is both more complex and less deterministic than pictured by the traditional accounts. The process is best captured by a *dynamic systems* (DS) approach [2]. The most important assumption of DS for this discussion is that motor patterns are 'softly assembled', rather than being hard-wired in the CNS. Soft assembly means that the actual trajectories of movement are determined by many contributing factors: the patterns of neural firing, but also the elastic qualities of the muscles, anatomical properties of the bones and joints, passive and mechanical forces acting on the body, and the energy delivered to the moving limbs and segments. Soft assembly also means that the movement can have no detailed iconic representation wired into the brain or spinal cord. Rather, movement patterns are assembled 'on-line', so to speak, in reference to, and in continual interaction with, the intentions of the subjects, and their perceptions of the task at hand, and the physical properties of their bodies and the environment. Within these constraints, some movement patterns – like walking – are very stable, while others – like tap-dancing – are so unstable that they must be continually practiced. Motor patterns change, and new forms arise in development only when the old patterns are destabilized and the system is free to explore and select new, more adaptive actions.

In the remainder of this paper, I outline a developmental sequence of learning to walk from the DS approach that integrates findings from my lab and others over the last decade. I then conclude with some implications of this approach for clinical practice.

Nature of Early Leg Pattern Generation

Considering their overall motor immaturity, it is remarkable that newborns and young infants produce highly patterned leg movements as spontaneous kicks and steps elicited by a treadmill. It is reasonable to conclude – as I indeed did conclude when I first studied these movements – that the rhythmical, alternating cycles of movements are manifestations of an innate human spinal locomotor program (central pattern generator, or CPG), or patterns of motorneuron firing sufficient to produce the essential elements of locomotion [3]. My further research has led me to believe that these early movements are precursors to later locomotion, but not in the sense that they specify the precise firing pattern of alternating flexors and extensors that characterize CPGs studied in other species. Rather, these early movements are the products of a system designed to learn to walk from interactions with the periphery. As such, they represent only the rough outline and the mechanisms for acquiring the specific details, which are carved in by function. Specifically:

(1) Patterned leg movements in newborn and young infants are the result of anatomical and neural structures that link the segments of one leg in a tight, co-active synergy. At the initiation of a leg flexion, both flexors and extensors contract [4]. The extension phase of the movement is passive, produced by gravity and the inertial and elastic properties of the limb [5]. Note, however, that this early pattern is not similar to walking either in the phasing of the joints, in the pattern of muscle contraction or in the interplay of passive and active torques that produce the movements.

(2) Coordination between the two legs is dynamic rather than obiligatory or rigid. This means that the movement of one leg is determined by the moving status of the other, and that the neural connections between them must transmit this information. We know this because the bilateral synergy is exquisitely sensitive to biomechanical manipulations that perturb the forces of one limb through changing its mass [6, 7], or its movement quality [8]. We also know that the stability of the coupling between the legs changes during development [9].

(3) Even in early infancy, the muscular contribution to the movement is modulated in response to changing passive forces acting on the limb [5]. This means that the muscle activation patterns could not be produced by a

rigid central pattern, but are continually modulated through lower level mechanisms such as stretch reflexes. Most important, these results indicate that the system is designed to *detect* and to *respond* to a dynamic force environment.

Developmental Changes in Locomotor Precursors

Given these initial characteristics, by what processes are these early patterns converted into later locomotion? Following Bernstein [10] and Edelman [11], I believe that locomotion (and other motor patterns) are carved into the system through continual activity: that is, as infants move and explore, the perceptual and motor consequences of their actions are used by the CNS to form continually more adaptive motor actions. In short, that the stable patterns seen in adults are not genetically predetermined but acquired through function from the rough outline provided by the initial structures. This view is consistent with very recent evidence pointing to the plasticity of sensorimotor mapping, not only in developing, but also in adult mammals [12]. While we, of course, cannot map the cortices of human infants, behavioral evidence supports this view:

(1) By 4–5 months, infants have broken out of the tight synergies of the newborn period to more flexible leg and foot motor patterns, including individual joint actions rather than synchronous flexions and extensions, and novel bilateral coordination patterns such as kicking both legs together. Reciprocally alternating muscle patterns appear only late in the first year [13].

(2) Over the first year, we found consistently more stable patterns of alternating treadmill stepping. This improvement is, at least in part, due to the diminishing dominance of flexor tone, which allows the legs to be dynamically stretched by the treadmill [2]. Strength in extensor muscles, in turn, may well increase through function, especially from standing and moving in gravity.

(3) Although infants step well on the treadmill by 7 months, and their steps are kinematically quite similar to adults, at the level of forces, they produce these steps differently, and less efficiently [14]. Thus, they must learn efficient patterns of walking as they in fact walk alone.

The Transition to Walking Alone

Although during the first year, infants have used their legs for a variety of functions – support while sitting, standing, crawling, exploring –

and have produced a variety of patterned movements, the requirements of static and dynamic balance impose difficult demands. As has been true throughout infancy, the babies 'soft-assemble' solutions with what they have available. Indeed, the notable characteristics of early walking, wide stance, long double support, short swing, high cadence, bent knees, flat-foot contact, and extensive co-contraction of antagonist muscles, can all be seen as ad hoc accommodations to the infants' instability and inability to balance on one foot in order to swing the other forward. The fact that steps all look more mature on the treadmill – including the presence of distinctive heel strike in a proportion of steps – argues that what limits mature walking is not immaturity of pattern generation, but the fact that the toddler has not yet discovered through practice and modulation, the most efficient and stable motor mode. Stability parameters improve dramatically in the first few months after the onset of walking [15] and reciprocal patterns of innervation do not appear until after stability is achieved [16]. It is reasonable to speculate that what is called CNS maturation are changes functionally imposed from 'outside-in' on the developing nervous system and not the other way around.

Implications for Therapy

A dynamic systems view has profound implications for therapy [17]. Autonomous neural maturation cannot be considered as a sufficient cause for developmental change. Rather, therapists should seek more system-wide, multidetermined bases for treatment, which focus equally on what the nervous system is *receiving* from the muscles and other senses. Patients with damaged or poorly developing nervous systems have much tighter constraints on movement and perception and their systems are much more limited in their abilities to explore and discover efficient movement solutions. A cycle can be established where disfunctional patterns are recruited, much like new walkers find opportunistic solutions to their instability, but unlike normal toddlers, these patients stay in their less-than-optimal patterns. Over time, these abnormal patterns may become self-sustaining and reinforced by caregiving practices. What is clear from the DS view, and from the current research on brain plasticity, is that intervention must begin while the system is still labile and before motor categories become stable maps in the brain. This may be difficult if, as in the case of infants with cerebral palsy, diagnosis is only made after abnormal patterns are evident. At that point, therapy must first disrupt the abnormal patterns to establish more functional ones. This points to a need for research on early diagnosis in at-risk populations.

References

1 McGraw MB: The Neuromuscular Maturation of the Human Infant. New York, Columbia University Press, 1943.

2 Thelen E, Ulrich BD: Hidden Skills: A Dynamic Systems Analysis of Treadmill Stepping during the First Year. Monogr Soc Res Child Dev 1991; Serial No 223, 56.

3 Grillner S, Wallen P: Central pattern generation for locomotion, with special reference to vertebrates. Annu Rev Neurosci 1985;8:233–262.

4 Thelen E, Fisher DM: The organization of spontaneous leg movements in newborn infants. J Motor Behav 1983;15:353–377.

5 Schneider K, Zernicke RF, Ulrich BD, Jensen JL, Thelen E: Understanding movement control in infants through the analysis of limb intersegmental dynamics. J Motor Behav 1990;22:493–520.

6 Thelen E, Fisher DM, Ridley-Johnson R: The relationship between physical growth and a newborn reflex. Infant Behav Dev 1984;7:479–493.

7 Thelen E, Skala K, Kelso JAS: The dynamic nature of early coordination: Evidence from bilateral leg movements in young infants. Dev Psychobiol 1987;23:179–186.

8 Thelen E, Ulrich BD, Niles D: Bilateral coordination in human infants: Stepping on a split-belt treadmill. J. Exp Psychol [Hum Percept] 1987;13:405–410.

9 Thelen E, Ridley-Johnson R, Fisher DM: Shifting patterns of bilateral coordination and lateral dominance in the leg movements of young infants. Dev Psychobiol 1983;16:29–46.

10 Bernstein N: Coordination and Regulation of Movements. New York, Pergamon Press, 1967.

11 Edelman GM: Neural Darwinism. New York, Basic Books, 1987.

12 Kaas JH: Plasticity of sensory and motor maps in adult mammals. Annu Rev Neurosci 1991;14:137–167.

13 Thelen E: Developmental origins of motor coordination: Leg movements in human infants. Dev Psychobiol 1985;18:1–22.

14 Ulrich BD, Jensen JL, Thelen E, Schneider K, Zernicke RF: Adaptive dynamics of the leg movement patterns of human infants. II. Treadmill stepping in infants and adults. 1991;submitted.

15 Bril B, Breniere Y: Postural requirements and progression velocity in young walkers; 1991;submitted.

16 Okamoto T, Goto Y: Human infant pre-independent and independent walking; in Kondo S (ed): Primate Morphophysiology, Locomotor Analyses and Human Bipedalism. Tokyo, University of Tokyo Press, 1985, pp 25–45.

17 Kamm K, Thelen E, Jensen JL: A dynamical systems approach to motor development. Phys Ther 1990;70:763–774.

Esther Thelen, Department of Psychology, Indiana University,
Bloomington, IN 47405 (USA)

Forssberg H, Hirschfeld H (eds): Movement Disorders in Children.
Med Sport Sci. Basel, Karger, 1992, vol 36, pp 174–181

A Neural Control Model for Human Locomotion Development: Implications for Therapy

Hans Forssberg

Nobel Institute for Neurophysiology, Department of Pediatrics,
Karolinska Institute, Stockholm, Sweden

Neural Control Models

The fast development of new techniques in neuroscience has allowed a detailed exploration of the neural mechanisms controlling various motor behaviors, from the molecular and cellular levels to the system and behavioral levels. Most of this work, especially at the lower levels, has been carried out in nonhuman species. For example, models of the locomotor system in invertebrates and lower vertebrates have been of great importance for understanding of the human nervous system.

In *lower vertebrates* (e.g. the lamprey) [Schotland, this vol.], the neural networks generating locomotor movements have been identified to individual spinal neurones and their membrane properties, transmitters and connections to other neurons in the network. In addition, spinal neurones providing sensory information from the moving body have been examined as well as their connections to the neurones in the locomotor network and the influence they have on the locomotor activity. The supraspinal control of the spinal networks, exerted by descending reticulospinal neurones, have also been elucidated.

In *higher vertebrates* (e.g. the cat) [1], electrophysiological and behavioral studies have explored a similar model, although the magnitude of the neurones involved and the complexity of the neurol networks have not allowed such a detailed characterization. The basic locomotor rhythm is produced by neural networks in the spinal cord producing alternating activity in flexor and extensor muscles. Sensory afferents from the moving limbs, (e.g. from the hip joint and the ankle muscles), provide a powerful influence on the central network and can modify the pattern. This modulation of the centrally generated pattern is of great importance to adapt the locomotor activity to the external environment. The complexity of the interaction between the central network and the sensory input can be exemplified by the stumbling corrective reaction [2]. This reaction is modified in phase with the step cycle, although the stimulus is the same. This creates different functional stumbling corrections for each phase of the step cycle. The phase-dependent modulation of the response is accomplished by central gating of the transmission in the reflex pathways controlled by the central networks for locomotion. There are several neural networks generating the locomotor pattern at least one network for each limb. The interaction between these networks determines the interlimb coordination, e.g. walk, trot and gallop. There might even be separate networks for each joint of a single limb. By shifting the coupling between the networks for the hip and for more distal joints, it is possible to walk backwards.

The spinal organization of central networks for locomotion, interacting with sensory neurones, allows a cat to walk with an almost normal locomotor pattern after a transaction of the spinal cord [3]. The produced locomotor activity supports the body weight and propels the body forward. However, supraspinal mechanisms are required to achieve a more purposeful locomotion; to induce activity in the spinal networks; to set the speed of the locomotion; to maintain equilibrium; to steer the direction of the locomotion; to avoid obstacles and to guide the placement of the paws, etc. Several centers in the brainstem have been shown to control the spinal networks via reticulospinal pathways. These centers can initiate and halt the locomotor activity as well as determine the speed. They are influenced by circuits in both motor cortex and basal ganglia. Other centers of the reticular system influence the muscle tone in the limbs, both during standing and locomotion, and are of great importance in controlling the mode of locomotion [4]. Cortical circuits are involved in fast corrections of the ongoing locomotor movements which serves to avoid visible obstacles [5]. The cerebellum is provided with information both from sensory afferents in the moving limb and activity in the spinal locomotor generating circuits [6]. This information can be used to activate the proper adjustments.

In *primates*, it has not been possible to demonstrate locomotion after spinal cord transection. One might therefore doubt that evidence for a spinal organization in other animals may have any relevance to human locomotion? However, stimulation of the locomotor centers in the brain stem has induced locomotion in monkeys [7]. A steretoyped alternating extensor-flexor activity has been recorded after complete spinal cord transection in humans [8] and the walking movements after incomplete spinal cord transection are improved after administration of drugs that are known to activate the spinal locomotor generating circuits in the cat [Barbaue, this vol.]. In the following sections, I will describe the development of locomotion in children and argue that the locomotor control in humans may be organized according to the same principles as in other mammals.

Table 1. Plantigrade determinants

1	Foot movement – heel strike
2	Knee movement – stance leg flexion
3	Intralimb coordination – out of phase
4	Pelvic movement – rotation, tilt, translation
5	Muscle activity – specific temporal pattern

From Saunders et al. [11] and Forssberg [12].

Phylogeny of Human Locomotion

The human species has evolved a bipedal, plantigrade gait, which is unique since it is not used by any other species. Analysis of hominid skeletons [9] and preserved footprints [10] suggest that this occurred about 3 million years ago. Although, modern apes may walk on two legs, their musculoskeletal system and the activation of their muscles during locomotion differ significantly from that of humans. Probably the plantigrade gait developed to improve the postural stability and to increase the efficiency.

There are several specific determinants for the bipedal, plantigrade gait (table 1) not present in the locomotion of other species [11, 12]. These determinants contribute to the reduction of the vertical oscillation of the body and to the increase in step length. The development of a prominent heel strike is of special interest. This is due to an active dorsiflexion of the foot, provided by contractions of the pretibial muscles and inhibition of the calf muscle activity during the end of the swing phase.

Ontogeny of Human Locomotion

Children go through several phases during their locomotor development (table 2). The first locomotor-like activity occurs already in the fetus at 10–12 gestational weeks [13]. These alternating leg movements are produced until birth, whereafter they can be elicited as stepping movements if the child is held erect over a horizontal surface [14]. It has been suggested that the fetal locomotor-like movements may play a role in positioning the fetus with the head in the birth canal prior to delivery, otherwise there is no obvious function during these early stages. The stepping movements usually fade away during the first months after birth although they continue to be present until the onset of supported locomotion in many children. The

Table 2. Stages of human locomotor development

1	Fetal locomotor-like movements
2	Infant stepping
3	Inactive period
4	Supported locomotion
5	Independent walking
6	Transformation to plantigrade gait

presence of locomotor activity during this phase also seems to be influenced by several factors such as daily training [15], different body positions and surrounding environment (e.g. submersion in water) [Thelen, this vol.].

Supported locomotion emerges at 7–9 months of age, whether infant stepping has been present or not. The movements during supported locomotion seems to be voluntary elicited and goal directed, while the infant stepping is externally induced by pulling the child slowly forward, i.e. sensory information from weight bearing and from stretching the hips. During supported locomotion, the child can support the body weight with one leg but still needs assistance to maintain equilibrium. During infant stepping, the child needs weight support as well. Between 9 and 18 months, the child starts to walk independently, i.e. without any external support. This event is often mentioned as a 'milestone', and is used to monitor the progress of locomotor development. This likely has nothing to do with the networks generating the locomotor activity but with the development of the postural control system.

Throughout all these phases, the infant has an immature locomotor pattern, i.e. they lack all of the plantigrade determinants (table 1) [12]. Flexor and extensor muscles are coactivated producing synchronized flexion-extension movements in all joints of the leg. The calf muscles are activated during the end of the swing phase, plantar flexing the foot before ground contact. This produces a digitigrade gait, in which the toes or the fore part of the foot is first placed on the ground. Following foot contact, there are short latency EMG-bursts in several leg muscles, indicating hypersensitive segmental stretch reflexes to be elicited at the impact of the foot.

The transformation from the infantile stepping pattern begins first after the establishment of independent locomotion, although some changes already occur during supported locomotion. There is a successive delay of the calf muscle activity with age. As a consequence, the heel is placed first on the ground between 18 and 24 months in the majority of children [16], while a prominent heel strike, including an active dorsiflexion until heel strike, does not occur until after 2 years of age [17]. The shaping and tuning of the specific muscle activation patterns also produces desynchronized joint movements characteristic of the plantigrade gait. The maturation of the gait pattern is mainly completed at 4 years of age, but the finding of higher energy expenditure up to 12 years of age compared to adults indicates that the final development may take an even longer time.

Locomotion Development in Children with Cerebral Palsy

During the early phases of locomotion, i.e. prior to independent locomotion, children with cerebral palsy (diplegia or hemiplegia) exhibit an immature locomotor pattern similar to that of nonimpaired children [18]. In the subsequent development, when children normally transform their locomotor pattern into a plantigrade gait, children with cerebral palsy retain the immature non-plantigrade pattern [19, 20, Berger this vol. Leonard this vol.]. All muscles are activated together in a uniform pattern with a high degree of co-activation. The sharp reflex spikes after foot contact is retained. The foot is placed on the toes or forepart of the foot and several children even walk on their toes. This is a result of the premature activation of the calf muscles during the swing phase. The absence of an enhanced calf muscle contraction during the end of the support phase results in a loss of the major propulsive force during plantigrade locomotion, which also is reflected in the initiation of the swing phase with a disturbed sequence of joint movements at lift-off.

Yet, although children with cerebral palsy do not develop a plantigrade gait, they develop and change their locomotion as compared with the original stepping movements. A variety of patterns may emerge, likely depending on the nature of the brain lesions and secondary musculoskeletal malformations.

Neural Control Model for Human Locomotion

The spontaneous, endogenous production of locomotor-like leg movements in the human fetus is present also in fetuses with cervical cord lesions [Prechtl, personal commun.] The infant stepping movements after birth are induced by appropriate somatosensory stimulation of the erect child given some weight on the legs and extending the hip joints. A similar afferent stimulation is effective in eliciting locomotion after spinal cord transection in cats [3]. Already Peiper, in 1963, demonstrated that anencephalic infants could perform stepping movements. All these findings are in agreement with a neural control excerted by autonomous spinal networks. These would evolve early during the fetal life to be spontaneously active before birth and to be induced by proper somatosensory stimulation after birth.

The inhibitory period, when stepping movements cannot usually be induced, probably reflects excitability changes in the spinal networks. Such inhibitory influence might be exerted by inactivity, a changing environment or by the postural control system since training [15] and submersion in water may retain the locomotor activity and since locomotor-like kicking may be exerted when the infant is supine [20; Thelen, this vol.]. Another possibility would be that an increased influence from supraspinal centers depresses the excitability level of the spinal networks while the proper connectivity is building up.

The emergence of voluntary, goal-directed locomotion might reflect the maturation of locomotor centers in the brainstem and that these have established proper contact with the spinal locomotor networks via the reticulospinal system. As mentioned above the onset of independent walking is probably the result of the maturing postural control system, e.g. cerebellum and vestibular structures. Several attempts to train locomotion in order to hasten the development of independent walking have failed. Similar negative results have been described for other motor tasks [21]. It seems as if the brain has to mature to a certain degree before it is ready to execute a certain skill. On the other hand, instructions and practice seem to be involved in the achievement of independent walking, since children deprived of normal human contact (e.g. Kaspar-Hause) may not develop bipedal gait [22].

The emergence of plantigrade gait is unique for the human species and can therefore not be implemented in the animal model for locomotion. The slow and gradual transformation of the locomotor pattern after the onset of independent walking suggests, however, that the original neural networks can be used and that they are gradually more and more influenced by other neural mechanisms thus changing the locomotor pattern. The nature of these underlying mechanisms are not clear. Thelen [this vol.] has suggested an ensemble of different subsystems, which under a dynamical period of practice organize themselves to achieve the most efficient pattern. However, I am skeptical to this model of self-organization for several reasons [17]. I believe that a considerable part of the development is predetermined and governed by the maturation of specific neural mechanisms and their activity, in conjunction with sensory feedback. The adaptation of the gait pattern to the bipedal position has probably taken place during evolution throughout the last 3 million years. The genetic code for brain development has then changed in a similar way as that for the musculoskeletal system. This rather consevative and rigid model, not allowing for large variations of the locomotor development, is also supported by the absence of plantigrade transformation in children with cerebral palsy. The early damage probably, directly or indirectly, influences the neural mechanisms responsible for this transformation.

Implications for Therapy

This conservative developmental model, with a strong anchorage in the development of neural systems, unfortunately, does not provide a very optimistic view for improving locomotion in children following brain damage with physical therapy. This seems also to be in agreement with current clinical experience. A child with cerebral palsy can be taught to walk in a more normal way, i.e. not on the toes and by placing the heel first. However, as soon as the child is not concentrating on the walk, the old immature pattern returns. This probably reflects two different levels of the motor system being used. During the training procedure, with intense mental concentration, higher, probably cortical structures, are used to voluntarily produce and control the locomotor movements. But as soon as the child starts focusing the attention on other issues, the original, autonomous locomotor network takes over. In order to see whether the locomotor networks could be 'reprogrammed' in cats, we transferred the lateral gastrocnemius muscle to become an ankle flexor. If the sensory information could be used to adapt the locomotor activity of the transferred muscle to its new function, the activity should be shifted from the support phase to the swing phase. This did not occur, even when small kittens were operated on shortly after birth and when they were tested after several years [23].

Hence, it seems inefficient to spend too much time and energy normalizing locomotion in the therapy, i.e. to establish a straight and plantigrade gait. Instead the therapist should focus on the functional level of locomotion, i.e. to find out the best way for the child with his or her constraints to move from one location to another, whether it is walking on the toes, walking with crutches or using a wheelchair.

References

1   Grillner S: Control of locomotion in bipeds, tetrapods, and fish; in Brooks VB (ed): Handbook of Physiology, vol 2. The Nervous System II, Motor Control. Bethesda, American Physiological Society, 1981, pp 1179–1236.

2   Forssberg H: Stumbling corrective reaction: A phase-dependent compensatory reaction during locomotion. J Neurophysiol 1979;42:936–953.

3   Forssberg H, Grillner S, Halbertsma J: The locomotion of the spinal cat. I. Coordination within a hindlimb. Acta Physiol Scand 1980;108:269–281.

4   Mori S: Contribution of postural muscle tone to full expression of posture and locomotor movements: Multi-faceted analyses of its setting brainstem-spinal cord mechanisms in the cat. Jpn J Physiol 1989;39:785–809.

5   Drew T: Motor cortical cell discharge during voluntary gait modification. Brain Res 1988;457:181–187.

6   Arshavsky YI, Orlovsky GN: Role of the cerebellum in the control of rhythmic movements; in Grillner S, Stein GS, Douglas G, et al (eds): Neurobiology of Vertebrate Locomotion, vol 45. Stockholm, Wenner-Gren International Symposium Series, 1985, pp 677–689.

7   Eidelberg E, Walden JG, Nguyen LH: Locomotor control in macaque monkeys. Brain 1981;104:647–663.

8   Bussel B, Roby-Brami A, Azouvi Ph, Biraben A, Yakovleff A, Held JP: Myoclonus in a patient with spinal cord transection. Possible involvement of the spinal stepping generator. Brain 1988;111:1235–1245.

9   Lovejoy CO: Evolution of human walking. Sci Am 1988;Nov:82–89.

10   White TD: Evolutionary implications of pliocene hominid footprints. Science 1980;208:175–176.

11   Saunders M, Inman V, Eberhart H: The major determinants in normal and pathological gait. J Bone Joint Surg [Am] 1953;35:543–558.

12   Forssberg H: Ontogeny of human locomotor control. I. Infant stepping, supported locomotion and transition to independent locomotion. Exp Brain Res 1985;57:480–493.

13   de Vries JIP, Visser GHA, Prechtl HFR: Fetal motility in the first half of pregnancy; in Prechtl HFR (ed): Continuity of Neural Functions from Prenatal to Postnatal Life Clinics in Developmental Medicine, No 94. Oxford, Spastics International Medical Publications, 1984, pp 46–64.

14   Peiper A: Cerbral Function in Infancy and Childhood. New York, Consultants Bureau, 1963.

15   Zelazo PR: The development of walking: New findings and old assumptions. J Mot Behav 1983;15:99–137.

16   Sutherland DH, Olshen RA, Cooper L, et al: The Development of Mature Gait. J Bone Joint Surg [Am] 1980;62:336–353.

17   Forssberg H: A developmental model of human locomotion; in Grillner S, Stein PSG, Stuart DG, Forssberg H, Herman, RM (eds): Neurobiology of Vertebrate Locomotion. Wenner-Gren International Symposium Series, vol 45. Hong Kong, MacMillan, 1986, pp 485–501.

18   Leonard CT, Hirschfeld H, Forssberg H: The development of independent walking in children with cerebral palsy. 1990;unpublished.

19   Berger W, Quintern J, Dietz JV: Pathophysiology of gait in children with cerebral palsy. Electroencephalogr Clin Neurophysiol 1982;53:538–548.

20   Thelen E, Bradshaw G, Ward JA: Spontaneous kicking in month-old infants: Manifestation of a human central locomotor program. Behav Neural Biol 1981;32:45–53.

21   Mc Graw MB: Neuromuscular development of the human infant as exemplified in the achievement of erect locomotion. J Pediatr 1940;17:747–771.

22   Koluchova, J: Severe deprivation in twins: A case study. J Child Psychol Psychiatry 1972;13:107–114.

23   Forssberg H, Svartenberg G: Hardwired locomotor network in cat revealed by a motor pattern to Gastrocnemius after muscle transposition. Neurosci Lett 1983;41:283–288.

Hans Forssberg, MD, PhD, Department of Pediatrics, Motor Control Lab. Q4, Karolinska Hospital, S–104 01 Stockholm (Sweden)

Forssberg H, Hirschfeld H (eds): Movement Disorders in Children.
Med Sport Sci. Basel, Karger, 1992, vol 36, pp 182–185

Normal and Impaired Development of Children's Gait

W. Berger

Department of Clinical Neurology and Neurophysiology, University of Freiburg, FRG

It is a widely accepted hypothesis that motor impairment in spasticity is based on increased muscle tone and that this muscle hypertonia is the consequence of enhanced motoneuron activity, coactivation and increased stretch reflexes. Investigations in adult patients with spasticity of cerebral or spinal origin could not confirm this interpretation but led to the conclusion that in functional movements such as gait or in corrective responses to perturbations the enhanced muscle tone is based on structural changes of the muscle fibers itself which are tonically activated at a low level. The functional extensor EMG activity was reduced and the enhanced monosynaptic stretch reflexes did not contribute significantly to the overall EMG activity [1–3]. The reciprocal activation was preserved [4].

Also in children with cerebral palsy the hypothesis underlying this motor disorder was that primitive reflexes persist and that muscle hypertonia is the consequence of an abnormally enhanced postural reflex activity [5]. Consequently, comparison with this group should give further insight into the pathophysiology of spasticity and motor impairment and, at last, a comparison with age-matched normal children had to be performed. In the course of these studies the very beginning of gait development was followed by means of treadmill walking and brought up the following new interpretations.

Reflex Changes during Development

The newborn stepping as an innate locomotor program in children is described by Forssberg and Wallberg [6] as a coactivation of all leg muscles which may be preprogrammed as the activity starts a little before the ground contact of the feet. These locomotor-like stepping movements last for about 10 weeks. The results described here are performed after this

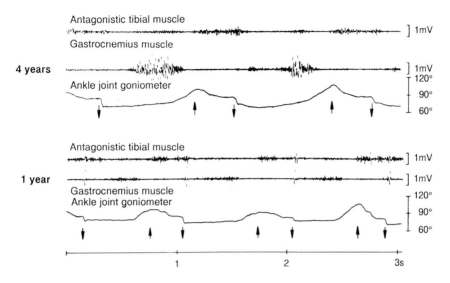

Fig. 1. Leg muscle EMG and ankle goniometer signals of two children representing early and mature stepping. Arrows indicate stance and swing phase of gait.

period by children from the beginning of free standing and by inducing steps on a moving treadmill [methods, see 7].

The typical features of immature gait were (fig. 1):

(i) A coactivation of antagonistic leg muscles during the stance phase of gait similar to the finding in the newborn stepping.

(ii) Large, solitary potentials 20–30 ms after ground contact with stretching of the gastrocnemius muscle.

(iii) Slow and tonic activity of gastrocnemius EMG.

These typical features of early gait pattern are changed in parallel to the ability of free walking to a reciprocal activation, suppression of the monosynaptic reflexes and an increase of gastrocnemius EMG activity during the second year of life. While the magnitude of tibialis anterior activation did not change substantially the final magnitude of gastrocnemius EMG was established around 5–6 years of age. From about 7 years of life no differences to the adult pattern could be observed. The conclusion was that the predominance of a centrally programmed innate pattern is modulated by spinal stretch reflexes under the control of supraspinal centers which have yet to mature. A mutual modulation of mono- and polysynaptic reflexes takes place in favor of the latter ones. This enables the child to compensate for irregularities of ground conditions in the form of a stronger extensor EMG.

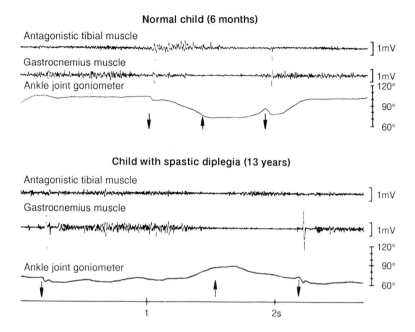

Fig. 2. Leg muscle EMG and ankle goniometer signals of a normal child and a child with cerebral palsy. Arrows as in figure 1.

These basic findings could be confirmed by corrective EMG responses following perturbations and by recording mechanically evoked potentials at the same time for afferent pathway control: close parallel changes with age in EMG responses and cerebral potentials could be demonstrated. Together with a suppression of monosynaptic reflexes a blocking of group I afferents and an increase of polysynaptic EMG responses took place [8]. It is suggested that maturation of normal gait pattern and compensatory EMG responses is achieved by the descending inhibition of group I afferents and facilitation of polysynaptic spinal reflexes via group II afferents.

Reflex Behavior in Cerebral Palsy

The gait pattern of children with cerebral palsy (8–16 years) showed the same characteristics as the pattern during early development with coactivation, reduced extensor EMG and the enhanced monosynaptic stretch reflexes [9]. These biphasic potentials were associated with digitigrade stepping as in the small healthy children around 1 year of age. In contrast to adult spastic patients a reciprocal pattern is not established. The corrective EMG responses following perturbations showed reduced EMG activity together with enhanced monosynaptic reflexes [7]. In contrast to the normal immature stage muscle tone is enhanced as in spastic adults. Similarities and differences of the gait pattern and reflex behavior of children with cerebral palsy and spastic adult patients and the comparison with healthy children during development of gait led to the following suggestions: coactivation and enhanced monosynaptic stretch reflexes represent a physiological stage during development. This does not lead to enhanced muscle tone but seems to be a mechanism to stiffen the legs and to support body weight for equilibrium control. In children with cerebral palsy this normal maturation does not take place due to an impairment of supraspinal centers. In spastic adult patients, however, a part regression to this early gait pattern follows the supraspinal lesion along with the preservation of the reciprocal mode of activation, once established. In both groups of patients, muscle hypertonia seems to be the consequence of altered muscle fibre properties.

References

1   Dietz V, Quintern J, Berger W: Electrophysiological studies of gait in spasticity and rigidity. Evidence that altered mechanical properties of muscle contribute to hypertonia. Brain 1981;104:431–449.

2   Berger W, Horstmann GA, Dietz V: Tension development and muscle activation in the leg during gait in spastic hemiparesis: the independence of muscle hypertonia and exaggerated stretch reflexes. J Neurol Neurosurg Psychiatry 1984;47:1029–1033.

3   Dietz V, Berger W: Normal and impaired regulation of muscle stiffness in gait: A new hypothesis about muscle hypertonia. Exp Neurol 1983;79:680–687.

4   Berger W, Horstmann GA, Dietz V: Spastic paresis: Impaired spinal reflexes and intact motor programs. J Neurol Neurosurg Psychiatry 1988;51:568–571.

5   Walshe FMR: On certain tonic or postural reflexes in hemiplegia, with special reference to the so called 'associated movements'. Brain 1923;46:1–37.

6   Forssberg H, Wallberg H: Infant locomotion: A preliminary movement and electromyographic study: in Berg K, Eriksson BO (eds): Children and Exercise. IX Int Series on Sport Sciences. Baltimore, University Park Press, 1980, pp 32–40.

7   Berger W, Altenmüller E, Dietz V: Normal and impaired development of children's gait. Hum Neurobiol 1984;34:163–170.

8   Berger W, Quintern J, Dietz V: Afferent and efferent control of stance and gait: Developmental changes in children. Electroenceph Clin Neurophysiol 1987;66:244–252.

9   Berger W, Quintern J, Dietz V: Pathophysiology of gait in children with cerebral palsy. Electroenceph Clin Neurophysiol 1982;63:538–548.

Dr. W. Berger, Department of Clinical Neurology and Neurophysiology,
Hansastrasse 9, D-W–7800 Freiburg (FRG)

Forssberg H, Hirschfeld H (eds): Movement Disorders in Children.
Med Sport Sci. Basel, Karger, 1992, vol 36, pp 186–198

Pathophysiological Profile of Gait in Children with Cerebral Palsy

P. Crenna[a], *M. Inverno*[b], *C. Frigo*[c], *R. Palmieri*[c], *E. Fedrizzi*[b]

[a]Istituto di Fisiologia Umana II, University of Milan; [b]Istituto Neurologico C. Besta; [c]Centro di Bioingegneria, Dip. di Elettronica, Fnd. Don Gnocchi, IRCCS, Milan, Italy

Up to the 1970s, attempts to quantitatively evaluate motor disorders were mainly based on measurements performed under static conditions (with the subject lying or sitting). The assumption was that static testing reliably predicted the interference of the observed abnormalities in everyday life motor behaviour. However, more recent studies demonstrated that results of static measurements can be poorly correlated with the performance of natural movements. As regards gait pathology, for instance, normal voluntary EMG output, observed in a given muscle under static conditions, may show low or no motor unit recruitment when the same muscle is activated 'automatically', possibly via different command pathways, during locomotion [1]. Discrepancies between predictions of static testing and actual gait performance have also been observed for muscle responses to stretch [2–4]. Such unexpected outcomes might be due to the variable mechanical effectiveness of the EMG activity evoked by lengthening of muscle throughout the step cycle. Again, they might be accounted for by unpredictable changes in the excitability of the myotatic arc, resulting from abnormal task-dependent and/or phase-dependent modulation during gait [5]. The aforementioned observations point to a substantial inadequacy of static testing on its own and call for complementary evaluation of natural motor functions, among which gait is certainly one of the most relevant.

Need for Pathophysiological Assessment of Gait Disturbances

Different strategies can be adopted for the analysis of gait. The most common approach involves collection of kinematic, dynamic and EMG recordings, to provide a quantitative description of the abnormal pattern of walking in terms of joint angles, joint torques and EMG phasing. Such an approach can be used for monitoring the evolution of the functional picture and for objective assessment of the effectiveness of treatments. Yet, it fails to provide insight to the mechanisms underlying the disturbed motor control. We feel that an alternative strategy, i.e. one based on the evaluation of pathophysiological information about the gait disorder, is necessary.

A pathophysiologically oriented analysis of gait is of particular interest in the case of children with cerebral palsy (CP). This is because motor impairments associated with brain damage occurring during ontogeny are often the result of multiple factors, both central (e.g. paresis) and peripheral (e.g. tendon retraction), which occur in varying proportions and may possibly change their relative contribution over time. Despite previous studies concerning the pathophysiology of gait in CP patients [6–9] to our knowledge, no attempts have been made to determine the contribution of different factors involved in abnormal gait in individual children. In our gait laboratory, we recently developed a new approach aimed at addressing the above issue. The method is based on the multifactorial analysis of gait (kinematics, dynamics, EMGs), and consists of a set of analytic routines, each devoted to the detection and quantization of a single pathophysiological component. The overall procedure produces a 'pathophysiological profile' of the gait of the individual patient. In this article we discuss the main features of the method and the results of preliminary studies on children with CP.

Methodological Guidelines for the New Approach

A central point in the present study was the isolation of a number of relevant pathophysiological factors which could potentially hinder locomotion in CP children. Accordingly, the following components were identified: (1) defective recruitment of motor units (paretic component); (2) abnormal velocity-dependent EMG recruitment during muscle stretch (spastic component); (3) nonselective activation of antagonistic muscles with loss of the normal reciprocal inhibitory pattern (co-contraction component); (4) changes in the mechanical properties of the muscle-tendon system (non-neural component).

When designing the recording protocol and the elaboration procedures, several basic requirements were satisfied:

(a) Analysis of various locomotor tasks, covering different velocities and levels of difficulty. With reference to a control condition (standing), data are recorded during overground walking at natural (most comfort-

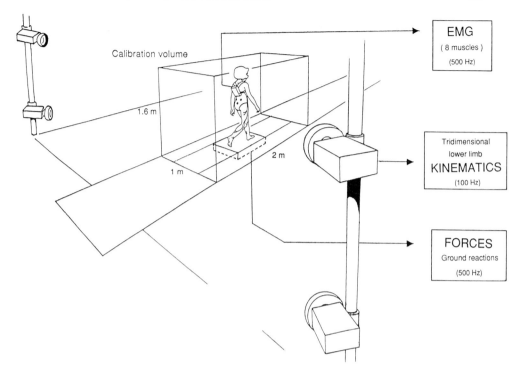

Fig. 1. Schematic view of the experimental set up used for multifactorial analysis of gait in cerebral palsied children.

able) speed, at maximal speed, stepping on the spot and alternate hopping on the spot. The use of different movement speeds results in different stretching velocities of the examined muscles, which in turn are expected to uncover abnormal velocity-dependent EMG responses. Analysis of locomotor tasks with various degrees of automatization and difficulty, which appear to require different settings of the segmental apparatus (e.g. different gating of Ia input from muscle spindles [10]), is expected to test locomotor function over a wider range of central control situations.

(b) Acquisition of multiple gait parameters during free and unconstrained motion. Three-dimensional lower limb kinematics are recorded similtaneously from both sides with a motion analyzer equipped with four 100 Hz cameras (ELITE). The system detects the instantaneous position of passive reflective markers (no wires) placed on relevant landmarks of lower limbs, and computes joint angles on the basis of anthropometric parameters. Dynamic variables (ground reactions and joint torques) are measured by means of a force plate (Kistler) hidden in the floor, and EMG signals are collected by surface preamplified electrodes from pairs of antagonistic muscles of thigh and leg, bilaterally. A schematic view of the recording set up is shown in figure 1.

(c) Data reduction. Efforts were made to process a minimal number of variables, relevant for the detection of the pathophysiological factors as defined above. At the same time, however, criteria for the assessment of the single factors have been established, requiring the convergence of kinematic, dynamic and EMG conditions. This 'redundancy' is expected to increase the reliability of the information extracted.

(d) Low complexity layout. For an easier clinical application, data processing will eventually produce a readable histogram-like presentation, containing the relevant information, i.e. the relative contribution of different pathophysiological factors, scaled in discrete levels.

Dissecting Out Single Pathophysiological Factors

Criteria for detection of the factors defined above were established for children with congenital hemiparesis, the pathology for which the method is currently being tested.

Paretic Component
Criteria for detection during gait include: (a) significant reduction of the EMG output (50% or less as compared to the homologous muscle on the contralateral non affected side) in the absence of activity on the antagonist; (b) congruent kinematic correlate in terms of abnormal excursion of the relevant joint. Items must be true for all the motor tasks examined.

An example of paresis is shown in figure 2, which reports the EMG activity of tibialis anterior (TA) and soleus (Sol), and the relative knee and ankle joint angles from the affected and contralateral limb of a hemiplegic child, walking at natural speed. A consistent decrease in TA activation (which can be quantified as the area of rectified-integrated signal) is particularly prominent around the ground contact on the affected limb. The congruent kinematic correlate is obvious in the ankle joint excursion, as increased plantar flexion in the late swing-early stance phase (arrow in fig. 2). At variance, the reduced recruitment in TA around the toe off instant (EMG from 50 to 70% of the step cycle) appears to maintain some functional effectiveness in clearing the foot off the ground, as indicated by the normal ankle dorsiflexion in the early swing phase on the affected side. The absence of any detectable push off burst on Sol muscle (EMG

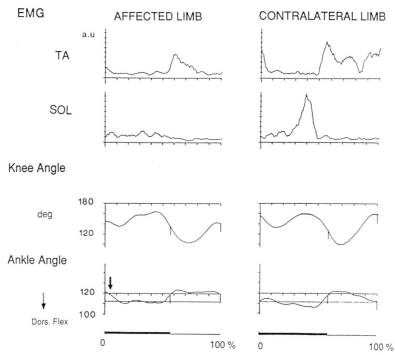

Fig. 2. Defective EMG recruitment and its kinematic correlates (paretic component) on the affected side of a 7-year-old hemiplegic child, walking at natural speed. Upper graphs: Rectified-integrated EMGs of TA and Sol. Lower graphs: Relative knee and ankle joint angles on the sagittal plane. The step cycle is normalized as the time interval between two subsequent ipsilateral ground contacts. Stance and swing phases are shown below as thick and thin lines, respectively.

recording in the second half of the stance phase) does not affect the ankle kinematics, due to the concurrent compensatory activation of gastrocnemii (not shown in fig. 2).

Spastic Component

Criteria for the assessment during movement include: (a) synchronous EMG recruitment during stretching of the relevant muscle, and (b) positive correlation between EMG amplitude and velocity of muscle stretching. Lengthening velocity is computed as the first derivative of muscle length, the latter being obtained from joint angles by means of geometrical muscle models [11].

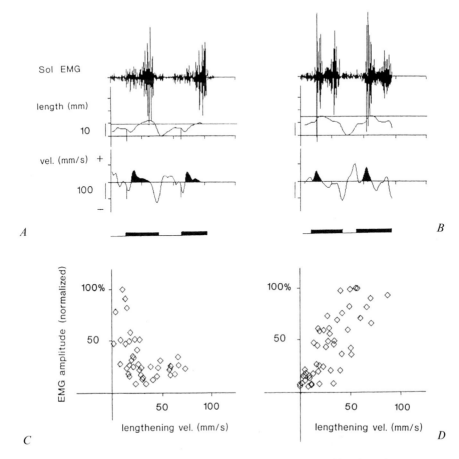

Fig. 3. Abnormal velocity-dependent EMG activity during stretching (spastic component) in the Sol muscle. Upper graphs: EMGs, relative muscle length (with reference to quiet standing) and velocity of muscle stretching (positive values) and shortening (negative values) in a normal *(A)* and hemiplegic child *(B)* during natural speed walking. Lower graphs: Relationship between lengthening velocity and EMG amplitude of Sol muscle (delayed by the latency of the Sol tendon reflex) calculated over three consecutive step cycles during the early stance stretching period (filled areas in the velocity traces) in the normal *(C)* and hemiplegic child *(D)*. Note the positive correlation in the CP patient.

The upper graphs in figure 3 compare EMGs, relative changes of muscle length, and velocity of muscle stretching (positive values) and shortening (negative values), for the Sol muscle of a normal (A) and hemiplegic child (B), walking at natural speed. A marked increase in the amplitude and degree of synchronization of the EMG activity recorded during the stretching phase which takes place after ground contact (filled areas in the velocity traces) is obvious in the hemiplegic patient (B). The abnormal velocity dependence of this EMG burst is confirmed in the lower graphs of figure 3. In fact, when over the same time windows, the lengthening velocity of Sol muscle is plotted versus the amplitude of Sol EMG (normalized to the maximal locomotor output and delayed by the latency of Sol tendon reflex), a positive correlation is observed in the patient (D), but not in the control (C). It is worth mentioning that a velocity-dependent strategy of recruitment on Sol muscle was actually observed in some normal children after ground contact, however the EMG amplitudes at maximal lengthening velocities never attained the levels measured in patients.

Co-Contraction Component

One criterion for the detection of co-contraction is a significant increase in the overlapping between EMGs of two antagonistic muscles. The degree of overlapping is quantified both temporally, as the percentage of the step cycle during which the antagonistic muscles are coactivated above a given threshold, and geometrically, as the area of rectified-integrated EMG over the same period, normalized to the mean locomotor activity of the two muscles [12]. Careful exclusion of artifactual co-contraction due to cross-talk is obviously a prerequisite for the detection of such a component.

Figure 4 reports examples of quantitative analysis of co-contraction between TA and Sol over single stride cycles in a normal child (A), and in two hemiplegic children with different degrees of motor impairment (B, C). Abnormal increase in temporal and geometrical overlappings is obvious in the 2 patients, even in the presence of a rather high detection threshold (20% maximal locomotor activity of each muscle).

Non-Neural Component

Assessment of the non-neural component necessitates a reduced joint excursion during passive mobilization (quantified by goniometry) in the absence of detectable articular pathologies. Criteria for the assessment during movement include: (a) reduced excursion of the relevant joint angle; (b) stepwise increase of torque during lengthening of the muscle-tendon considered; (c) abnormal relationship between joint torque and joint angle, and (d) absence of correlation between changes in the EMG output and the above biomechanical phenomena on the muscle examined.

Typical kinematic and dynamic features of the gait of a hemiplegic child with shortening of the Achilles tendon are shown in figure 5. A clear-cut block of the ankle dorsiflexion in the early stance phase (arrow in the ankle angle graph) is associated with a steep increase of the ankle joint torque over the same period (arrow in the torque graph). In the absence of

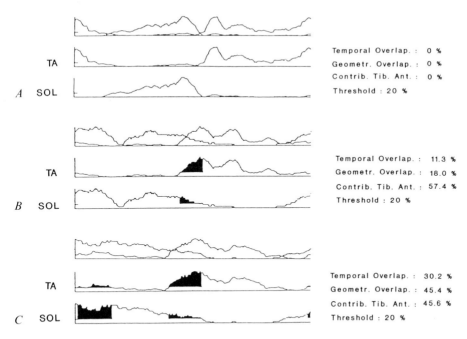

Fig. 4. Quantitative analysis of co-contraction between TA and Sol in a normal 8-year-old child *(A)* and in two hemiplegic children of the same age *(B, C)*. Each set of traces reports from top to bottom the rectified integrated EMG of Sol and TA superimposed, EMG from TA alone and EMG from Sol alone, over a single step cycle. Filled areas mark the periods during which both muscles are activated above a threshold corresponding to 20% of their maximal locomotor output (co-contraction periods).

congruent EMG recruitment in the calf muscles, this behaviour can be accounted for by an increased passive stiffness of the Achilles tendon-calf muscle system. Note that the limited dorsiflexion of the ankle results in a marked hyperextension of the knee (well evident in the knee angle excursion), and subsides only in concomitance with the knee flexion before the toe off. The blocked extension of the knee during the swing phase (arrow in the knee angle graph) is the kinematic expression of a partial retraction of the lateral hamstrings.

Assessing Discrete Levels of Impairment

To provide quantitative evaluation of the interference of the different pathophysiological factors in gait performance, discrete levels of impair-

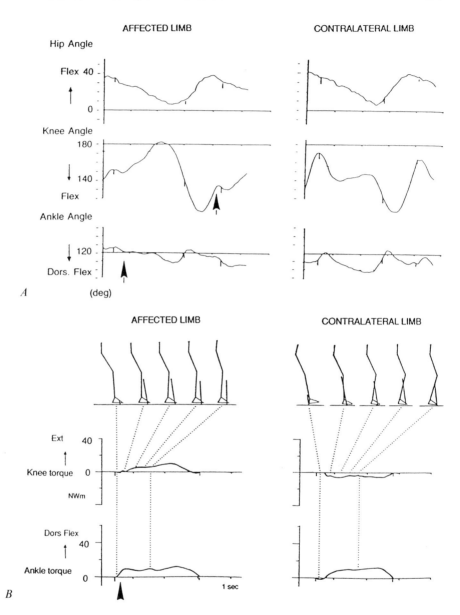

Fig. 5. Effects of Achilles tendon retraction on kinematic and dynamic parameters of walking in an 8-year-old hemiplegic child. *A* Relative hip, knee and ankle joint angles on the sagittal plane. *B* Knee and ankle joint torques calculated for the stance phase of the same stride. Stick diagrams of lower limbs and ground reaction vectors (superimposed) are also shown for the early stance phase.

ment must be assigned. In our pilot analysis two levels were considered and were expressed in arbitrary units. Levels 1 and 2 indicate lower and higher degree of gravity, respectively. Examples of scaling applied to the distal muscles (Sol and TA) are listed below.

Paresis. Level 1 is assigned when the set of criteria defined for its detection (see above) is true for specific phases of the step cycle. Level 2 requires all items to be true for the whole step cycle. Such a scaling rule was derived from the observation that recruitment of TA was usually absent around contact (pre-contact burst), when the knee is extended, but was rarely affected in swing phase (early swing burst), when the flexion synergy of the lower limb is likely to lower the excitability threshold of the ankle dorsiflexors to the central command. Similarly, activation of Sol was frequently defective in the second half of the stance phase (push off burst), but not in early stance.

Spasticity. Level 1 exists when criteria for detection are true only for maximal walking speed (and hopping), when the highest velocities of muscle stretching are expected to occur. Level 2 exists when the same items are true also for natural walking speed (and stepping), indicating a lower threshold for pathological muscle responses to stretch.

Co-Contraction. On the basis of data obtained in normal children (mean age 7 years), level 1 is assigned when temporal overlapping is >5% and <10% and geometrical overlapping is >10% and <20%. Level 2 implies values higher than 10% and 20% for temporal and geometrical overlapping, respectively.

Non-Neural Component. Level 1 is attained when joint excursion during passive mobilization is reduced by 10° to 20°, while level 2 requires a more severe limitation of joint excursion (>20°). In both cases all criteria defined for detection during gait must be true.

The Pathophysiological Profile

Examples of pathophysiological profiles obtained in 2 children with congenital hemiparesis (ages 7 and 8 years), using the above scaling levels are shown in figure 6. It appears that several factors can be present simultaneously in the same patient and each patient has gait with a distinct profile. This indicates there is consistent intersubject variability, even within the same clinical group. The profile could be dominated by the spastic,

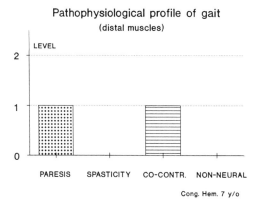

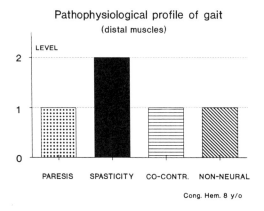

Fig. 6. Examples of pathophysiological profiles of gait calculated in two hemiparetic children for distal muscles (TA and Sol).

co-contraction, or non-neural component. Rather unexpectedly, the paretic component was rarely prominent, and most often attained its lowest scaling level.

Increased co-contraction was apparent on the paretic side, but could also be revealed on the contralateral 'healthy' side, especially at the highest walking speeds. This suggests that co-contraction is not necessarily derived from a loss of selectivity in MN recruitment, as a result of decreased reciprocal inhibition and/or disturbed centrally-generated locomotor program. Alternatively, this could be a protective strategy aimed at stiffening a certain joint, to compensate for postural instability or paresis. Analysis of rhythmic tasks requiring different postural or equilibrium demand (e.g. free walking vs. hopping) could help distinguish the two conditions.

In certain cases, analysis of the degree of co-contraction, together with phasing of the activity of representative muscles within the step cycle, could provide information concerning disturbed organization of the locomotor program. In fact, EMG features reminiscent of those described for the immature digitigrade gait could be observed in some hemiparetic children (fig. 4C). For distal muscles EMG markers of immaturity include: (a) pre-contact activation of triceps surae (TS); (b) short latency (monosynaptic) response to stretch on TS after ground contact; (c) absence of forward thrust burst on TS; (d) persistent activity of TS in early swing, and (e) subcontinuous activation of TA in stance [6, 13–16]. Kinematic features include forefoot or footflat ground contact, and ankle movement in phase with the knee movement [16]. A prominent dynamic hallmark is the absence of typical push off peak in the vertical component of the ground reaction [16]. Features of the immature digitigrade gait and of the early unsupported locomotion have been reported in CP patients by Leonard et al. [8, 9], who documented their persistence after the puberal age. These observations suggest the possible introduction of an additional pathophysiological component, i.e. the primitive, immature one. The latter of course will always be associated with a higher incidence of co-contraction, and possibly with increased excitability of the stretch reflex.

A final point worth mentioning concerns intra-subject variability of the observed findings. We found that when the full recording session was performed twice within a 10-day interval, the overall profile of a patient's gait was consistently reproducible. After longer periods, however (1 year), dramatic changes in single components (e.g. non neural c) could be detected, again suggesting the possible fluctuation in the incidence of pathophysiological mechanisms during development. We feel that knowledge of these changes might be a valuable step towards more in-depth understanding of the history of disturbed motor control during development. In this context, the 'pathophysiological profile' could also be used as a tool for more rational planning of patient-tailored, therapeutic and rehabilitation procedures, and possibly as a predictor of the functional evolution.

References

1   Knutsson E: Analysis of gait and isokinetic movements for evaluation of antispastic drugs or physical therapies; in Desmedt JE (ed): Motor Control Mechanisms in Health and Disease. New York, Raven Press, 1983, pp 1013–1034.
2   Knutsson E: Restraint of spastic muscles in different types of movements; in Feldman RG, Young RR, Koella WP (eds): Spasticity; Disordered Motor Control. Chicago, Year Book, 1980, pp 123–132.

3   Dimitrijevic ML, Lenman JAR: Neural control of gait in patients with upper motor lesions; in Feldman RG, Young RR, Koella WP (eds): Spasticity: Disordered Motor Control. Chicago, Year Book, 1980, pp 101–121.

4   Crenna P, Frigo C: Monitoring gait by a vector diagram technique; in Delwaide PJ, Young RR (eds): Clinical Neurophysiology in Spasticity. Amsterdam, Elsevier, 1985, pp 109–124.

5   Crenna P, Frigo C: Changes in the excitability of the H-reflex arc during walking and stepping in man. Exp Brain Res 1987;66:49–60.

6   Berger W, Quintern J, Dietz V: Pathophysiology of gait in children with cerebral palsy. Electroenceph Clin Neurophysiol 1982;53:538–548.

7   Berger W, Altenmueller E, Dietz V: Normal and impaired development of children's gait. Hum Neurobiol 1984;3:163–170.

8   Leonard CT, Hirshfeld H, Forssberg H: The development of independent walking in children with cerebral palsy. Dev Med Child Neurol 1991;33:567–577.

9   Leonard CT, Hirshfeld H, Forssberg H: Gait acquisition and reflex abnormalities in normal children and children with cerebral palsy; in Amblard A, Berthoz A, Clarac F (eds): Posture and Gait: Development, Adaptation and Modulation. Amsterdam, Elsevier, 1988, pp 33–45.

10 Llewellyn M, Yang JF, Prochazka A: Human H-reflexes are smaller in difficult beam walking than in normal treadmill walking. Exp Brain Res 1990;83:22–28.

11 Frigo C, Pedotti A: Determination of muscle length during locomotion. Biomechanics 1987;VI-A:355–360.

12 Rodano R, Bulgheroni M, Crenna P: Quantitative assessment of co-contraction between antagonistic muscles during rhythmic movements in man. Proceedings of the Italian ISEK Meeting 1991. Functional Neurol, (in press).

13 Statham L, Murray MP: Early walking patterns of normal children. Clin Orthop 1971;79:8–24.

14 Okamoto T, Kamamoto M: EMG study of the learning process of walking in infants. EMG Clin Neurophysiol 1972;12:149–158.

15 Sutherland DH, Olsen R, Cooper L, Woo SLY: The development of mature gait. J Bone Joint Surg 1980;62:354–363.

16 Forssberg H: Ontogeny of human locomotor control I. Infant stepping, supported locomotion and transition to independent locomotion. Exp Brain Res 1985;57:480–493.

Prof. P. Crenna, Istituto di Fisiologia Umana II, University of Milan,
I–20133 Milano (Italy)

Forssberg H, Hirschfeld H (eds): Movement Disorders in Children.
Med Sport Sci. Basel, Karger, 1992, vol 36, pp 199–208

Postural Control: Acquisition and Integration during Development

Helga Hirschfeld

Nobel Institute for Neurophysiology, Karolinska Institute, Stockholm, Sweden

Introduction

We are constantly influenced by the force of gravity. Postural control refers to the actions of sensorimotor systems organized toward contending with this force. In this review I will mainly discuss mechanisms involved in maintenance of equilibrium in static positions and during movements.

The ability to maintain a certain posture involves: (i) generation of muscle activity supporting body weight against gravity; (ii) control of body segments in relation to each other, and (iii) control of the body in relation to the environment, in which the center of mass must be maintained within the limits of the support base. Displacement of the body is detected by information from the somatosensory, vestibular and visual systems. Activation of these systems during a perturbation of the equilibrium induce postural reactions which return the body to equilibrium. Recognizing the difficulties of estimating the spatial orientation of each body segment it is proposed that the postural control system may use an internal model of posture as a reference [1]. This internal model consists of information regarding the metric properties and mechanical characteristics of myosceletal system for a particular posture. There are two principal means by which body equilibrium is perturbed: (1) An *external* force is applied to the body or the support surface moves. (2) An *internal* force is applied during a self-induced movement. The postural adjustment will occur after the perturbation in response to an external force. In contrast, the postural adjustment will precede (anticipate) the equilibrium perturbation when a voluntary movement (internal force) perturbs the equilibrium.

Postural Responses to External Perturbations

During the last two decades movable platforms with built-in force sensors have been used to quantify postural responses following support surface perturbations. A sudden translation of the platform backward evokes a forward body sway of the standing subject. Muscle activity on the dorsal aspect of the body counteracts the forward fall. The activity begins in the muscles closest to the support base (calf muscle) and radiates upward to thigh and trunk, moving the body backward to its initial position [2, 3]. The recruitment of muscles during a particular postural response is dependent on the support base conditions, e.g. if a similar perturbation is applied with the support base shorter than foot length, the ventral thigh and trunk muscles are activated first producing a horizontal shear force moving the center of mass backward [4]. If the subject instead uses the hand for support, the postural response in the trunk and lower extremities is suppressed [5].

Recently we studied postural responses after perturbations of seated subjects (straight-legged sitting on the platform). Two different perturbations, forward translation and upward rotation of the legs, were used. Both perturbations gave the subject the impression of falling backward. Responsible for this impression was the pelvis rotation posteriorly instantly with the platform movement onset, while hip joint, trunk and head moved differently after translation and rotation. The pattern of muscle activity in hip and trunk muscles on both the ventral and dorsal aspect of the body was essentially the same with only small variability between translation and rotation and subjects (fig. 1A). The early onset of pelvis rotation posteriorly (some 10 ms after perturbation onset) supports the hypothesis that one important information source for generating the postural response is the shift of the center of gravity backward (fig. 2A). In contrast, perturbations causing the upper body to sway forward evoked only weak postural responses. This is probably due to the much higher stability in the direction with a long distance to the border of the support base. The stability in the backward direction as during standing is much less, due to the very short distance to the border of the support base requiring rapid invariant postural patterns.

Children able to stand independently have similar postural responses as adults when perturbed on a movable platform [6, 7]. Children just able to sit independently exhibit directionally specific postural responses which are very similar to the adult pattern after perturbation of the support surface [Hirschfeld and Forssberg, unpubl.]. A platform translation forward, causing a backward sway of the trunk, was counteracted by muscle activity in hip flexors followed by activity in trunk and neck flexors (fig.

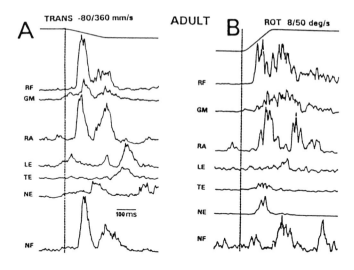

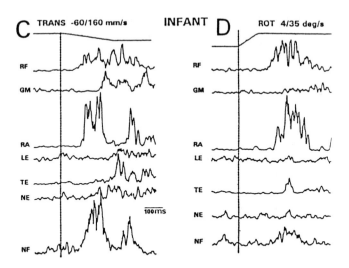

Fig. 1. Ensemble-averaged leg and trunk EMGs (3 trials) for one adult *(A, B)* and one 7-month-old child *(C, D)* during forward translation and rotation (legs up). The vertical line indicates platform movement onset. RF = Rectus femoris muscle; GM = gluteus maximus; RA = rectus abdominus; LE = lumbar extensors; TE = thoracal extensors; NE = neck extensors; NF = sternocleidomastoideus.

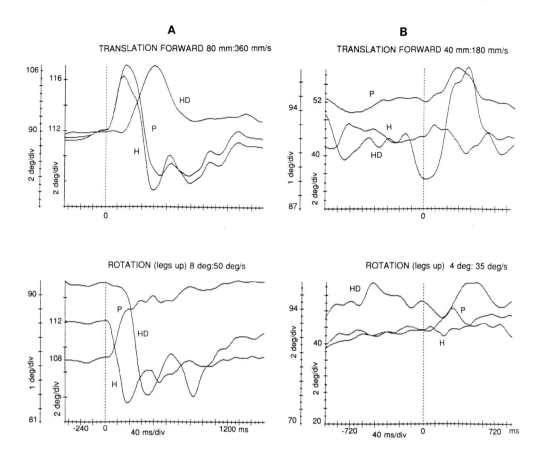

Fig. 2. Kinematics of head, pelvis and hip joint for one trial of translation, respectively rotation (legs up) for one adult (*A*) and one child 7-month-old (*B*). Angular displacement of head (HD) and pelvis (P) were calculated relative to the horizontal axis (X) and the hip joint angle (H) was calculated in the sagittal plane. The vertical dotted line with zero value denotes platform movement onset. The movements were recorded with an image processing system (Elite, BTS, Italy), samplings frequency 100 Hz.

1C). A similar response was also seen after platform rotation (legs up, fig. 1D). However, the latency to the onset of muscle activity was almost twice that of adults. Children also showed similar kinematics of the postural response of head, pelvis and hip joint, although large head and trunk oscillations occurred during resting (fig. 2B; notice the large oscillations of head and trunk during unperturbed sitting and the backward rotation of the head after pelvis rotation).

Postural Responses to Self-Induced Movements

Movement of a body segment perturbs the equilibrium by its reaction force (especially if rapid) and by shifting the center of mass. Postural muscular activity is generated in advance to initiation of the movement (anticipatory) and counteracts the following equilibrium disturbance. It has been suggested that the performance of any voluntary movement involves a precise interaction between the anticipatory postural activity and the voluntary action. For example when raising the arms forward [8, 9] or pulling on a stiff handle [5, 10] particular postural muscle activity patterns of the lower limb and trunk are initiated before the arm muscle activity. When adults rise from sitting to standing a backward displacement of the center of foot pressure occur prior to the rising movement. In this case the postural response occurs in the same limb as the voluntary movement. The displacement is evoked by a spatiotemporal muscle sequence in which soleus inhibition is followed by tibialis anterior activity [11].

Everyday motor activities as well as advanced athletic skills are often performed during locomotion and require interaction between various motor systems. The central mechanisms controlling equilibrium when voluntary movements are performed during locomotion must take into consideration the dynamically changing biomechanics in conjunction with the performance of the voluntary action. Recent studies on subjects walking on a treadmill while pulling a handle have shown that although the voluntary movement is unchanged, the onset, temporal sequence, shape and amplitude of the postural activity in various muscles are continuously modulated with respect to the ongoing locomotor activity [6, 12]. This phase-dependent modulation of the postural response suggests an internal representation of the body at different levels of the CNS that is continuously updated with respect to ongoing locomotor movement. This phase-dependent modulation may be due to central gating of the descending motor commands, exerted by the central locomotor network and peripheral reflex interactions [13].

Haas et al. [14] studied the development of the integration between voluntary actions and postural control in a tip toe rising task. Four-year-old children (the youngest age at which they are able to follow the instructions) were able to appropriately integrate voluntary and postural control strategies. Tibialis anterior is activated (forward shift of center of gravity projection) prior to the activation of the calf muscles. It is possible that children use anticipatory postural strategies earlier, although we do not have adequate tools for testing. We studied the development of integration between locomotion, postural control and voluntary movement in 6–14 year-old children when pulling a handle while walking on the treadmill [15]. All children used an anticipatory strategy in which the postural activity in the leg muscles preceded the arm muscle activity. However, there were age-dependent defferences in the temporal sequences of the leg muscles in the postural response. In addition, the youngest children did not execute pulls during the early part of the support phase, resulting in long delays between the onset of postural and arm muscle activity onset. This may reflect difficulties in the interaction of the locomotor pattern for the arm (ipsilateral forward arm movement) and the voluntary pull when the direction of the locomotor pattern in the arm and pull are out of phase. This difficulty disappeared in the older age group (10 years). Further, calf muscle activity prior to heel strike was present in postural responses during the swing phase (6 years) and during the transition to stance phase (6, 10 and 14 years) while it never occurred in adults. The occurrence of calf muscle activity prior to heel strike suggests an immature (non-plantigrade) neural representation of the gait and parallels the earlier shift of the calf muscle activity during development of plantigrade gait [16, Forssberg, this vol.]. The results suggest a continuous development of these integrative motor systems up to adolescence.

Impaired Postural Control in Children with Cerebral Palsy

Nashner et al. [17] studied postural responses in children with different types of cerebral palsy during perturbations while standing on a movable platform. The temporal order of muscle activity was changed relative to normals. The spastic hemiplegic group activated proximal muscles (far away from the support base) prior to distal muscles and demonstrated a high degree of co-activation between antagonists in the hemiplegic leg, while the less-involved leg showed postural responses within normal values. Preliminary results of platform perturbations during sitting have shown that children with spastic diplegia also have impaired direction specificity of the postural responses [Hirschfeld, Brogren and Forssberg, unpubl.]. Perturbations evoking backward body sway elicited similar muscle activity patterns as following forward body sway. The postural response was characterized by strong coactivation in hip and neck muscles (fig. 3). In spite of this, the postural response was sufficient to prevent a fall.

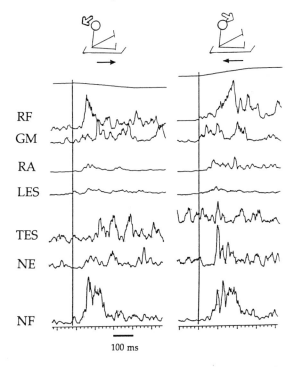

Fig. 3. Ensemble-averaged leg and trunk EMGs (6 trials) for one 11-year-old child with cerebral palsy (spastic) during platform translation forward (160:360 mm/s) and platform translation backward. The vertical line denotes platform movement onset. For abbreviation of muscles see figure 1.

When children with cerebral palsy were instructed to pull on the handle following an auditory signal, the activity started in the arm muscles followed by postural activity with a proximal to distal order in the spastic leg [17]. Hence, the pull was not anticipated by postural activity, instead the postural activity was compensatory after the voluntary movement. It is likely that the anticipatory processes involve cortical structures which may be damaged in children with cerebral palsy [18, 19].

Considerations for Assessment and Treatment

A typical example from clinics is the testing of different 'postural reflexes' such as righting reactions [20] in infants. The therapist changes the position of one body segment (external force), and the other segments will follow in order to maintain alignment of body parts in relation to each

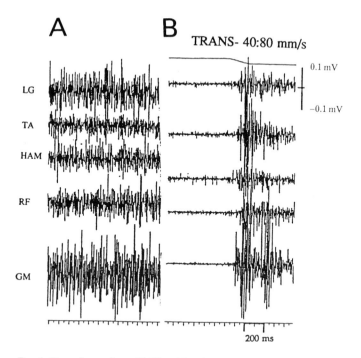

Fig. 4. Recordings of raw EMGs of five leg muscles (left leg) of one 12-year-old child with cerebral palsy when standing with hand-support on a walking aid *(A)* and when standing in a standing-shell on the platform *(B)*. The upper trace indicates the platform movement. LG = Lateral gastrocnemius muscle; TA = tibialis anterior; HAM = biceps femoris; RF = rectus femoris; GM = gluteus maximus.

other and to gravity. Other examples include testing tonic neck reflexes in which head position changes the postural tone in muscles in a predictive way, or testing equilibrium reactions evoked by pushing a body part or tilting the support surface. However, the presence of those reactions under test conditions does not give any information about if and how these reflexes or reactions are integrated in motor performance. During motor performance the postural reflex is admixed with the voluntary movement in order to increase strength and efficiency [21]. A classic example is the combination of the asymmetric tonic neck reflex with the voluntary action of the baseball player when throwing a ball [22].

Although children with cerebral palsy used inappropriate muscle sequences when external forces perturbed the equilibrium, they managed to avoid falls [17]. Our management of cerebral palsy should be aimed at optimizing the childs own strategies instead of trying to 'normalize' postural responses. We should consider that using the hands for support suppresses postural responses in legs and trunk and influence the interactions between voluntary movement and postural control. The integration of postural control and voluntary movement is an important prerequisite for performance of goal directed movements. One major goal of treatment should be to enable the child to perform purposeful movements.

I would like to close this chapter with a practical treatment solution, based on the present knowledge of postural control. We know that the distribution of postural tone depends both on the neural lesion and on biomechanical constraints. We cannot change the neural lesion but we can change the biomechanics. As demonstrated in figure 4A when the subject with a spastic diplegia stands with support on a walking aid, all tested leg muscles are continuously active. When freely upright standing was provided by a standing-shell, postural tone is minimized to normal values (fig. 4B; the standing-shell is a body-shaped orthosis of orthoplast, reaching up to the middle of the thorax; the feet are aligned with the hip joints; the center of gravity projects in front of the ankle joint). Horizontal translations while standing in the standing-shell on the platform-evoked postural responses with proximal to distal sequence order similar to those reported by Nashner et al. [17]. The child did not fall. When standing on the floor, in this supported posture, the child has the opportunity to practice interaction between posture and movement when catching or throwing a ball, etc. Although we provide mechanical help to maintain upright posture, we offer to the damaged CNS the possibility to optimize an internal model of upright posture and to develop strategies for voluntary actions, integrated with the postural control system. The next step in our clinical research program is to evaluate the long-term effects of using the standing-shell as a therapeutic aid.

References

1   Lestienne FG, Gurfinkel VS: Posture as an organizational structure based on a dual process: A formal basis to interpret changes of posture in weightlessness. Prog Brain Res 1988;76:307–313.
2   Nashner LM: Adapting reflexes controlling the human posture. Exp Brain Res 1976;26:59–72.
3   Nashner LM: Fixed patterns of rapid postural responses among leg muscles during stance. Exp Brain Res 1977;30:13–24.
4   Horak FB, Nashner LM: Central programming of postural movements: Adaptation to altered support-surface configurations. J Neurophysiol 1986;55:1369–1381.
5   Cordo PJ, Nashner LM: Properties of postural adjustments associated with rapid arm movements. J Neurophysiol 1982;47:287–302.

6   Nashner LM, Forssberg H: Phase-dependent organization of postural adjustments associated with arm movements while walking. J Neurophysiol 1986;55:1382–1394.

7   Shumway-Cook A, Woollacott MH: The growth of stability: Postural control from a developmental perspective. J Motor Behav 1985;17:131–147.

8   Belenkii VY, Gurfinkel VS, Paltsev YeI: Elements of control of voluntary movements. Biofizika 1967;12:135–141.

9   Zattara M, Bouisset S: Posturo-kinetic organisation during the early phase of voluntary upper limb movement. 1. Normal subjects. J Neurol Neurosurg Psychiatry 1988;51:956–965.

10 Woollacott MH, Bonnet M, Yabe K: Prepartory process for anticipatory postural adjustments: Modulation of leg muscles reflex pathways during preparation for arm movements in standing man. Exp Brain Res 1984;55:263–271.

11 Crenna P, Frigo C: A motor programme for the initiation of forward-oriented movements in man. J Physiol 1991, in press.

12 Hirschfeld H, Forssberg H: Phase-dependent modulations of anticipatory postural activity during human locomotion. J Neurophysiol 1991;66:12–19.

13 Forssberg H: Stumbling corrective reaction: A phase-dependent compensatory reaction during locomotion. J Neurophysiol 1979;42:936–953.

14 Haas G, Diener HC, Rapp H, et al: Development of Feedback and Feedforward Control of Upright Stance. Dev Med Child Neurol 1989;31:481–488.

15 Hirschfeld H, Forssberg H: Development of integrative motor functions for voluntary perturbations during locomotion. J Neurophysiol 1992, submitted.

16 Forssberg H: Ontogeny of human locomotor control. I. Infant stepping, supported locomotion and transition to independent locomotion. Exp Brain Res 1985;57:480–493.

17 Nashner LM, Shumway-Cook A, Marin O: Stance posture control in select groups of children with cerebral palsy: Deficits in sensory organization and muscular coordination. Exp Brain Res 1983;49:393–409.

18 Paltsev YI, Elner AM: Preparatory and compensatory period during voluntary movement in patients with involvement of the brain of different localization. Biophysics 1967;12:161–168.

19 Traub MM, Rothwell JC, Marsden CD: Anticipatory postural reflexes in Parkinson's disease and other akinetic-rigid syndromes and in cerebellar ataxia. Brain 1980;103:393–412.

20 Milani-Comparetti A, Gidoni EA: Routine developmental examination in normal and retarded children. Dev Med Child Neurol 1967;9:631–638.

21 Hellebrandt FA, Houtz SJ, Partridge MJ, et al: Tonic neck reflexes in exercises of stress in man. Am J Phys Med 1956;35:144–159.

22 Fukuda T: Studies on human dynamic postures from the viewpoint of postural reflexes. Acta Otolaryngol Suppl (Stockh) 1961;161:1–52.

Helga Hirschfeld, PT, PhD, The Nobel Institute for Neurophysiology, Karolinska Institute, S–104 01 Stockholm (Sweden)

Forssberg H, Hirschfeld H (eds): Movement Disorders in Children.
Med Sport Sci. Basel, Karger, 1992, vol 36, pp 209–216

Role of the Vestibular System in Motor Development: Theoretical and Clinical Issues

Anne Shumway-Cook

Department of Physical Therapy, Northwest Hospital, Seattle, Wash., USA

A fundamental question of concern to both developmental theorists and clinicians involved in the habilitation of children, concerns the role of the vestibular system in the development of motor coordination. A common assumption in developmental theory suggests that an intact vestibular system is critical to normal motor development and coordination [Ornitiz, 1983; Baloh, 1984]. Consistent with this presumption is the belief that abnormal vestibular function is the basis for many developmental disorders, including developmental delays [Kantner et al., 1976; Pignataro et al., 1979], motor dyscoordination [Kaga et al, 1981; Raphin, 1974], and learning disabilities [Ayres, 1972; de Quiros, 1976; Ottenbacher, 1982].

Based on these two assumptions, clinical methods to assess and treat vestibular dysfunction have been developed and applied to children with a wide variety of developmental disorders [Ayres, 1972; de Quiros, 1976; Eviatar and Eviatar, 1978; Harris, 1981; Montgomery, 1985]. Clinicians relying on therapeutic strategies which focus on the vestibular system should ask, what is the evidence supporting the assumption that vestibular dysfunction is a key factor in developmental movement disorders? This paper will discuss theoretical and clinical issues concerning the role of the vestibular system in motor development.

Vestibular Function and Motor Development

Does the vestibular system play a critical role during development? The vestibular system is one of the first sensory systems to mature prenatally, and is anatomically complete and functioning at birth [Ornitz, 1983]. Normally, vestibulo-ocular inputs are critical to eye-head coordination essential for stabilizing gaze, while vestibulo-spinal inputs, along with

Table 1. Vestibular function and gross motor milestones[1]

| | Head control (month) | | | Walking (month) | | |
	n	x	range	n	x	range
Normal children	30	3.4	3–3.8	30	12.4	11–12
Hearing impaired						
Normal vestibular	22	3.7	3–7	18	13.7	11–20
Reduced vestibular	38	5.3	3–9	51	21.4[2]	10–48
Absent vestibular	6	7.3	6–12	5	25.6	18–41

[1] Summary of studies by Rapin [1974] and Kaga et al. [1981].
[2] Three children with absent vestibular function walked at a normal age.

visual and somatosensory inputs, are essential to maintaining postural stability [Baloh, 1984; Nashner, 1985]. A number of research studies have suggested that loss of vestibular function may affect *early* stages of motor development, but have little long-term effect on most aspects of motor proficiency.

Studies by Kaga et al. [1981] and Raphin [1974] were consistent in showing that some, but not all, children with vestibular deficits showed motor delays early in development. In these studies the acquisition of head control and independence in walking was compared in hearing impaired (HI) children with and without vestibular deficiencies. Vestibular sensitivity was assessed through neuro-otologic tests of vestibulo-ocular function (rotational chair or caloric stimulation).

Table 1 summarizes results from both studies. Presented is the average age (x) and range in months, in which children achieved independence in head control, and walking. Results from both studies showed that most HI children with vestibular deficits showed delays in the acquisition of these motor milestones. All children with vestibular hyposensitivity did eventually acquire the motor skills, albeit later than their age-matched peers. Raphin [1974] reported that 3 children with absent vestibular function walked at a normal age, suggesting that not all children with hypoactive vestibular function show developmental delays.

These authors suggest that during maturation the central nervous system (CNS) effectively compensates for loss of vestibular afferent inputs with alternative senses such as vision and somatosensation. Thus, while decreased vestibular function may delay the acquisition of motor skills early in life, few residual delays are seen in older children.

Results from our studies with older children support the assumption that early loss of vestibular function appears to have little long-term effect on most

Table 2. Vestibular function and motor proficiency in children aged 7–12 years.

	Mean and SD for Bruininks-Oseretsky gross motor subtests			
	balance	strength	speed	bilateral coordination
Normal	14 ± 5*	19 ± 5	21 ± 4	17 ± 3
Hearing impaired				
Normal vestibular	14 ± 5	15 ± 4	13 ± 6	14 ± 4
Reduced vestibular	6 ± 6	14 ± 4	12 ± 7	14 ± 4
Absent vestibular	2 ± 2	16 ± 2	12 ± 7	15 ± 3

* Normal standardized subtest score = 15 ± 5.
Adapted from Horak et al. [1988].

aspects of motor proficiency, except for selected aspects of balance control [Horak et al., 1988; Shumway-Cook et al., 1986; Crowe and Horak, 1988].

We examined the effects of vestibular dysfunction occurring early in life on motor proficiency in children aged 7–12 years. Children were classified according to vestibular function based on neuro-otologic tests of vestibulo-ocular (rotational chair testing) and vestibulo-spinal (posturography testing) function. Motor proficiency was tested using the gross motor subtests (balance, running speed, bilateral coordination, and strength) from the Bruininks-Oseretsky Test (BOT) of Motor Proficiency [Bruininks, 1978].

Table 2 presents the results from the BOT summarizing motor proficiency in the 30 HI and 54 normal children classified according to vestibular status. The HI children with decreased vestibular function (n = 20) were normal on most aspects of motor proficiency including running speed and agility, bilateral coordination and strength subtests, but performed poorly on balance tests. Among the HI population, the lowest scores on the BOT were found in the 4 children with bilateral absent vestibular function.

In further tests of postural control in these same HI children, we found the affects of vestibular dysfunction on balance control were context dependent. In many situations children with reduced or absent vestibular function demonstrated balance skills which were functionally equivalent to children with an intact vestibular system. However, in conditions where both visual and somatosensory information were inaccurate or unavailable, children with reduced or absent vestibular function were unable to maintain postural orientation and lost balance [Shumway-Cook, 1989; Shumway-Cook et al., 1987].

These results suggest that with the exception of select balance skills, motor proficiency in older children (ages 7–12) is largely unaffected by early loss of vestibular function.

Rate-Limiting Components in Early Development

Why might reduced vestibular function disproportionately affect the acquisition of motor skills during development? Several developmental theorists have suggested the importance of rate-limiting components during development [Thelan et al., 1989; Woollacott and Shumway-Cook, 1991; Kamm et al., 1991]. Rate-limiting components limit the pace at which an independent behavior emerges, since emergence of that behavior must await the maturation of the slowest critical component. In addition, since development is discontinuous, loss or alteration of a rate-limiting parameter may affect the emergence of a behavior differentially depending on when in the emergence of a skill the loss occurs.

The research reviewed in this paper suggests that maturation of vestibular function may be a rate-limiting component to the acquisition of motor skills early in development. Thus, children with reduced vestibular function affecting postural control show delays early in the development of motor skills. However, vestibular dysfunction itself may not be the most important rate-limiting component to motor development.

A more significant rate-limiting component to postural control and motor development may be the capacity of the maturing CNS to develop compensatory strategies to early loss of vestibular function. Compensatory strategies in part determine the rules for combining remaining sensory inputs for gaze, postural and perceptual functions.

Despite vestibular loss, some children develop normally, perhaps because they form compensatory strategies early in development. It is also possible that an inability to develop appropriate compensatory strategies for organizing remaining sensory inputs may be responsible for the profound developmental delays and dyscoordination found in children with combined vestibular dysfunction and CNS pathology [Raphin, 1974; Horak et al., 1988]. In adults, CNS pathology delays compensation for acute vestibular loss, and as a result symptoms of vertigo and disequilibrium persist [Monnier et al., 1970; Pfaltz and Kamath, 1983]. In addition, in contrast to children with isolated vestibular pathology, children with central sensory organization problems (inability to effectively organize normal vestibular inputs with visual, somatosensory inputs for postural control) have severe problems in all aspects of motor proficiency [Shumway-Cook et al., 1987].

Compensating for a sensory loss appears to require: (1) the availability of other senses; (2) central sensory processes which determine the rules for organizing remaining senses, and (3) applying these rules in active behavior [Fentress, 1989]. Of great significance to pediatric therapists is the understanding that experience can help the process of organizing remaining senses and coordinating senses to action, potentially changing the speed and timing of developmental movement sequences [Bles et al., 1983; Igarashi et al., 1988].

Clinical Implications

Several approaches have been developed to treat symptoms of vestibular pathology and facilitate CNS compensation for loss of vestibular function.

Many physical and occupational therapists treating children with vestibular dysfunction stimulate the vestibular system with devices such as swings, scooter boards and hammocks [Ayres, 1972; Chee et al., 1978; Sellick and Over, 1980]. This type of generalized vestibular stimulation is directed at improving 'vestibular processing' in order to enhance development globally by improving cognitive, perceptual and motor skills. Generalized vestibular stimulation is not necessarily specific to vestibulo-ocular versus vestibulo-spinal function.

An alternative approach to nonspecific vestibular stimulation involves the use of therapeutic strategies which are specific to symptoms of vestibular system pathology. Symptoms can include vertigo, disruption of gaze stabilization, imbalance, and gait ataxia. However, symptoms and functional problems will be different in each patient, since symptoms vary depending on the underlying vestibular pathology and the degree of CNS compensation. Thus, therapeutic goals and exercises are individualized for each patient [Shumway-Cook and Horak, 1989, 1990; Herdman, 1990].

Specific exercise protocols are used to reduce position and movement provoked vertigo, improve visual-vestibular interactions for stabilizing gaze, and enhance sensory and motor strategies underlying postural control in sitting, standing and walking. In addition, distinct strategies have been developed to enhance use of remaining vestibular inputs versus promote the substitution of remaining senses as needed [Shumway-Cook and Horak, 1990; Herdman, 1990].

How might a more specific rehabilitation approach be applied to children with vestibular dysfunction? Therapeutic interventions in children with vestibular dysfunction need to be specific to underlying pathology and associated symptoms. Some types of vestibular deficits require exercises which *decrease* the systems' sensitivity to inputs, i.e. habituation exercises. Other problems benefit from exercises which enhance the use of remaining vestibular function, or alternatively focus on the development of compensatory strategies involving substituting alternative senses during gaze and postural tasks. For example, in children with partial loss of vestibular function the goal of therapy may be to improve processing within the vestibular system, while children with complete loss of vestibular function may require sensory substitution strategies.

Will therapy directed at specific underlying pathology and resultant problems be more effective than nonspecific stimulation approaches in minimizing the affects of vestibular deficits on gaze and postural functions? This remains an important question for future research.

Summary and Conclusions

This paper has addressed the question does the vestibular system play a critical role during the development of motor proficiency? Research reviewed here suggests the answer is more complicated than a simple yes or no, possibly because the question itself is rather limited. Broadening the focus of questions asked would benefit both researcher and clinician concerned with the relationship between vestibular function and the development of coordinated action.

Alternative broader questions ask: How will changes in vestibular sensitivity alter the emergence of coordinated action at various stages in development? Will vestibular dysfunction affect the development of both gaze-stabilizing functions and postural control similarly? How do children compensate for degraded information from one sense during the course of development? What therapeutic strategies can enhance children's capacity to develop appropriate compensatory strategies? Finally, will the formation of compensatory strategies early in development minimize or prevent delays? Issues related to the interaction between the degree and timing of sensory loss on development, and the effect of therapeutic interventions, are critical questions for future research.

References

Ayres A: Sensory Integration and Learning Disorders. Los Angeles; Western Psychological Services, 1972.
Baloh R: Dizziness, Hearing Loss and Tinnitus: The Essentials of Neuro-otology. Philadelphia; Davis, 1984.

Bles W, deJong J, deWit G: Compensation for labyrinthine defects by use of a tilting room. Acta Otolaryngol (Stockh) 1983;95:576–582.

Bruininks R: Bruininks-Oseretsky Test of Motor Proficiency, Examiner's Manual. Circle Pines, American Guidance Service, 1978.

Chee F, Kreutzberg J, Clark D: Semicircular canal stimulation in cerebral palsied children. Phys Ther 1978;58:1071–1075.

Crowe T, Horak F: Motor proficiency associated with vestibular deficits in children with hearing impairments. Phys Ther 1988;68:1493–1499.

de Quiros J: Diagnosis of vestibular disorders in the learning disabled. J Learn Disabil 1976;9:39–47.

Eviatar L, Eviatar A: Neurovestibular examination of infants and children. Adv Oto-Rhino-Lar 1978;23:169–191.

Fentress JC: Developmental roots of behavioral order: systemic approaches to the examination of core developmental issues; in Thelan E, Gunnar J (eds): Systems and Development: The Minnesota Symposium in Child Psychology, vol 22, Hillsdale, Erlbaum, 1989, pp 35–76.

Harris N: Duration and quality of the prone extension position in four-, six-, and eight-year old normal children. Am J Occup Ther 1981;35:26–31.

Herdman S: Assessment and treatment of balance disorders in the vestibular-deficient patient; in Duncan P. (ed): Balance: Proceedings of the APTA Forum. Alexandria, ATPA, 1990.

Horak F, Shumway-Cook A, Crowe T, Black FO: Vestibular function and motor proficiency of children with impaired hearing, or with learning disability and motor impairments. Dev Med Child Neurol 1988;30:64–79.

Igarashi M, Ishikawa M, Yamane H: Physical exercise and balance compensation after total ablation of vestibular organs. Prog Brain Res 1988;76:395.

Kaga K, Suzuki J, Marsh R, Tanaka Y: Influence of labyrinthine hypoactivity on gross motor development of infants; in Cohen B (ed): Vestibular and Oculomotor Physiology. New York, Annals New York Academy of Science, 1981.

Kamm K, Thelen E, Jensen J: A Dynamical systems approach to motor development; in Rothstein J (ed): Movement Science. Alexandria, APTA, 1991.

Kantner R, Clark D, Allen L, Chase M: Effects of vestibular stimulation in nystagmus response and motor performance of the developmentally delayed infant. Phys Ther 1976;59:414–421.

Lacour M, Xerri C: Vestibular compensation: New perspectives; in Flohr H, Precht W (eds): Lesion Induced Neuronal Plasticity in Sensorimotor Systems. New York, Springer, 1981.

Monnier I, Belin I, Pole P: Facilitation, inhibition and habituation of the vestibular response. Adv Otorhinolaryngol 1970;17:28–55.

Montgomery P: Assessment of vestibular function in children. Phys Occup Ther Pediatr 1985;2:33–55.

Nashner LM: Strategies for organization of human posture; in Igarashi M, Black FO (eds): Vestibular and Visual Control of Postural and Locomotion Equilibrium. Basel, Karger, 1985.

Ornitz E: Normal and pathological maturation of vestibular function in the Human Child; in Romand R (ed): Development of Auditory and Vestibular Systems. New York, Academic Press, 1983.

Ottenbacher K: Patterns of post-rotary nystagmus in three learning-disabled children. Am J Occup Ther 1982;36:657–663.

Pfaltz C, Kamath R: Central compensation of vestibular dysfunction: Peripheral lesions. Adv Otorhinolaryngol 1983;30:335–440.

Pignataro O, Rossi L, Gaini R, Oldini C, Sambataro F, Nino L: The evolution of the vestibular apparatus according to the age of the infant. Int J Pediatr Otorhinolaryngol 1979;1:165–170.

Raphin I: Hypoactive labyrinthins and motor development. Clin Pediatr 1974;13:922–937.

Sellick KJ, Over R: Effects of vestibular stimulation on motor development of cerebral palsied children. Dev Med Child Neurol 1980;22:476–483.

Shumway-Cook A: Equilibrium deficits in children; in Woollacott M, Shumway-Cook A (eds): Posture and Gait Across the Lifespan. Columbia, University of South Carolina Press, 1989.

Shumway-Cook A, Horak F: Vestibular rehabilitation: An exercise approach to managing symptoms of vestibular dysfunction. Semin Hearing 1989;10:196–235.

Shumway-Cook A, Horak F: Rehabilitation strategies for patients with vestibular deficits. Neurol Clin 1990;8:441–457.

Shumway-Cook A, Horak F, Black F: Contribution of the vestibulo-spinal system to development of postural coordination. Soc Neurosci Abstr 1986;12:1301.

Shumway-Cook A, Horak F, Black F: A critical examination of vestibular function in motor-impaired learning-disabled children. Int J Pediatr Otorhinolar 1987;14:21–30.

Shumway-Cook A, Woollacott M: The growth of stability: postural control from a developmental perspective. J Motor Behav 1985;17:131–147.

Thelen E, Ulrich JB, Jensen J: The developmental origins of locomotion; in Woollacott M, Shumway-Cook A (eds): Posture and Gait Across the Lifespan. Columbia, University of South Carolina Press, 1989.

Anne Shumway-Cook, PhD, PT, Department of Physical Therapy, Northwest Hospital, Seattle, WA (USA)

Forssberg H, Hirschfeld H (eds): Movement Disorders in Children.
Med Sport Sci. Basel, Karger, 1992, vol 36, pp 217–224

Spasticity Control in the Therapy of Cerebral Palsy[1]

Carol L. Richards, Francine Malouin

Physiotherapy Department, Faculty of Medicine, Laval University, and Neurobiology
Research Centre, Hôpital de l'Enfant-Jésus, Quebec City, Que., Canada

Introduction

The treatment of children with spastic cerebral palsy (SCP) has been
driven by the belief that spasticity is the root of the movement problem.
The premise has been that better control of spasticity should lead to the
expression of improved voluntary control. The combination of this belief
with the hierarchical model of motor control that has dominated the
approach to therapy further emphasized the role of abnormal or primitive
reflexes as the key to the movement disorder. There is a paucity of research
pertaining to the genesis and treatment of spasticity in SCP and furthermore much of the available research on treatment efficacy is fraught with
methodological concerns that limit the applicability of the findings [1]. It is
now generally accepted that spasticity should be considered as a component of the upper motor neuron syndrome (UMS) in SCP that also
includes to varying degrees, the diminished capacity to activate muscles to
produce voluntary movements (paresis), abnormal coactivation of antagonists and spasms. Moreover, because the UMS in SCP is the result of the
interaction of a brain injury on a maturing nervous system subjected to
deficient learning conditions, the UMS is not identical to that observed
after injury to the adult CNS and results of studies in patients with
spasticity onset as adults are not directly transferable to SCP. The purpose
of this paper is, first, to briefly review what is known about the role of
spasticity in the UMS specific to CP, and secondly, to propose physical
therapy treatment strategies based on current neuroscience principles using
locomotion as an example.

[1] This work was supported by grants from the Canadian National Health Research and
Development Program.

Is the Emphasis on Spasticity Control Justified?

When clinicians describe the hypertonia of SCP they usually include spasticity with other manifestations of increased tone such as spasms, abnormal movements and muscle hypoextensibility [4–6]. The most widely practiced therapy for SCP remains, despite the lack of conclusive evidence for its efficacy, the neurodevelopmental approach [5]. The rationale for this approach is that more normal movement patterns should emerge if the spasticity that is believed to inhibit these movements can be controlled and is largely based on a reflex or hierarchical theory of motor control [6]. Limited success with this approach, particularly in severely disabled cases, has led to the use of pharmacological agents and to the development of various surgical procedures to correct the muscle imbalances (lengthenings, tenotomies, nerve blocks), or to interrupt the neural pathways thought to be involved (dorsal rhizotomies).

This spasticity dominated approach to therapy has come under criticism for several reasons including: poor documentation of its efficacy and its archaic theoretical base incompatible with current neurophysiological concepts. A key question is how spasticity relates to voluntary motor control. Dorsal rhizotomies for spasticity control provide a rare opportunity to examine the interaction between spasticity and voluntary control. In some cases the reduction of spasticity after rhizotomy has unveiled a profound underlying muscle weakness [7] while in others, suppression of clonic beats in the muscle activations during gait revealed the pathological timing of the activations [8]. This muscle weakness, that can apparently be reduced with training over time after surgery, has been attributed to inadequate activation of muscles [9] although the role of postsurgical suppression remains to be elucidated. The apparent trainability of underlying weak muscles when spasticity is reduced also remains to be confirmed in long-term studies [7]. Other evidence points to abnormal coactivation of antagonists as a key factor in the motor disorder. Indeed, recent studies using transcranial magnetic stimulation suggest faulty corticospinal connections [10] while H reflex studies have demonstrated impairments in reciprocal inhibition both prior to and during voluntary movement [11] in SCP that could contribute to the coactivation of antagonists. The possible contribution of active restraint caused by hyperactive stretch reflexes in the antagonist enhanced by mechanisms involved in the voluntary contraction of agonists [12–14] could also be involved in the muscle coactivations observed during gait [4, 15, 16] and voluntary movements [13, 14]. The interrelationship, if any, between the reciprocal excitation [18, 20] and reflex overflow [20] described in SCP at rest with the coactivation observed during voluntary contractions remains to be clarified.

Evaluations of the effects of antispastic therapies have been fraught by methodological concerns including the difficulty of setting up randomized controlled clinical trials with a sufficient number of subjects and the choice of pertinent outcome measures [1]. Moreover, when evaluating the effect of a therapy on spasticity, it is not enough to measure spasticity at rest because spastic reflexes may be enhanced during functional movements [12, 21]. For example, we [19] found that a single 30-min session of prolonged stretch of the triceps surae (TS) by standing on a tilt table significantly reduces (for up to 35 min) reflex activation in the TS at rest and improves the capacity to activate the TS during static contractions (fig. 1) but did not change the activation profile of the TS during walking [16]. An improved activation pattern during walking may require a more intense task-specific stretching paradigm of the TS that allows for gait training while the muscle is being stretched. We are currently attempting to determine the effects of such long-term stretch imposed by an ankle-foot-orthosis during task-specific training in a group of SCP infants within the context of a modified time series design.

In conclusion, spasticity is viewed as but one of the manifestations of the lesion in CP that contributes to the total UMS. The relationship between hyperactive stretch reflexes evaluated at rest and functional behavior remains to be deciphered. It cannot be taken for granted, however, that spasticity always masks good voluntary control. Given the heterogeneity of the lesions in SCP, the most logical approach is to assume that mechanisms such as hyperactive stretch reflexes, weakness of agonists and excessive coactivation of antagonists may contribute in varying degrees to the disturbed motor control [8, 12, 21] in the individual patient. Consequently, determination of the key factor by quantitative methods is crucial to the choice of therapy [21].

Disturbed Motor Control in Spastic Cerebral Palsy and Physical Therapy Strategies

Research in the neurosciences over the last 20 years has identified both central nervous system and behavioral changes following CNS injury. The role of processes such as neural shock resolution, denervation hypersensitivity, sprouting and unmasking, support the hypothesis that the CNS is a dynamic system capable of reorganization [22]. The current thinking is that recovery of function can be best promoted by a therapy that begins early after injury, is sufficiently intense, is task-specific, provides an enriched environment and is motivational [22, 23]. The reflex or hierarchical motor control theories have been largely replaced by a more interactive systems

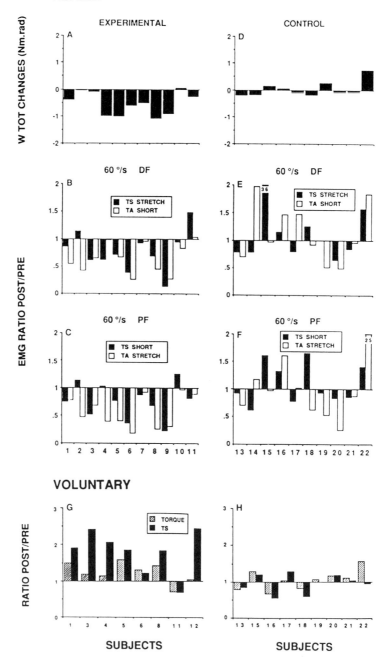

approach [6] which removes the emphasis on one aspect of the motor disorder such as spasticity. As an example, strategies for the training of locomotion in SCP will be proposed.

Physical therapy promoting appropriate skill acquisition should be started in the very young infant when the developing neuromuscular system is still very plastic. The reflex stepping at birth that usually disappears within the first months, possibly in part as proposed by Thelen et al. [24] because of insufficient strength to produce the movements as the infant gains weight, can apparently be retained with training [25]; moreover, specific exercises for 5-month-old infants can lead to increased response rates of stepping and placing and longer standing times [26]. These results suggest that it is possible to use reflex and postural responses very early as a precocious method of locomotor training. In practice, supporting an infant over a treadmill [24] while providing weight and balance support will promote stepping. It can also be postulated that by decreasing the biomechanical and equilibrium demands, the high degree of leg muscle coactivation seen in infant stepping [17, 27], unsupported early normal walkers [27, 28] and SCP [4, 15–17] will be reduced to allow the emergence of a more normal reciprocal pattern. The much improved reciprocal activation of the TS and tibialis anterior activation profiles observed when a 4-year-old diplegic child walked with the support of a walker [30] confirms this postulate. Such treadmill training in SCP infants would provide them with the missing or delayed locomotor practice and experience needed to guide the neuromotor development. Furthermore, it is possible that enriched locomotor experience could promote neural changes to limit the expression of the motor disorder. In light of these considerations we propose a task-specific locomotor training strategy that is interactive with appropriate weight and equilibrium support combined with manual and verbal assistance from a therapist to guide the foot and leg movements. Such a program could be carried out on a treadmill capable of very slow speeds with a weight and equilibrium support system [31]. This task-specific

---

Fig. 1. Comparison of the individual changes in neuromuscular responses to passive movements at 60°/s (A–F) and the muscle activation and torque produced during voluntary static contractions (G and H) in an experimental and a control group of children with spastic cerebral palsy. Bars in A and D represent differences between pre- and post-test values for the total energy (Wtot). Bars in B, C, E and F represent the concomitant changes in EMG, calculated as post/pre ratios of EMG responses in the triceps surae (TS: dark columns) and tibialis anterior (TA: open columns) during passive dorsiflexion (DF) and plantar flexion (PF) and bars in G and H the torque (stripped) and TS activation (dark) calculated as post:pre ratios, respectively. Modified from Tremblay et al. [19] with permission.

training must be sufficiently intense and started early enough to encourage the development of new patterns of locomotor control. The feasibility and preliminary findings on efficacy of such a training strategy are presently under study within the context of a pilot randomized clinical trial.

As the infants get older and can participate more consciously to the therapy, other strategies can be used to encourage the learning task. Results from biofeedback studies suggest the potential of electromyographic or position feedback to reduce reflex activity [3] and abnormal movements [3, 32, 33]. For example, we have observed that verbal cues while treadmill walking can result in a dramatic 'normalization' of both movement and muscle activation profiles in a 5-year-old diplegic child [unpubl. results]. The challenge for therapy is to find ways to help the child integrate this capacity into spontaneous locomotor movements. The use of biofeedback may prove to be particularly effective when abnormal coactivation of antagonists is the dominant abnormality.

Conclusion

It is imperative to develop therapeutic strategies based on current scientific concepts of development and recovery of sensorimotor function and motor learning. The efficacy of these strategies and intensity and precocity of therapy onset must then be tested in appropriate clinical trials with pertinent outcome measures. To date, physical therapy has mainly been directed to the modulation of disability. New strategies should also attempt to modulate the impairment in the very young infant or be specifically adapted to complement surgical or pharmacological interventions.

References

1   Campbell SK: Efficacy of physical therapy in improving postural control in cerebral palsy. Pediatr Phys Ther 1990;2:135–140.
2   Katz RT, Rymer WZ: Spastic hypertonia: Mechanisms and measurements. Arch Phys Med Rehabil 1989;70:144–155.
3   Neilson PD, McCaughey J: Self-regulation of spasm and spasticity in cerebral palsy. J Neurol Neurosurg Psychiatry 1982;45:320–330.
4   Berger W, Quintern J, Dietz V: Pathophysiology of gait in children with cerebral palsy. EEG Clin Neurophysiol 1982;53:538–548.
5   Bobath B: Motor development, its effect on general development, and application to the treatment of cerebral palsy. Physiotherapy 1971;57:526–532.
6   Horak F: Assumptions underlying motor control for neurological rehabilitation; in Contemporary Management of Motor Control. Proceedings of the II STEP Conf. Alexandria, Foundation for Physical Therapy, 1991, pp 11–27.

7   Giuliani CA: Dorsal rhizotomy for children with cerebral palsy: Support for concepts of motor control. Phys Ther 1991;71:248–259.

8   Cahan LD, Adams JM, Perry J, Becker LM: Instrumental gait analysis after selective dorsal rhizotomy. Dev Med Child Neurol 1990;32:1037–1043.

9   Sahrmann SA, Norton BJ: Relationship of voluntary movement to spasticity in the upper motor neuron syndrome. Ann Neurol 1977;2:460–465.

10   Brouwer B, Ashby P: Do injuries to the developing human brain alter corticospinal projections? Neurosci Lett 1990;108:225–230.

11   Leonard CT, Moritani T, Hirschfeld H, Forssberg H: Deficits in reciprocal inhibition of children with cerebral palsy as revealed by H reflex testing. Dev Med Child Neurol 1990;32:974–984.

12   Knutsson E: Analysis of spastic paresis. Proc Xth World Congr Physical Therapy, Sydney, 1987, pp 626–633.

13   Corcos DM, Gottlieb GL, Penn RD, Myklebust B, Agarwal GC: Movement deficits caused by hyperexcitable stretch reflexes in spastic humans. Brain 1986;109:1043–1058.

14   Milner-Brown HS, Penn R: Pathophysiological mechanisms in cerebral palsy. J Neurol Neurosurg Psychiatry 1979;42:606–618.

15   Knutsson E: Muscle activation patterns of gait in spastic hemiparesis, paraparesis and cerebral palsy. Scand J Rehabil Med 1980;Suppl 7:47–52.

16   Richards CL, Malouin F, Dumas F: Effects of a single session of prolonged plantarflexor stretch on muscle activations during gait. Scand J Rehabil Med 1991;23:103–111.

17   Leonard CT, Hirschfeld H, Forssberg H: Gait acquisition and reflex abnormalities in normal children and children with cerebral palsy; in Amblard B, Berthoz A, Clarac F (eds): Posture and Gait: Development, Adaptation and Modulation. Amsterdam, Elsevier Press, 1988, pp 33–45.

18   Myklebust BM, Gottlieb GL, Penn RD, Agarwal GC: Reciprocal excitation of antagonistic muscles as a differentiating feature of spasticity. Ann Neurol 1982;12:367–374.

19   Tremblay F, Malouin F, Richards CL, Dumas F: Effects of prolonged muscle stretch on reflex and voluntary muscle activations in children with spastic cerebral palsy. Scand J Rehabil Med 1990;22:171–180.

20   Leonard CT, Hirschfeld H, Moritani T, Forssberg H: Myotatic reflex development in normal children and children with cerebral palsy. Exp Neurol 1991;111:379–382.

21   Knutsson E, Richards C: Different types of disturbed motor control in gait of hemiparetic patients. Brain 1979;102:405–430.

22   Bach-y-Rita P: Brain plasticity as a basis for therapeutic procedures; in Bach-y-Rita P (ed): Recovery of Function: Theoretical Considerations for Brain Injury Rehabilitation. Baltimore, University Park Press, 1980, pp 225–263.

23   Carr JH, Shepherd RB: A Motor Relearning Program for Stroke. Rockville, Aspen, 1987.

24   Thelen E, Ulrich BD, Jensen JL: The developmental origins of locomotion; in Woollacott MH, Shumway-Cook A (eds): Development of Posture and Gait Across the Lifespan. Columbia, University of South Carolina Press, 1989, pp 25–47.

25   Zelazo PR, Zelazo NA, Kolb S: 'Walking' in the newborn. Science 1972;177:1058–1059.

26   Leonard E, Zelazo P: Facilitating bipedal locomotion in high risk infants. Phys Ther 1988;68:839.

27   Forssberg H: Ontogeny of human locomotor control. I. Infant stepping, supported locomotion and transition to independent locomotion. Exp Brain Res 1985;57:480–493.

28   Kazai N, Okamoto T, Kumamoto M: Electromyographic study of supported walking of infants in the initial period of learning to walk; in Komi PV (ed): Biomechanics V-A. Champaign, University Park Press, 1976, pp 311–318.

29 Okamomo T, Kumamoto M: Electromyographic study of the learning process of walking in infants. Electromography 1972;12:149–159.
30 Richards CL, Malouin F, Dumas F, Wood-Dauphinee S: New rehabilitation strategies for the treatment of spastic gait disorders; in Patla A (ed): Adaptability of Human Gait: Implications for the Control of Locomotion. Amsterdam, Elsevier, 1991, pp 387–411.
31 Visintin M, Barbeau H: The effects of body weight support on the locomotor pattern of spastic paraparetic patients. Can J Neurol Sci 1989;16:315–325.
32 Malouin F, Trahan J, Parrot A, Gemmel M: Comparison of two strategies of biofeedback withdrawal in head position training in cerebral palsy children. Physiother Can 1986;38:337–342.
33 Malouin F: Application of a new method for the evaluation of therapy in patients with abnormal head posture and movement control. Proc Xth World Congr Physical Therapy, Sydney, 1987, pp 842–846.

Carol L. Richards, PhD, PT, Department of Physiotherapy, Laval University,
Neurobiology Research Centre, Hôpital de l'Enfant-Jésus, 1401-18e rue,
Quebec City, PQ G1J 1Z4 (Canada)

Forssberg H, Hirschfeld H (eds): Movement Disorders in Children.
Med Sport Sci. Basel, Karger, 1992, vol 36, pp 225–233

Spasticity: Exaggerated Reflexes or Movement Disorder?

V. Dietz

Department of Clinical Neurology and Neurophysiology,
University of Freiburg, FRG

Spasticity produces numerous physical signs. These have little relationship to the patient's disability which is due to impairment by a movement disorder. On the basis of the clinical signs a widely accepted conclusion was drawn for the pathophysiology and treatment of spasticity: exaggerated reflexes are responsible for muscle hypertonia, and, consequently, the movement disorder. Drug therapy, therefore, is usually directed to reduce the activity of stretch reflexes. The function of these reflexes during natural movements and the connection between exaggerated reflexes and movement disorder is frequently not considered.

Clinical observations have already given rise to doubts about such a direct relationship: (1) following an acute stroke, tendon reflexes can be exaggerated early, while spastic muscle tone develops over weeks; (2) in healthy subjects a connection between the excitability of reflexes and motor performance is not known. *Electrophysiological* investigations of natural movements have not revealed any causal relationship between exaggerated reflexes and movement disorder. The neurophysiological background of spasticity arising from these studies and their therapeutic consequences will now be considered.

Pathophysiology

The neuronal regulation of functional movements, such as gait, is achieved by a complex interaction of spinal and supraspinal mechanisms: the rhythmic activation of leg muscles by spinal interneuronal circuits is modulated and adapted to the actual needs by a multisensory afferent input. The *spinal programming* as well as the *reflex activity* are under *supraspinal* control. Disturbances of this supraspinal control lead to characteristic gait impairments seen in cerebellar and extrapyramidal disorders as well as in spastic paresis [1]. The electrical leg muscle activity which results from a close interaction between these different mechanisms, is transferred to a functionally modulated muscle tension by the *mechanical muscle fibre properties* [2].

Central Programming

Clinical signs of spasticity, especially disorders of muscle tone, are more pronounced during active movements than under a relaxed condition. Therefore, investigations of the modulation and coordination of leg muscle activity during gait can provide more insight into the pathophysiological mechanisms underlying spastic movement disorder. Several findings suggest that the central programming in spastic patients is basically preserved. Gait analysis shows that neither the timing nor the reciprocal mode of activation of the antagonistic leg muscles differs between healthy subjects and patients with severe spasticity [3].

A similar observation concerns the compensatory leg muscle activation following feet displacement during stance [4]: the timing of the triphasic pattern, which is assumed to be centrally programmed [5], is preserved in patients with spastic paresis. These findings are in accordance both with earlier [6, 7] and more recent investigations [8] of various functional movements in patients with spasticity.

In *conclusion*, the reciprocal mode of leg muscle activation during gait as well as the triphasic activity pattern underlying the compensation of feet displacement is preserved in spasticity. This indicates an intact central programming.

Proprioceptive Reflexes

Exaggerated reflexes are frequently thought to be responsible for the spastic movement disorder, without considering the functional significance of the different reflex mechanisms involved in the regulation of complex movements. The analysis of the compensatory responses following feet displacement during stance in patients with spastic hemiparesis due to a cerebral lesion gives us more information about the behavior of mono- and polysynaptic reflexes during functional movements [4, 9, 10]: in the gastrocnemius of the unaffected leg, a small monosynaptic reflex potential is followed by a strong polysynaptic EMG response; in the spastic leg, the monosynaptic reflex potential is larger, the functionally essential polysynaptic reflex response, however, is absent. Reduction or absence of the compensatory polysynaptic reflex response has also been described for the tibialis anterior [11] and the forearm muscles [12] in patients with spasticity of spinal and cerebral origin. In all these investigations the overall activity of the spastic muscle is reduced compared to the healthy muscle, despite exaggerated monosynaptic reflexes. The duration of symptoms has little influence on this behavior [13].

In patients with predominant spasticity and little paresis, due to a chronic spinal lesion, the activity in the calf muscles during gait is slightly reduced in amplitude and less modulated compared to the healthy subject. This observation is most probably due to the impaired function of the reflexes. Corresponding to the loss of EMG modulation during gait, a fast regulation of motoneuron discharge, which characterizes the normal muscle, is absent in spasticity [13, 14]. In patients with spastic hemiparesis due to a cerebral lesion, the strength of EMG activity on the affected leg is reduced compared to the unaffected one, corresponding to the degree of paresis [9, 15].

The exaggeration of tendon reflexes in spasticity is probably due to a reduced presynaptic inhibition of group Ia afferent [16–18]. No evidence exists for (1) enhanced gamma-motoneuron activity and, consequently, increased input from group Ia afferent [19, 20]; (2) a reduced Renshaw-cell inhibition [21], or (3) a 'sprouting' of Ia fibers at the motoneuron [22] as possible sources of an increased activity of motoneuron in spasticity.

A lack of both, inhibition of monosynaptic and facilitation of polysynaptic spinal reflexes, is also described for small healthy children [23, 24]. Inhibition and facilitation of spinal reflexes obviously depend on the control of supraspinal motor centers, which is impaired in spasticity and has yet to mature in small children.

In *conclusion*, exaggerated stretch reflexes in spasticity are associated with an absence or reduction of the functionally essential polysynaptic reflexes. When supraspinal control of spinal reflexes is impaired (spasticity) or immature (small children) the inhibition of monosynaptic reflexes is missing in combination with a reduced facilitation of polysynaptic reflexes.

Reflex Effects and Muscle Tone

In patients with spastic hemiparesis a basically different tension development of triceps surae takes place during the stance phase of gait [9, 15]: in the unaffected leg, the tension development correlates with the modulation of EMG activity (the same is true in healthy subjects), while in the spastic leg, tension development is connected to the stretching period of the tonically activated (with small EMG amplitude) muscle. There is no visible influence of monosynaptic reflex potential on muscle tension. A similar discrepancy between the resistance to stretch and the level of EMG activity is described for upper limb muscles of spastic patients [25–27]. It should be noted, however, that the tension development during the relatively slow functional movements of the patients has little relationship to the muscle stiffness felt by a clinical examiner during fast passive limb movements.

Investigations of functional movements in spastic patients have led to the conclusion that spastic muscle tone can hardly be explained by an increased activity of motoneuron. Instead, a transformation of motor units occurs, with the consequence that regulation of muscle tension takes place on a lower level of neuronal organization. Such a transformation of motor units is functionally meaningful, as it enables the patient to support the body weight during gait; fast active movements, however, become impossible. The time interval of several weeks between the occurrence of an acute stroke and the development of spastic muscle tone is needed for such a muscle transformation [13]. It is misleading to uncritically apply animal findings in pathophysiological and therapeutic considerations, as there are basic differences in the development of muscle tone: an acute rigor appears in the decerebrate cat, while in patients with an acute supraspinal lesion connected with paresis muscle tone develops slowly over a period of weeks.

There are additional findings which support the suggestion that changes in the mechanical muscle fibre properties occur in spasticity: (1) contraction times in hand muscles [28] as well as in the triceps surae [11] are prolonged; (2) torque motor experiments applied to the triceps surae indicate a peripheral contribution to spastic muscle tone [29]; (3) histochemistry and morphometry of spastic muscle reveal specific changes of muscle fibres [13, 30].

In *conclusion*, tension development during gait does not depend on exaggerated monosynaptic stretch reflexes. The overall leg muscle activity is reduced in patients with spasticity of spinal and cerebral origin. According to electrophysiological and histological findings, a transformation of motor units takes place following a supraspinal lesion with the consequence that regulation of muscle tone is achieved on a lower level of neuronal organization which enables the patients to walk.

Therapeutic Consequences

The alteration to a simpler regulation of muscle tension following paresis due to a supraspinal lesion is basically *advantageous* for a patient; it enables him to support the body during gait and, consequently, to achieve mobility. Rapid movements are, however, no longer possible due to the missing modulation of muscle activity. In an immobilized patient following severe spinal or supraspinal lesions, these transformation processes can overshoot, with unwelcome sequelae. The therapeutic consequences of the pathophysiological aspects of spastic movement disorder will be discussed in the next section.

Drug Therapy

The aim of antispastic therapy is to reduce spastic muscle tone without affecting the voluntary force [31]. Antispastic therapy is believed to reduce the excitability of spinal reflexes and, consecutively, to ameliorate spastic symptoms. Different sites of action are attributed to the various drugs: (1) increased presynaptic inhibition of group I afferents, i.e. reduction of monosynaptic reflex activity (baclofen, diazepam); (2) inhibition of excitatory interneurons, which are interconnected in spinal reflex pathways (tizanidine, glycine); (3) reduced susceptibility of peripheral receptors (dantrolene, phenotiazine) and reduced muscle contraction amplitude (dentrolene).

An effect of antispastic drugs listed under the first two points can hardly be expected considering the behavior of mono- and polysynaptic reflexes during spastic gait. Clinical studies have shown, indeed, that the activity of stretch reflexes become reduced, but that this effect is not connected with a significant improvement of functional movements (tizanidine [32]; diazepam [33]; baclofen [34]). These findings correspond to the experimental observation that abolishing hyperactive stretch reflexes of patients with spasticity does not result in an improvement of motor function [35, 36]. With higher doses of these drugs, an improvement of spastic symptoms (such as muscle spasms and clonus) may be observed. These changes are, however, usually connected with a disabling paresis during movement performance (baclofen, tizanidine [37–39]). According to electrophysiological studies of spastic gait under antispastic medication [unpubl. observation] this effect is due to the reduction, not only of monosynaptic reflexes, but also of the tonic EMG activity in the leg extensor muscles during the stance phase. Because the latter activity is necessary to maintain muscle tone which supports body weight during gait, its reduction results in the development of paresis.

Similar considerations also apply to the peripherally acting drug, dantrolene. Because there is, without the drug, no difference in contraction amplitudes between spastic and healthy muscles [11, 28], a drug influence on contraction amplitude means muscle paresis. This corresponds to the clinical experience [40]: an effective treatment of muscle tone usually leads to the appearance of paresis which hampers active physiotherapy. This, together with the side effects of these drugs, frequently leads to a short-term limitation of drug therapy [41].

Beyond the pathophysiological arguments, these observations and consequences are not so surprising, given the testing conditions applied for antispastic drugs: (1) Effects of the antispastic drugs are usually not tested during functional movements with recording of biochemical and electrophysiological parameters. (2) Dependent on the condition, drug effects are observed not only on mono- and polysynaptic reflexes but also on other neuronal mechanisms (for example on Renshaw cell or fusimotor activity). The interaction of these effects on motor function can hardly be controlled (baclofen and diazepam) [42, 43]. (3) Differential drug effects have been described for the decerebrate and the spinalized cat (tizanidine) [44].

The therapeutic consequence of the arguments established above for a cautious application of antispastic drugs concerns primarily *mobile* patients, as they require spastic muscle tone for compensation and physiotherapy should predominantly treat them to improve movement performance. This conclusion is, however, not valid for *immobilized* patients. In these cases increasing paresis must not be disadvantageous, but can even be helpful for the application of physiotherapy and for the improvement of symptoms such as painful spasms and clonus. In these patients with severe diplegia, oral antispastic drugs are usually not well tolerated in the long term and their effect is unsatisfactory. It has been shown in recent years that the intrathecal application of baclofen can efficiently reduce the painful symptoms with tolerable side effects [31, 45, 46]. The latter authors followed the application of baclofen by implanted pump systems over 2 years and did not observe a loss of efficiency.

In *conclusion*, according to clinical and electrophysiological investigations, the therapy of spastic symptoms by presently available antispastic drugs makes no sense in mobile patients: (1) a diminution of exaggerated reflexes is not followed by an improvement in movement performance; (2) a drug-induced reduction of muscle tone is connected with the development of paresis. In immobile patients antispastic drugs might be of some value by diminishing painful sequelae of spasticity.

Physiotherapy

According to the neurophysiological background, physiotherapy should represent the most conclusive mode of treatment for mobile as well as immobilized patients although this suggestion is not based on hard data. Both active and passive manipulative forms of physiotherapeutic treatment are of great importance for both groups of patients. On the one hand, residual motor functions have to be mobilized and trained. On the other hand, contractures of muscle and joints, which can hardly be treated when already established, must be prevented at an early stage. Physiotherapy within a water-filled pool seems to be promising, as recent immersion experiments revealed profound effects on postural reflexes [47]. Specially built motor-driven bicycles provide an active and passive training which can be performed at home. It seems less important which mode of physiotherapy is applied to the patients. A superiority of one specific physiotherapeutic method or 'school' over another has never been demonstrated. In addition, although some of physiotherapy 'schools' claim a neurophysiological background, their physiotherapeutic techniques are usually restricted to influence inhibition or facilitation of reflexes and do not take into account more recent concepts of motor physiology. It is most reasonable to apply a pragmatic approach, tailoring the physiotherapeutic program to needs of an individual patient, in order to achieve a maximum improvement for the activities of daily living.

In *conclusion*, at present a pragmatic form of physiotherapy represents the best approach for an adequate treatment of spasticity.

References

1   Dietz V: Human neuronal control of functional movements. Interaction between central programs and afferent input. Physiol Rev 1992;72 in press.
2   Gollhofer A, Schmidtbleicher D, Dietz V: Regulation of muscle stiffness in human locomotion. Int J Sport Med 1984;5:19–22.
3   Dietz V, Quintern J, Berger W: Electrophysiological studies of gait in spasticity and rigidity. Evidence that altered mechanical properties of muscle contribute to hypertonia. Brain 1981;104:431–449.
4   Berger W, Horstmann GA, Dietz V: Spastic paresis: impaired spinal reflexes and intact motor programs. J Neurol Neurosurg Psychiatry 1988;51:568–571.
5   Dietz V, Quintern J, Sillem M: Stumbling reactions in man: Significance of proprioceptive and pre-programmed mechanisms. J Physiol (Lond) 1987;386:149–163.
6   Altenburger H: Eletrodiagnostik; in Bumke O, Förster O (eds): Handbuch der Neurologie, Algemeine Neurologie III. Berlin, Springer, 1973, pp 968–1019.
7   Wacholder K, Altenburger H: Beiträge zur Physiologie der willkurlichen Bewegung, X Mitteilung, Einzelbewegungen. Pflügers Arch Physiol 1926;214:642–661.
8   Knutsson E, Richards C: Different types of disturbed motor control in gait of hemiparetic patients. Brain 1979;102:405–430.
9   Berger W, Horstmann GA, Dietz V: Tension development and muscle activation in the leg during gait in spastic hemiparesis: The independence of muscle hypertonia and exaggerated stretch reflexes. J Neurol Neurosurg Psychiatry 1984;47:1029–1033.
10   Nashner LM, Shumway-Cook A, Martin O: Stance posture controls in select groups of children with cerebral palsy: Deficits in sensory organization and muscular coordination. Exp Brain Res 1983;49:393–409.
11   Dietz V, Berger W: Interlimb coordination of posture in patients with spastic paresis. Impaired function of spinal reflexes. Brain 1984;107:965–978.
12   Cody FWJ, Richardson HC, MacDermott N, Ferguson IT: Stretch and vibration reflexes of wrist flexor muscles in spasticity. Brain 1987;110:433–450.
13   Dietz V, Ketelsen UP, Berger W, Quintern J: Motor units involvement in spastic paresis: Relationship between leg muscle activation and histochemistry. J Neurol Sci 1986;75:89–103.

14   Rosenfalck A, Andreassen S: Impaired regulation of force and firing pattern of single
      motor units in patients with spasticity. J Neurol Neurosurg Psychiatry 1980;43:907–
      916.

15   Dietz V, Berger W: Normal and impaired regulation of muscle stiffness in gait: A new
      hypothesis about muscle hypertonia. Exp Neurol 1983;79:680–687.

16   Burke D, Ashby P: Are spinal 'presynaptic' inhibitory mechanisms suppressed in
      spasticity? J Neurol Sci 1972;15:321–326.

17   Delwaide PJ: Human monosynaptic reflexes and presynaptic inhibition; in Desmedt JE
      (ed): New Developments in Electromyography and Clinical Neurophysiology, vol 3.
      Human Reflexes, Pathophysiology of Motor Systems, Methodology of Human Refl-
      exes. Basel, Karger, 1973, pp 508–522.

18   Iles JF, Roberts RC: Presynaptic inhibition of monosynaptic reflexes in the lower
      limbs of subjects with upper motoneuron disease. J Neurol Neurosurg Psychiatry
      1986;49:937–944.

19   Hagbarth KE, Wallin BG, Löfstedt L: Muscle spinal response to stretch in normal and
      spastic subjects. Scand J Rehabil Med 1973;5:156–159.

20   Vallbo ÅB, Hagbarth KE, Torebjörk HE, Wallin BG: Somatosensory, proprioceptive,
      and sympathetic activity in human peripheral nerves. Physiol Rev 1979;59:919–957.

21   Katz R, Pierrot-Deseilligny E: Recurrent inhibition of alpha-motoneurons in patients
      with upper motor lesions. Brain 1982;105:103–124.

22   Ashby P: Discussion; Emre M, Benecke R (eds): Spasticity. The Current Status of
      Research and Treatment. Carnforth, Parthenon, 1989, pp 68–69.

23   Berger W, Altenmueller E, Dietz V: Normal and impaired development of children's
      gait. Hum Neurobiol 1984;3:163–170.

24   Forssberg H: Ontogeny of human locomotor control. I. Infant stepping, supported
      locomotion and transition to independent locomotion. Exp Brain Res 1985;57:480–
      493.

25   Lee WA, Boughton A, Rymer WZ: Absence of stretch reflex gain enhancement in
      voluntarily activated spastic muscle. Exp Neurol 1987;98:317–335.

26   Powers RK, Campbell DL, Rymer WZ: Stretch reflex dynamics in spastic elbow flexor
      muscles. Ann Neurol 1989;25:32–42.

27   Powers RK, Marder-Meyer J, Rymer WZ: Quantitative relations between hypertonia
      and stretch reflex threshold in spastic hemiparesis. Ann Neurol 1988;23:115–124.

28   Young JL, Mayer RF: Physiological alterations of motor units in hemiplegia. J Neurol
      Sci 1992;54:401–412.

29   Hufschmidt A, Mauritz KH: Chronic transformation of muscle in spasticity: A periph-
      eral contribution to increased tone. J Neurol Neurosurg Psychiatry 1985;48:676–685.

30   Edström L: Selective changes in the size of red and white muscle fibres in upper motor
      lesions and parkinsonism. J Neurol Sci 1970;11:537–550.

31   Latash ML, Penn RD, Carcos DM, Gottlieb GL: Short-term effects of intrathecal
      baclofen in spasticity. Exp Neurol 1989;103:165–172.

32   Lapierre Y, Bouchard S, Tansey C, Gendron D, Barkas WJ, Francis GS: Treatment of
      spasticity with tizanidine in multiple sclerosis. Can J Neurol Sci 1987;14:513–517.

33   Bes A, Eyssette M, Pierrot-Deseilligny E, Rohmer F, Warter JM: A multi-centre,
      double-blind trial of tizanidine, a new antispastic agent, in spasticity associated with
      hemiplegia. Curr Med Res Opin 1988;10:709–718.

34   Corston RN, Johnson F, Godwin-Austen RB: The assessment of drug treatment of
      spastic gait. J Neurol Neurosurg Psychiatry 1981;44:1035–1039.

35   Thach WT, Montgomery EB: Motor systems; in Pearlman AL, Collins RC (eds):
      Neurobiology of Disease. Oxford, Oxford University Press, 1990, pp 168–196.

36 Landau WM: What is it? What is it not? In Feldman RG, Young RR, Loella WP (eds): Spasticity: Disordered Motor Control. Miami, Symposia Specialists, 1980, pp 17–24.
37 Bass B, Weinshenker B, Rice GP, Noseworthy JH, Cameron MG, Hader W, Bouchard S, Ebers GC: Tizanidine versus baclofen in the treatment of spasticity in multiple sclerosis patients. Can J Neurol Sci 1988;15:15–19.
38 Hoogstraten MC, van der Ploeg RJ, van der Burg W, Vreeling A, van Marle S, Minderhoud JM: Tizanidine versus baclofen in the treatment of spasticity in multiple sclerosis patients. Acta Neurol Scand 1988;75:224–230.
39 Stien R, Nodal HJ, Oftedal SI, Slettebo M: The treatment of spasticity in multiple sclerosis: a double-blind clinical trial of a new antispastic drug tizanidine compared with baclofen. Acta Neurol Scand 1987;75:190–194.
40 Meyler WJ, Bakker H, Kok JJ, Agoston S, Wesseling H: The effect of dantrolene sodium in relation to blood levels in spastic patients after prolonged administration. J Neurol Neurosurg Psychiatry 1981;44:334–339.
41 Anderson TP: Rehabilitation of patients with completed stroke; in Kottka FJ, Stilwell GK, Lehmann JF, (eds): Krusen's Handbook of Physical Medicine and Rehabilitation. Philadelphia, Saunders, 1982, pp 583–603.
42 Davidoff RA: Antispasticity drugs: Mechanisms of action. Ann Neurol 1985;17:107–116.
43 Pedersen E: Clinical assessment and pharmacologic therapy of spasticity. Arch Phys Med Rehabil 1974;55:344–356.
44 Chen DF, Blanchetti M, Wiesendanger M: The adrenergic agonist tizanidine has differential effects on flexor reflexes of intact and spinalized rat. Neuroscience 1987;23:641–647.
45 Muller H, Zierski J, Dralle D, Börner U, Hoffmann O: The effect of intrathecal baclofen on electrical muscle activity in spasticity. J Neurol 1987;234:348–352.
46 Ochs G, Struppler A, Meyerson BA, Linderoth B, Gybels J, Gardner BP, Teddy P, Jamous A, Weinmann P: Intrathecal baclofen for long-term treatment of spasticity: A multicentre study. J Neurol Neurosurg Psychiatry 1989;52:933–939.
47 Dietz V, Horstmann GA, Trippel M, Gollhofer A: Human postural reflexes and gravity. An underwater simulation. Neurosci Lett 1989;106:350–355.

V. Dietz, MD, Department of Clinical Neurology and Neurophysiology, Hansastrasse 9, D-W–7800 Freiburg (FRG)

Forssberg H, Hirschfeld H (eds): Movement Disorders in Children.
Med Sport Sci. Basel, Karger, 1992, vol 36, pp 234–246

New Experimental Approaches in the Treatment of Spastic Gait Disorders

Hugues Barbeau, Joyce Fung

School of Physical and Occupational Therapy, McGill University,
Montreal, Que., Canada

Introduction

Spastic paretic gait is characterized by a spectrum of problems including hyperactive spinal reflexes, altered muscle activation patterns, and the inability to cope with weight bearing, balance and speed during walking. Conventional treatment efforts have focused on normalizing muscle tone by the use of antispastic medication [1], corrective surgery [2] or physical means such as passive stretching [3] and orthotic devices [4]. While abnormal muscle tone may be corrected in the static or resting position, the response very often cannot be carried over to a dynamic situation such as locomotion. Even in gait rehabilitation, the traditional approach is to progress from standing to walking while correcting individual problems, rather than retraining all the dynamic components simultaneously in a task-specific manner. Despite an intensive rehabilitation regime, many individuals with a central nervous system lesion have persistent gait deviations.

Thus, the purpose of this paper is to propose new rehabilitation approaches to improve locomotion in spastic paretic patients. Preliminary results are presented to show that such new treatment strategies can restore locomotor function in spastic paretic subjects who have previously obtained maximal benefit from conventional therapies. The implications of these new experimental approaches in the treatment of children with spastic gait dysfunction are also discussed.

Results

Normal Gait
The kinematic and EMG pattern during treadmill walking from a representative normal subject is presented to provide a template against

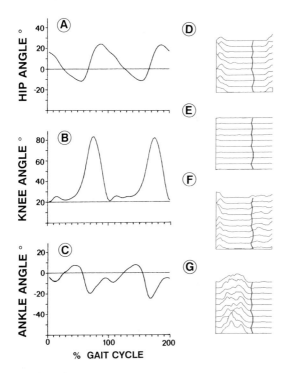

Fig. 1. The kinematic (*A*–*C*) and EMG (*D*–*G*) profiles of a normal subject walking on the treadmill at a comfortable speed of 0.90 m s^{-1}. Illustrated are 2 consecutive cycles of hip (*A*), knee (*B*) and ankle (*C*) angular displacements, normalized to the gait cycle from one foot floor contact (0%) to the next (100%). All angles were calculated with respect to the neutral standing position (0°), with flexion or dorsiflexion taken as upward displacements, and extension or plantarflexion taken as downward displacements. Also shown are 10 consecutive cycles of EMG activity in the MH (*D*), VL (*E*), TA (*F*), and GA (*G*) normalized to 100% of the gait cycle. Solid line across the cycles depicts stance-swing transition.

which the pathological gait profiles and the effects of new experimental approaches are compared. The profiles of hip, knee and ankle sagittal angular excursions for a representative normal subject, during two consecutive step cycles, is shown in figure 1A–C. Briefly, the hip joint (fig. 1A) had its maximum flexion just prior to heel strike, after which it was extended until push-off, when it was flexed to bring the leg forward for the next heel strike. The knee joint (fig. 1B) had two excursions of flexion and extension during one stride. Just after heel strike, the knee was slightly flexed during load acceptance, after which it was held in extension as the contralateral leg moved forward. Then it was flexed prior to, and after toe-off, providing foot-floor clearance early in swing, before the leg was extended forward for the next heel contact. The ankle joint (fig. 1C) had two excursions of flexion and extension displacements in one stride as well. At heel strike, the ankle joint was held in neutral position, then plantarflexed slightly until the foot was in total contact with the ground, after which it was dorsiflexed as the leg rotated over the foot. A greater excursion of plantarflexion occurred prior to, and after push off, followed by a dorsiflexion to provide foot-floor clearance at mid-swing.

Figure 1D–G shows the normal EMG pattern, during ten consecutive step cycles, for the knee and ankle flexor and extensor muscles. The medial hamstrings (MH) were active in late swing to decelerate the swinging leg, and remained active during early and midstance, to provide knee stability and hip extension, respectively. A knee extensor muscle, vastus lateralis (VL), usually starts its activity in late swing, peaks just after heel-strike to provide knee stability during weight acceptance and remains active throughout midstance. As observed in figure 1E, this muscle may not be active in normal subjects during locomotion. The tibialis anterior (TA) was reciprocally active to the gastrocnemius (GA). It peaked immediately after heel contact to lower the foot gently to the ground, after which it was generally silent until toe-off, at which point it was activated again, in order to dorsiflex and clear the foot off the treadmill belt during midswing. As a plantarflexor, GA was active during stance, initially being stretched by the forward rotation of the leg at the ankle, and then shortened between 40 and 60% of the stride to generate a push-off momentum.

Effects of Interactive Locomotor Training

Figure 2 shows an example of the effects of 6 weeks of interactive locomotor training on the kinematic pattern in a spastic paretic subject (26 years old) who had sustained a traumatic, chronic spinal cord (C_{7-8}) injury. The interactive locomotor training was performed on a treadmill, with the subject mechanically supported in a comfortable overhead harness at different percentages of body weight support (BWS) using a strain gauge transducer [5]. As the subject walks on the treadmill with a reduced load on the lower extremities, gait deviations can instantly be corrected and proper muscle activation can be facilitated during both the stance and swing phases [6]. Optimal BWS is initially provided and progressively reduced until the subject can walk at full weight bearing (0% BWS) with minimal gait deviations, coping comfortably with the adjustable treadmill speed. In the present example, the spastic paretic subject was trained for 6 consecutive weeks, 4–5 times/week 1 h per session with intermittent rest periods.

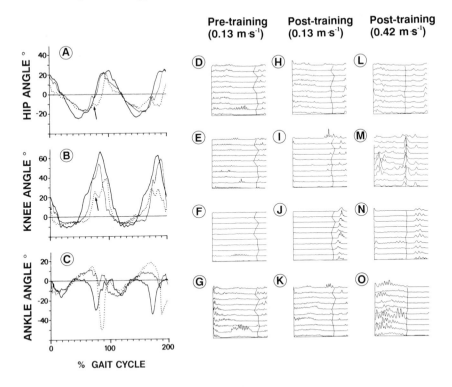

Fig 2. The effects of interactive locomotor training on the kinematic (*A–C*) and EMG (*D–O*) profiles of a spastic paretic subject during treadmill walking. Illustrated are angular displacements of the hip (*A*), knee (*B*) and ankle (*C*) normalized across 2 consecutive gait cycles in: pretraining evaluation at minimal speed of 0.13 m s^{-1} (dotted line); post-training evaluation at 0.13 m s^{-1} (thin solid line); and post training evaluation at 0.42 m s^{-1} (bold solid line). Arrows indicate 'hiking' response at the hip and knee. EMG activity from MH, VL, TA and GA were normalized across 10 consecutive cycles in: pretraining evaluation at 0.13 m s^{-1} (*D–G*); post-training evaluation at 0.13 m s^{-1} (*H–K*); and post-training evaluation at 0.42 m s^{-1} (*L–O*). Solid line across the cycles depicts stance-swing transition.

During the pre-training evaluation, the subject presented with severe spasticity in extension and had much difficulty coping with the weight and treadmill speed. Being a nonfunctional walker overground, he could barely be evaluated at full weight bearing on the treadmill only when the walking speed was as low as 0.13 m s^{-1}. The kinematic pattern showed mainly a knee hyperextension during the loading phase (from 10 to 60% of the gait cycle) with a lack of flexion during the swing period (peaking at 30° and 40°; fig. 2B, dotted line). Hip hiking (an upward thrust of the hip and pelvis to assist swinging the limb through, fig. 2A, arrows) was also present at the stance-swing transition. Foot-floor contact was made with the plantarflexed forefoot (12°; fig. 2C). A marked plantarflexion up to 50° during the beginning of swing was the result of foot drag on the surface of the treadmill belt. The EMG patterns during the pretraining session, illustrated in figure 2D–G, showed prolonged activity in MH and VL during the first half of the stance period. Minimal or no activity was present in the TA, while activity and clonus were present in the GA during the early stance and swing period. Following 6 weeks of locomotor training, marked changes could be observed in both the kinematic profiles (fig. 2A–C, thin line) and EMG patterns (fig. 2H–K). At the same treadmill speed of 0.13 m s^{-1}, a symmetrical and smooth kinematic pattern with increased hip and knee flexion could be observed. A marked decrease of the hip hiking at the stance-swing transition was also noticeable. Heel contact was now clearly present, and a marked decrease of the toe drag during the swing phase could be observed. As illustrated in figure 2J, a burst of TA activity became present during the swing phase, with better EMG timing in the GA. Interestingly, this spastic paretic subject could now walk at a much faster speed of 0.42 m s^{-1}, with a smoother gait pattern and a near normal amplitude of excursion at the three joints (compare the bold line in fig. 2A–C, with the normal pattern illustrated in fig. 1). The main defect which remained was the knee flexion at foot-floor contact and the absence of yield during the loading phase of stance. The lack of ankle dorsiflexion could also be observed. The appearance of clonus in GA became evident at that treadmill speed, but did not impede locomotion (fig. 2O). An inconsistent burst of activity in the TA at foot-floor contact could also be observed (fig. 2N). The temporal pattern was characterized by a more regular pattern with low variability of the stance-swing transition (as indicated by the solid line across the cycles in figure 2L–O), which is similar in many aspects to the normal gait pattern (compare fig. 2L–O with fig. 1D–G; the stance duration was around 60%, swing duration 40%, and the variability of the stance-swing transition was similar).

Functionally, this initially wheelchair-bound spastic paretic patient could now walk overground at 0.23 m s^{-1} with two Canadian crutches for a distance up to 50 m. Moreover, a marked improvement in his endurance could be noted, as indicated by the walking tolerance on the treadmill, which was 5 min before training and more than 10 min after training.

The Combined Effects of Pharmacological Intervention and Interactive Locomotor Training

Figure 3 shows an example of the combined effects of two new experimental medications, cyproheptadine (a serotonergic antagonist) and

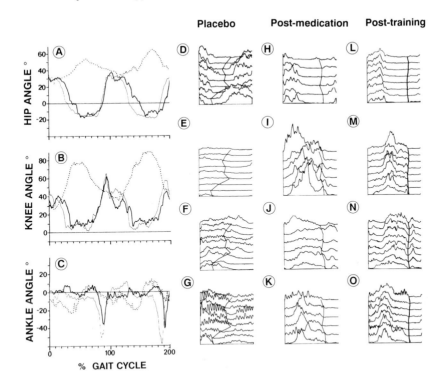

· *Fig 3.* The combined effects of pharmacological intervention and interactive locomotor training on the kinematic (*A – C*) and EMG (*D – O*) profiles of a spastic paretic subject during treadmill walking. Illustrated are angular displacements of the hip (*A*), knee (*B*) and ankle (*C*), normalized across 2 consecutive gait cycles, during the placebo (dotted line), post-medication (thin solid line) and post-training (bold solid line) evaluations. EMG activity from MH, VL, TA and GA were normalized across 6–10 consecutive gait cycles, during the placebo (*D – G*), post-medication (*H – K*), and post-training (*L – O*) evaluations. Solid line across the cycles depicts stance-swing transition.

clonidine (a noradrenergic agonist), together with an interactive locomotor training program, in a chronic spastic paretic subject. This subject (23 years old) had sustained a traumatic (C$_{7-8}$) spinal cord injury due to motor vehicle accident. He had no isolated voluntary movements in either lower limb, whether tested lying or side-lying. Limited by severe spasticity, this subject could stand with support but was unable to take steps independently overground.

During the placebo evaluation (fig. 3A–C; dotted line), this spastic paretic subject required maximum body weight support (≈ 50% BWS) and manual assistance to initiate stepping on the treadmill. His gait pattern was characterized by a flexed posture and a marked flexion profile in the hip and knee indicating the total incapacity to bear weight on the lower extremity even at the minimal treadmill speed. Furthermore, this subject frequently encountered flexor spasms as soon as the foot was lifted off the treadmill, giving rise to an excessive flexion in the hip and knee (up to 60° and 80°, respectively) during swing. It can be seen from figure 3D–G that the EMG profiles in this subject, during the placebo evaluation, were characterized by abnormal timing and clonic discharge. The MH showed a major burst of activity corresponding to the flexor spasm while TA showed a prolonged tonic burst throughout the gait cycle. GA showed similar tonic activity as TA, with clonus present during both stance and swing. Minimal activity was present in VL, possibly due to the incapacity to cope with weight acceptance during stance. Moreover, there was a marked variation of the stance-swing transition and prolonged swing duration due to flexor spasms, as indicated by the solid line across the cycles in figure 3D–G.

Following the administration of clonidine (0.20 mg/day) in combination with cyproheptadine (24 mg/day), the patient gained the ability to walk unassisted and independently at full weight bearing on the treadmill at the speed of 0.26 m s^{-1}. With the improved ability to cope with weight, there was a marked decrease in flexion at both the hip and knee joints during stance (fig. 3A, B, thin line). Concurrent with the disappearance of flexor spasm, the excessive flexion of both joints in swing was also markedly diminished. The angular profiles now approximated a near normal gait pattern, except for the marked knee flexion during early stance, the lack of heel contact at foot floor contact and the presence of toe drag at the beginning of swing (50–60°, fig. 3C, thin line). This may be responsible for the tonic TA activation seen in figure 3J. With the ability to walk full weight bearing, a prolonged EMG activation of VL muscle now occurred throughout stance during single limb support. Such a pattern of EMG activity, described as 'crutch spasticity', can be related to loading as well as tonic stretch reflex activation [7]. The abnormal burst of MH activity, corresponding to the flexor spasm, became silent and was replaced by a functional burst in early stance. Another important change was the more appropriate timing of GA, now limited to the stance phase with a marked reduction of the clonus. This resulted in a more regular stance-swing transition, as indicated by the solid line across the cycles in figure 3H–K. Following a further 3 weeks of interactive gait training, this spastic paretic subject showed minimal changes except for the decrease in toe drag at the end of stance and the attainment of a more regular locomotor pattern (see stance-swing transition in fig. 3L–O). It seems that patients who, despite taking the medications, still have difficulty coping with weight bearing, would benefit more from the interactive training program. However, this needs to be further investigated.

Functionally, this spastic paretic subject could walk independently overground with a walker following medication, and with Canadian crutches following locomotor training. This was remarkable since this patient was wheelchair-bound at the beginning of the study. Moreover, the patient showed a marked improvement in his endurance, from being able to take only 6–10 steps with maximal BWS and manual assistance during the placebo evaluation, to a much longer period, 5–8 min continuously and independently at full weight bearing following locomotor training.

Effects of Conditioning Cutaneomuscular Stimulation

Figure 4 shows an example of the effect of cutaneomuscular stimulation on the joint angular displacements in a chronic spastic paretic subject. The conditioning stimulus, consisted of an 11-ms train of three 1-ms pulses at 200 Hz, was delivered to the medial plantar region, stimulating the cutaneomuscular afferents (intensity ranging from 2.5 to $3.0 \times$ sensory threshold). This severely impaired subject (27 years old) had severe clinical signs of spasticity and marked gait deficits due to traumatic (C_{7-8}) spinal cord injury sustained 4 years ago. Overground walking was laborious or unstable, hence limited to 5–10 steps. Treadmill walking could be extended to 15–20 steps per trial, when the speed was lowered to 0.10 m s^{-1} and when the subject was provided with a safety body harness and handrails for support.

With the conditioning stimulation appropriately timed to occur just before or during swing, this spastic paretic subject reported greater ease at swinging the limb through and a decreased effort to walk. An example is shown in figure 4, depicting the joint angular displacements from 3 gait cycles, before, during, and after cutaneomuscular stimulation. The prestimulus cycle shows the typical gait pattern of ground contact made with the forefoot, with the hip and knee held in flexion, and ankle in plantarflexion. The hip and knee progressively extended to reach neutral position in midstance, and the knee was locked briefly in extension. This together with the coincident burst of VL activity is commonly referred to as 'crutch spasticity' [7], an adaptation of the loading of one limb in order for the other to swing through. The hip continued to extend until late stance as the limb was brought backwards together with the moving treadmill belt while the knee yielded slightly in flexion. The ankle plantarflexion in late stance was a passive consequence of the knee yield while the hip was extended, as evidenced by the lack of triceps surae activity (not illustrated), hence minimal push-off force could be generated for the swing phase. Most effort came from trunk extension and resistance was encountered as the plantarflexed foot dragged along the treadmill. The swing phase was

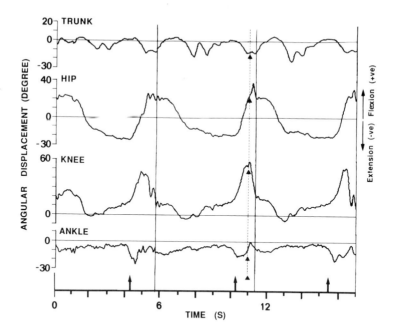

Fig 4. The effects of conditioning cutaneomuscular stimulation of the sole on the kinematic profiles of a severely impaired spastic paretic subject walking on the treadmill at a speed of 0.10 m s^{-1}. Three consecutive cycles of the trunk, hip, knee and ankle angular displacements are illustrated. Upward arrows on the time scale indicate stance-swing transition in each cycle. The conditioning stimulation, consisting of an 11 ms train of three 1 ms pulses at 200 Hz, was delivered in the midswing of the second cycle *(*indicated by dotted vertical line joined by filled triangles*).*

relatively short, and the angular excursion of the hip and knee show some oscillations before the foot land on the ground. The second cycle shows essentially the same features throughout the stance phase. However, with the conditioning cutaneomuscular stimulation timed to occur in midswing (dotted line joined by filled triangles in fig. 4), a clear increase in hip flexion and ankle dorsiflexion was noted. This led to proper foot floor clearance and the subject reported that less effort was required to initiate swing. The foot also landed without the oscillation shown in the previous cycle. In the poststimulation cycle, all the features in the kinematic profiles essentially reverted to those observed in the pre-stimulation cycle, and the subject once again reported difficulty in swinging through.

Discussion

The rationale for the proposed gait rehabilitation approaches are based on spinal animal studies and preliminary human studies. Following a complete spinal cord transection, the adult spinal cat could be trained to recover a locomotor pattern which was similar in many respects to the intact cat[8]. The training consisted of an intensive program of daily treadmill walking exercise during which the cat was supported at the tail. There was a close interaction between the experimenter and the spinal cat such that the cat was allowed to walk with only the amount of weight that it could bear, without accentuating gait deficits such as toe drag. The amount of weight supported through the tail was gradually reduced until the cat could walk fully supporting its hindquarters in digitigrade locomotion with minimal gait deficits. This novel training strategy is presently being extended to treat spastic paretic gait. In a preliminary study done on seven spinal cord injured subjects, it was shown that providing BWS during treadmill walking can facilitate the expression of a more normal gait pattern [9]. As the demand of loading and balance decreased, there was also an increase in speed and step length. The advantage of such an intensive locomotor training approach is that all the different dynamic components of gait, as well as external influences such as loading, speed, support and balance, can be addressed simultaneously. By providing BWS, even the severely impaired patients can be assisted to walk on the treadmill at a minimal speed. These patients normally have difficulty in standing between parallel bars and conventional gait training cannot be instituted until a much later stage. The proposed interactive locomotor training program can be initiated in the acute stage as permitted by the patients' conditions. However, as a first step, only chronic patients who reached a plateau in their rehabilitation were included in the present preliminary studies to avoid the confounding influence of natural recovery. Since preliminary results presented in this paper seem very promising, this training approach will be further tested by ongoing research studies to evaluate its efficacy in different neurological conditions including cerebral vascular accident and spinal cord injury.

The use of experimental medications such as cyproheptadine (5-HT antagonist) and clonidine (NA agonist) was also based on animal studies [10, 11]. Following a chronic, complete spinal cord transection in the adult cat, in which all the descending systems have degenerated, monoaminergic (5-HT and NA) agents that act on the receptors below the transection site were shown to modify spinal reflex activity and modulate the locomotor pattern. Separate clinical trials utilizing a randomized, double-blind, placebo-medication, cross-over design, have established the effectiveness of each of these medications in reducing clinical signs of spasticity and improving the locomotor function of spastic paretic patients [12, 13]. Recently, another clinical trial utilizing a single-subject, randomized, block design has been undertaken to compare and contrast the effects of each of these new medications to the conventional antispastic medication, baclofen, and the results are pending. Eventually, investigations will be undertaken to see if any combination of medications will be superior and offer optimal results. A recent preliminary study [14] has shown that the combined medications of cyproheptadine and clonidine could restore locomotor function in 2 chronic spinal cord injured subjects who were previously wheelchair-bound. Their locomotor patterns and endurance were further improved after a period of interactive locomotor training. As supported by the results presented in this paper, the approaches involving pharmacological intervention and interactive locomotor training should be considered in conjunction. Ongoing research studies have been undertaken to identify the patient population who would benefit from such a combined approach.

Injury to the central nervous system which interrupts descending input to the spinal cord often results in exaggerated activity of segmental reflexes which may impair movement. In normal subjects, the soleus H-reflex is deeply modulated during walking [15, 16]. The reflex is largely monosynaptic and related to the stretch reflex, which is functionally important for the control of locomotion. More recently, it has been shown in 21 spastic paretic subjects that the pattern of soleus H-reflex modulation during walking can vary considerably from being relatively normal to a complete absence of modulation [17]. The absence of reflex modulation may contribute to some abnormal features of spastic gait, such as clonus in stance and toe drag in swing. Thus, it would seem beneficial to have methods which can lower or modulate the reflex activity so that a normal pattern of modulation can emerge. This could be achieved in part by conditioning cutaneomuscular stimulation. Preliminary results have shown that, in the moderately and severely impaired spastic paretic subjects, cutaneomuscular stimulation delivered to the medial plantar region at a conditioning-test delay of 45 ms can selectively inhibit the soleus H-reflex in both the early stance and swing phases during walking [18], thereby producing a near normal reflex modulation pattern. Functionally, the conditioning stimulus in midswing can lead to a decrease in toe drag and limb stiffness, as reported in the example presented in this paper. This approach has much potential to be incorporated as a regime of functional electrical stimulation for gait retraining. The long term application as well as its effects in conjunction with the proposed approaches have yet to be investigated.

Although the new experimental approaches presented in this paper have only been investigated in adult spastic paretic subjects, it is envisaged that the concepts can be generalized to retrain gait in children with cerebral palsy. Many of the adult spastic gait features presented are also common to cerebral palsied children. However, cerebral palsy, which is caused by an injury to the immature brain occurring prenatally, perinatally or postnatally, is further complicated by the ongoing development of the child. Although the lesion is non-progressive, the clinical picture of disordered movement and posture will change as the child grows, since the nervous system continues to develop in the presence of the lesion. Thus, treatment strategies have to be adapted and considered in the context of these developmental factors. The proposed experimental approaches, namely interactive locomotor training, pharmacologic intervention and cutaneomuscular stimulation, provide a dynamic, comprehensive and integrative alternative for the treatment of gait disorders. Research is underway to examine these individual and combined approaches, and to identify the optimal period following lesion to initiate such intervention. The application of these approaches to children with movement disorders remains to be investigated.

Acknowledgment

This project is supported by the Medical Research Council of Canada. J. Fung received a studentship from the Rick Hansen Man in Motion Legacy Fund for spinal cord research. H. Barbeau is a Chercheur-Boursier supported by the Fonds de la Recherche en Santé du Québec.

References

1 Young RR, Delwaide PJ: Drug therapy: Spasticity. Engl J Med 1981;394:28–33, 96–99.
2 Close JRE: Motor Function in the Lower Extremity. Springfield, Thomas, 1964.
3 Odeen I, Knutsson E: Evaluation of the effects of muscle stretch and weight load in patients with spastic paraplegia. Scand J Rehabil Med 1981;13:117–121.
4 Tremblay F, Malouin F, Richards CL, Dumas F: Effect of prolonged muscle stretch on reflex and voluntary activations in spastic cerebral palsy. Scand J Rehabil Med 1990;22:171–180.
5 Barbeau H, Wainberg W, Finch L: Description and application of a system for locomotor rehabilitation. Med Biol Eng Comput 1987;25:341–344.
6 Finch L, Barbeau H: Hemiplegic gait: New treatment strategies. Physiother Can 1985;38:36–41.
7 Knutsson E: Analysis of gait and isokinetic movements for evaluation of antispastic drugs or physical therapies; in Desmedt JE (ed): Motor Control Mechanisms in Health and Diseases. New York, Raven Press, 1983, pp 1013–1034.
8 Barbeau H, Rossignol S: Recovery of locomotion after chronic spinalization in the adult cat. Brain Res 1987;412:84–95.

9   Visintin M, Barbeau H: The effects of body weight support on the locomotor pattern of
    spastic paretic patients. Can J Neurol Sci 1989;16:315–325.
10 Barbeau H, Julien C, Rossignol S: The effects of clonidine and yohimbine on locomo-
    tion and cutaneous reflexes in the adult chronic spinal cat. Brain Res 1987;437:83–96.
11 Barbeau H, Rossignol S: The effects of serotonergic drugs on the locomotor pattern and
    on cutaneous reflexes of the adult chronic spinal cat. Brain Res 1990;514:55–67.
12 Wainberg M, Barbeau H, Gauthier S: The effects of cyproheptadine on locomotion and
    on spasticity in spinal cord injured patients. J Neurol Neurosurg Psychiatr 1990;53:754
    763.
13 Stewart JE, Barbeau H, Gauthier S: Modulation of locomotor patterns and spasticity
    with clonidine in spinal cord injured patients. Can J Neurol Sci 1991;in press.
14 Fung J, Stewart JE, Barbeau H: The combined effects of clonidine and cyproheptadine
    with interactive training on the modulation of locomotion in spinal cord injured
    subjects. J Neurol Sci 1990;100:85–93.
15 Capaday C, Stein RB: Amplitude modulation of the soleus H-reflex in the human during
    walking and standing. J Neurosci 1986;6:1308–1313.
16 Crenna P, Frigo C: Excitability of the soleus H-reflex arc during walking and stepping
    in man. Exp Brain Res 1987;66:49–60.
17 Yang JF, Fung J, Edamura M, Blunt R, Stein RB, Barbeau H: H-reflex modulation
    during walking in spastic paretic subjects. Can J Neurol Sci 1991;18:443–452.
18 Fung J, Barbeau H: The effects of conditioning musculo-cutaneous stimulation on the
    H-reflex during walking in spastic paretic subjects. Soc Neurosci Abstr 1990;16:1262.

Hugues Barbeau, PhD, Associate Professor, School of Physical and Occupational
Therapy, 3654 Drummond Street, Montreal, PQ H3G 1Y5 (Canada)

Forssberg H, Hirschfeld H (eds): Movement Disorders in Children.
Med Sport Sci. Basel, Karger, 1992, vol 36, pp 247–254

Dorsal Rhizotomy as a Treatment for Improving Function in Children with Cerebral Palsy[1]

Carol A. Giuliani

Division of Physical Therapy, School of Medicine, University of North Carolina
at Chapel Hill, N.C., USA

Selective posterior rhizotomy (SPR) has become a popular surgical treatment for improving the care and function of children with spastic cerebral palsy. Several authors describe reduced spasticity and improved function after SPR [1–4]. Careful examination of these results suggests that although SPR reduces spasticity immediately after surgery, abnormal movement persists and movement patterns improve gradually. The cause of improvement is unclear but appears related to compliance with an intense exercise program, orthotic use, subject characteristics, and family support. I believe the research results and anecdotal reports of the effects of SPR may provide valuable insight into the movement problems of children with spastic cerebral palsy (CP). The problems identified suggest that treatment concepts of exercise training, motor control, and motor learning are indicated.

Rationale for Selective Posterior Rhizotomy

Interestingly the rationale for this surgery lacks a sound neurophysiologic basis, and the results of the surgery are inconclusive. The rationale for performing a SPR is based on the clinical assumption that spasticity is the underlying cause of disordered movement. Many clinicians believe that reducing or eliminating spasticity will improve motor control and increase capacity for improved function. However, the relationship of spasticity to movement is unclear and is dependent on the investigator's definition of spasticity [5, 6]. Furthermore, there have been no experimental studies that have attempted to understand the mechanisms related to functional change after surgery.

[1] This research was supported in part by Maternal Child Health, PHHS Grant 149.

Children with cerebral palsy often activate muscles in abnormal sequences, with inappropriate amounts of force, and frequently are unable to produce necessary postural adjustments [7]. These control problems are often attributed to hypertonia and spasticity. However, the persistence of abnormal movement patterns after spasticity has been reduced with SPR support the hypothesis that tone and spasticity alone cannot explain movement dysfunction in children with CP [8].

According to Young and Wiegner [9]: 'spasticity is often a dramatic symptom, but even if there were a treatment to eliminate spasticity . . . one would not expect it to restore function in most patients.' In a recent editorial, Landau and Hunt [10] presented compelling evidence that even when spasticity was reduced by surgery or drugs there was no evidence of improved function. It is possible that spasticity is not the cause of movement dysfunction, but that the mechanisms associated with spasticity and voluntary movement control are interactive.

Effects of Selective Dorsal Rhizotomy

Selective posterior rhizotomy is not a new concept to decrease spasticity [1, 11, 12–14]. Early use of rhizotomy for patients with spasticity was abandoned because of the associated sensory loss [12]. Modifications by Fasano et al. [3] and Peacock and co-workers [11, 15] described a method for testing and sectioning only aberrant posterior rootlets, a procedure which reduced spasticity and preserved sensation. This electrophysiologic testing appears to be a more scientific approach to SPR, however, the reliability of the testing is unproven and the validity of the method is contested by other surgeons and scientists.

Several authors reported decreased F wave, H reflexes, and SEPs [16–18] after SPR that confirmed the clinical observation of reduced spasticity. Reports of decreased spasticity and improved function after SPR have been favorable [1–4, 11, 19–26]. Most authors agree, however, that maximal functional improvement was dependent upon an intensive exercise program after SPR [2, 3, 15, 21]. For a 2 to 6 month period after SPR the children were weak [4, 15, 19, 20–24]. The spasticity appeared to be masking underlying weakness rather than underlying control as Bobath and Bobath [27] suggested. Once the spasticity and tone decreased as a result of SPR, the weakness was revealed, and the importance of parameters such as strength and motor control became apparent. According to Peacock and other surgeons, underlying strength is an important criteria for selecting subjects and for predicting favorable outcome [1, 3, 4, 15].

Strength testing has been problematic for patients with spasticity. Forces produced by a spastic muscle during a standard strength test may not measure the subject's ability to control and grade forces for coordinated functional movement. Several therapists, however, suggest that testing voluntary movements that require controlling speed, trajectory, and direction are valid methods for assessing functional strength in children with CP [26, 28].

In an ongoing longitudinal study of the effects of SPR in children with CP, we are measuring the changes in range of motion, reaching, sit to stand, sitting and standing posture, and locomotion [29]. Children are videotaped twice pre-operatively, at 6 weeks after surgery, and then at selected intervals for 2 years. Preliminary data were reported on several children, and data collection and analyses continue [22, 23, 29].

Consistent with other reports, all children showed increased ROM and decreased spasticity at the first test after surgery. This increased ROM appeared related to improved posture in long sitting and increased ankle dorsiflexion and knee extension in standing. Changes in sit to stand, reaching, and walking occurred gradually. Movement trajectories during sit to stand became smoother and more curvilinear, and had a greater horizontal component than before surgery. Visual observations suggested that patients became increasingly independent and required less assistance from the therapist for standing, sit to stand, and walking. Although patients improved in functional ability, there were periods when kinematic values and movement time increased rather than decreased. Review of the video records during these periods suggested that the apparent regression in control was associated with an improved level of function. The trajectories and velocity curves from early successful attempts of sit to stand without therapist assistance were more irregular than the trials recorded with therapist assistance. As children became more skilled in the independent mode, the trajectories became smoother and movement time decreased.

Gait parameters of walking velocity, stride length, double limb support, and passive ROM improved within 2–3 months after surgery, but the same abnormal movement patterns of the limbs were observed before and after surgery. For example, all children had adequate passive range of motion at the ankle, but during gait they continued to have a forefoot strike pattern that exaggerated when they walked faster, and during play. However, the children could place their foot flat during gait when they were instructed, attended to the task, and walked slowly. It appears that SPR initially improves ROM and static posture more than it improves movement patterns.

Knee buckling during standing was observed in most subjects after surgery and suggested lower limb weakness. The mechanism for this weakness may be a direct reduction of input to motoneuron pools as a result of the reduced peripheral input from dorsal roots. This weakness may result from a decreased number of motor units recruited and a decreased firing rate. The other possibility is that the weakness is a *revealed* weakness, rather than a weakness *created* by reduced dorsal root input. That is, the weakness is not new but is unmasked once the spasticity and tone are reduced. Bobath [30] suggested that weakness of the agonist muscle resulted from spasticity (hyperactive stretch reflex) of the antagonist. This concept led Bobath to propose that normalizing muscle tone, or reducing spasticity would unmask the voluntary capability for movement. Following SPR spasticity is reduced in the antagonist, but what is unmasked is weakness of the agonist.

There is evidence for neuromuscular changes contributing to weakness in adult patients with spastic hemiparesis from cerebrovascular accident (see Bourbonnais and Vanden Noven [31] for a recent review) and in children with spastic cerebral palsy [32–34]. These reports provide evidence for a reduced number, size, and activity level of muscle fibers in children with spastic cerebral palsy. This evidence supports the concept that children with CP are weak and probably are using what little muscle force they have available. Strength is the capacity of a muscle to produce the grade tension appropriately for maintaining posture and producing coordinated movement [35]. We understand that muscle forces alone cannot account for abnormal movement patterns, however, muscle activity does contribute to the force and the timing of force required to produce coordinated movement.

Several researchers provided evidence of mechanical changes in passive muscle properties that many contribute to abnormal movement patterns [33, 34, 36–38]. Dietz and Berger [34] reported increased plantar flexion tension within reduced gastrocnemius EMG amplitude. The authors concluded that passive rather than active antagonist tension was responsible for limited ankle dorsiflexion in patients with cerebral palsy.

In addition to weakness and changes in passive muscles properties, there is some suggestion of abnormal spinal circuitry in children with cerebral palsy. Myklebust et al. [39] believe that motor dysfunction in children with cerebral palsy results from damage to immature supraspinal structures that impress a secondary disorder on a developing spinal cord. Abnormal patterns of reciprocal excitation, reciprocal innervation, and changes in agonist control have been reported in children with cerebral palsy [18, 39, 40]. Myklebust et al. [39] report reciprocal excitation of the TA in response to a soleus muscle stretch which suggests a functionally disordered spinal circuitry. Kundi et al. [18] reported that children with cerebral palsy had abnormal somatosensory evoked potentials (SEPs) before posterior rhizotomy. After posterior selective rhizotomy, H reflexes and dorsal cord potentials from SEPs were depressed, but the SEPs recorded over the cortex did not change. These investigators concluded that the somatosensory disorder is the spinal cord below the cervical level. These observations and a recent report by Brouwer and Ashby [40] provide additional evidence for the hypothesis that CP may be a disorder of spinal circuitry as well as a disorder of the brain. The belief that problems of movement control in children with cerebral palsy result from released supraspinal control is at best an over simplification of the complexities of this disorder.

Our data and reports from others indicate that the patterns, rate, and amount of improvement vary among subjects with SPR. Subject differences may be related to the degree of underlying control, functional ability, amount of therapy, family support, intelligence, and patient motivation. In addition to subject characteristics, outcome may be related to the surgical procedure itself. Surgical reports confirm the variability in spinal level, distribution of rootlets, and number of rootlets severed in each patient. Unfortunately, there are no reports relating the number or distribution of rootlets severed to functional outcome. Also, we cannot rule out the effects of maturation on the changes observed after surgery. Considering the cost and risk involved continued study using a control group design should be used to examine the contribution of the surgery as well as these other important factors.

Increases in functional ability after surgery may be the result of several mechanisms, and the increased joint range observed in standing and sitting may be the result of decreased spasticity and tone. The persistence of abnormal patterns in the presence of reduced spasticity and increased range of motion suggests the influence of learned abnormal movement patterns. It is feasible that a period of learning, exercise, and practice is necessary for the continued development of normal movement patterns. This is consistent with the reports from several authors that an intensive period of physical therapy after surgery is required for maximum functional improvement [15, 21, 24]. We believe that a period of time is required for children to adjust to the increased ROM and reduced muscle stiffness after SPR and to learn new movement patterns.

Conclusions

Scientists studying movement in children with CP should be aware that the assumptions that spasticity is the underlying cause of disordered movement and that reducing or eliminating the spasticity will improve movement are unfounded. Research focused on reducing spasticity should include an examination of functional correlates. Reducing spasticity may increase range of motion, but may unmask underlying weakness rather than underlying control. If there is weakness in children with cerebral palsy then more emphasis should be placed on improving strength. Many therapists are reluctant to use strengthening for fear that it will increase spasticity and produce abnormal movement patterns. In a recent report, adults with head trauma and severe spasticity improved their performance significantly on a side-to-side tapping task after weight-lifting [41]. Also Kolobe [42] reported that upper extremity strengthening exercises (push-ups) for children with spastic cerebral palsy improved function and did not increase spasticity.

I believe that the results from SPR research support the application of motor control concepts to improve movement function in children with CP. I suggest that the functional potential of patients receiving SPR are maximized by using exercise programs that include strengthening, practice, and feedback for learning new patterns of movement.

References

1   Peacock WJ, Arens LJ: Selective Posterior rhizotomy for the relief of spasticity in cerebral palsy. South Afr Med J 1982;62:119–124.
2   Tippets RH, Walker ML, Liddell KL: Long-term follow-up of for relief of spasticity in cerebral palsied children. Dev Med Child Neurol 1989;59(suppl):19.
3   Fasano V, Broggi S, et al: Long-term results of posterior functional rhizotomy. Acta Neurochir 1980;30(suppl):435–439.
4   Abbott R, Forem SL, Johann M: Selective posterior rhizotomy for the treatment of spasticity. Child's Nerv Syst 1989;5:337–346.
5   Sahrmann SA, Norton BJ: The relationship of voluntary movement to spasticity in the upper motor neuron syndrome. Ann Neurol 1977;2:460–465.
6   Giuliani CA: Should we measure spasticity, tone and other ugly terms? In Krebs D (ed): Proceedings of the Neurology Forum on Neurological Physical Therapy Assessment. Washington, Neurology Section of the American Physical Therapy Association, 1989, pp 25–27.
7   Sutherland DH: Gait Disorders in Childhood and Adolescence. Baltimore, Williams & Wilkins, 1984.
8   Campbell SK: Central nervous system dysfunction in children, in Campbell SK (ed): Pediatric Neurologic Physical Therapy. New York, Churchill Livingstone, 1984, pp 1–12.
9   Young RR, Wiegner AW: Spasticity. Clin Orthop Rel Res 1987;219:50–62.
10 Landau WM, Hunt CC: Dorsal rhizotomy, a treatment of unproven efficacy. J Child Neurol 1990;5:174–178.
11 Peacock WJ, Staudt LA: Spasticity in cerebral palsy and the procedure. J Child Neurol 1990;5:179–185.
12 Foerster O: On the indications and results of the excision of posterior spinal nerve roots. Med Surg Gynecol Obstet 1913;16:493–474.

13 Bischof W: Die longitudinal Myelotomie. Zentralblat Neurochir 1951;11:79–88.

14 Sherrington S: Decerebrate rigidity and reflex coordination of movements. J Physiol 1898;22:319–337.

15 Peacock WJ, Arens LJ, Berman B: Cerebral palsy spasticity. Selective posterior rhizotomy. Pediatr Neurosci 1987;13:61–66.

16 Cahan LD, Kundi MS, McPherson D, et al: Electrophysiologic studies in for spasticity in children with cerebral palsy. Appl Neurophysiol 1987;50:459–462.

17 Cahan LD, Beeler L, McPherson D, et al: Clinical electrophysiologic and kinesiologic studies of selective dorsal rhizotomy. Dev Med Child Neurol 1988;57(suppl):4–5.

18 Kundi M, Cahan L, Starr A: Somatosensory evoked potentials in cerebral palsy after partial dorsal root rhizotomy. Arch Neurol 1989;46:524–529.

19 Fasano V, Broggi G, Barolat-Romana G, et al: Surgical treatment of spasticity in cerebral palsy. Child's Brain 1978;4:289–305.

20 Irwin-Carruthers SH, Davids LM, Van Rensburg CK, et al: Early physiotherapy in selective posterior rhizotomy. Fisioterapie 1985;41:45–49.

21 Laitinen L, Nilsson S, Fugl-Meyer A: Selective posterior rhizotomy for the treatment of spasticity. J Neurosurg 1983;58:895–899.

22 Kobetsky S, Mason D. Giuliani CA: The effects of dorsal rhizotomy on standing posture and the temporal characteristics of gait in children with cerebral palsy. Dev Med Child Neurol 1989;59:20–21.

23 Farley B, Giuliani CA, Mulvaney T: The effects of dorsal rhizotomy on the kinematic characteristics of reaching and sit to stand. Dev Med Child Neurol 1989;59(suppl):20.

24 Perry J, Adams J, Cahan LD: Foot floor contact patterns following selective dorsal rhizotomy. Dev Med Child Neurol 1989;59(suppl):19–20.

25 Vaughan CL, Berman B, Staudt LA, et al: Gait analysis of cerebral palsy children before and after rhizotomy. Pediatr Neurosci 1988;14:297–300.

26 Wilson J: Outpatient based physical therapy for children with cerebral palsy undergoing selective dorsal rhizotomy; in Park TS, Phillips LH, Peacock WJ (eds): State-of-the-Art Reviews in Neurosurgery: Management of Spasticity in Cerebral Palsy and Spinal Cord Injury. Philadelphia, Hanley & Belfus, 1989, pp 417–429.

27 Bobath B, Bobath K: Motor Development in Different Types of Cerebral Palsy. London, Heineman Medical Books, 1981.

28 Haley SM, Inacio CA: Evaluation of spasticity and its effect on motor function; in Glenn MB, Whyte J (eds): The Practical Management of Spasticity in Children and Adults. Philadelphia, Lea & Febiger, 1990, pp 70–98.

29 Giuliani CA, Mulvaney T: Dorsal rhizotomy for children with cerebral palsy: Support for concepts of motor control. Physical Ther 1991;71:248–259.

30 Bobath B: Abnormal Postural Reflex Activity Caused by Brain Lesions, ed 2. London, Heineman Medical Books, 1981.

31 Bourbonnais D, Vanden Noven S: Weakness in patients with hemiparesis. Am J Occup Ther 1989;43:313–319.

32 Castle ME, Reyman TA, Schneider M: Pathology of spastic muscle in cerebral palsy. Clin Orthop 1979;142:223–233.

33 Milner-Brown HS, Penn R: Pathophysiological mechanisms in cerebral palsy. J Neurol Neurosurg Psychiatry 1979;42:606–618.

34 Dietz V, Berger W: Normal and impaired regulation of muscle stiffness in gait: a new hypothesis about muscle hypertonia. Exp Neurol 1983;79:680–687.

35 Smidt GL, Rogers MW: Factors contributing to the regulation and clinical assessment of muscular strength. Phys Ther 1982;62:1283–1290.

36 Tardieu C, Lespargot A, Tabary, et al: Toe-walking in children with cerebral palsy:
    contributions of contracture and excessive contraction of the triceps surae muscle. Phys
    Ther 1989;69:656–662.

37 Hufschmidt A, Mauritz KH: Chronic transformation of muscle in spasticity: A periph-
    eral contribution to increased tone. J Neurol Neurosurg Psychiatry 1985;48:676–685.

38 Tang A, Rymer WZ: Abnormal force EMG relations in paretic limbs of hemiparetic
    human subjects. J Neurol Neurosurg Psychiatry 1981;44:690–698.

39 Myklebust BM, Gottleib GL, Penn RD: Developmental abnormalities of the spinal cord
    in cerebral palsy. Reciprocal excitation of antagonistic muscles as a differentiating
    feature in spasticity. Ann Neurology 1982;12:367–374.

40 Brouwer B, Ashby P: Corticospinal projections: Do they differ in patients with cerebral
    palsy. Dev Med Child Neurol 1989;59(suppl):22.

41 Hall CD, Light KE: Heavy resistive exercise effect on reciprocal movement coordination
    of close-head injured subjects with spasticity. Neurol Rep 1990.

42 Kolobe THA: The use of upper extremity proprioceptive neuromuscular facilitation
    techniques with children with spastic diplegia. APTA Combined Sections Meeting, New
    Orleans, 1990.

Carol A. Giuliani, PhD, PT, Division of Physical Therapy,
School of Medicine, University of North Carolina at Chapel Hill,
Chapel Hill, NC 27599-7135 (USA)

Forssberg H, Hirschfeld H (eds): Movement Disorders in Children.
Med Sport Sci. Basel, Karger, 1992, vol 36, pp 255–263

Discussion Section IV

*Eva Brogren, Gunilla Leinsköld, Eva Maresova, Ulla Myhr,
Marianne Salén, Inger Wadell*

During the fourth session of the Sven Jerring symposium, research in
the areas of locomotion, spasticity and postural control were presented.
The aim was to focus on how contemporary knowledge in recently acquired research can be implemented in treatment. The reflex/hierarchical
model of motor control, containing assumptions that form the basis for
different treatment methods, e.g. Bobath, Vojta and Sensory Integration,
was discussed. What other assumptions might be useful in treatment? A
system/task model has been proposed as a more appropriate model on
which to establish neurological treatment techniques [Horak, this vol.].
Can the assumptions of the system/task model provide us with a theoretical
basis more apt to elucidate questions arising in treatment? The members of
the task-force group have tried to mirror the discussion that was generated
in the session, but have also added questions emanating from the group.

Locomotion

Grillner discussed how locomotion is generated from innate neural
circuits within the spinal cord, called central pattern generators (CPGs)
[Schotland, this vol.]. Such 'hard-wired' circuits are also used in other
innate motor behavior such as swallowing and breathing. An important
feature of CPGs is that they can generate a basic pattern without sensory
or descending input. However, during normal movements sensory information plays an important role in modifying and adapting the activity to the
environment. Autonomous CPGs probably exist in some form in human
locomotion but has not yet been demonstrated [Forssberg, this vol.].

Cioni showed that motility in the fetus can be observed in the 8th to
9th gestational weeks prior to the afferents having made synaptic contact
with the alpha motor neurones. This means that movements are not elicited

by simple reflexes but endogenously triggered and generated by networks of neurones in the spinal cord. Therefore, the assumption of the reflex/hierarchical model, that the reflex serves as the basic functional unit in movements, has to be re-evaluated. In contrast, the central nervous system can be viewed as an acting system and not only as a reacting one.

The development of gait, from digitigrade (landing on toes or foot flat) to plantigrade (adult-like heel strike), exemplifies how different parts of the CNS interact to form adult walking. Forssberg described the determinants of plantigrade gait which produce an energy-efficient locomotion. In children with cerebral palsy the development of plantigrade gait does not take place, probably due to impaired supraspinal influences on the neural circuits generating the basic locomotor pattern [Leonard, Forssberg, Berger, this vol.]. Even intensive and long-term treatment of these children has not resulted in a normal locomotor pattern. Facilitation, e.g. giving sensory stimulation on an automatic basis, has been an often-used technique in treatment, thinking this would provide a possibility to learn a normal walking pattern. Instead, treatment should be focused on the purpose of walking. Forssberg expressed a similar point of view during the discussion: 'We can never teach children with cerebral palsy to walk normally, but we can teach them the best way to get from one point to another.' In the reflex/hierachical model, infant stepping is considered to be a reflex and to disappear when higher brain centers mature. This example of a rigid sequence in development has influenced many treatment strategies. Developmental milestones are often followed in therapy in order to achieve independent locomotion. This view appears to be outdated. Infant stepping responses are an integrated part of adult walking and could therefore be used as a resource in therapy.

The Bobath concept represents a recommendation to follow developmental sequences, but this recommendation is not imperative [Mayston, this vol.]. In Vojta therapy, however, children are not considered mature enough to stand and walk until they master reflex turning and reflex creeping [Aufschnaiter, this vol.].

Currently, it is not considered possible to change basic mechanisms involved in motor control in children with CP. The goal of treatment should rather be to analyze and treat the constraints of locomotion. These could be caused by contractures, isolated weakness, abnormal muscular co-contraction, hypermobility, etc. There are obviously many secondary complications that can be treated. Perhaps a child with cerebral palsy can walk more efficiently if biomechanical constraints are changed and he is provided with an ankle-foot orthosis. It is important to evaluate similar feasible treatment interventions. As mentioned earlier the basic locomotor pattern in walking is influenced by afferent input [Forssberg, this vol.].

Many orthopedic complications also give an abnormal sensory input and influence compensatory movement strategies. Might orthopedic surgery (e.g. lengthening of muscles and tendons), though it amplifies the muscular weakness, provide a new prerequisite for motor learning? The increased range of motion makes it possible for the child to stand foot flat with feet wide apart, offering a larger support base. In this way interaction between movement and postural control will be facilitated.

Widén-Holmqvist brought up a question concerning locomotor training and learning. In the initial stage of learning, motivation and understanding of the goal is very important [Gentile, this vol.]. Levitt stressed the importance of starting treatment by something the patient eagerly wants to achieve. Physical therapists working with children have all experienced that most children have a strong motivational drive in trying to learn how to walk. Maybe this emanates from the fact that we are genetically determined to walk in an upright position. The Bobath concept and Sensory Integration stress the importance of stimulating the child's motivation, whereas the Vojta method does not.

Widén-Holmqvist also focused on the difference between learned and performed movement. Learned movement can be defined as a permanent change in behavior, whereas performed movement is unstable, indicating that the child has to concentrate on performing the motor activity. Follow-up studies on adults after stroke have shown that 80% of the patients can walk, but they don't use this ability in activities outside their own home. Can this be an example of performed but not learned motor behavior? Can this lack of learning be due to factors such as high energy cost, walking speed, limited attention span or deficit in short-term memory, making it difficult to do many things simultaneously? Or do we structure the training incorrectly, making it difficult to go from performance to learning? These questions are also relevant for motor learning in children with neurological deficits. If we keep the patient in training for an extended period, we have to confirm, out of health economic reasons, that the patient has achieved some important function in the end.

Giuliani suggested that physical therapists have just been working on performance. If we concentrated the treatment on learning and somehow measured learning, maybe we would have a better result. Do we teach abilities that are indispensable for the child and can be carried over? An important factor is also how much time the child spends practicing. Are we convinced that the child knows what he is doing? Can he practice on his own, or is he relying on 45 min of training per week? Does the patient have the optimal range of motion, does he have the strength? We should also ask if it is useful to practice activities on a cognitive level that normally are performed automatically, like walking and balance reactions. Thelen suggested that learning normally starts at a cognitive stage and with time becomes autonomous. She discussed a 'dynamic system approach'. This means that motor patterns are softly assembled rather than 'hard wired' in the CNS. Soft assembly means that the actual trajectories of movements are determined by many contributing factors; neural firing, elastic qualities of the muscles and tendons, anatomical properties of bones and joints, passive and mechanical forces acting on the body, and, finally, the energy delivered to the moving limbs and segments. Movement patterns are assembled 'on-line' in reference to and in continual interaction with the intentions of the subject and his perceptions of the actual task and the physical properties of his body and the environment. Some movement patterns, like walking, are very stable. Others, such as tap dancing, are so unstable that they must be continually practiced. Motor patterns change and new forms arise in development only when the old patterns are destabilized and the system is free to explore and select new and more adaptive actions. Thelen emphasized the sensory input during development. She concluded that normal movements have to be taught before 'abnormal' movement patterns are fixed. This statement brings up the question if we should treat a child that shows no sign of cerebral palsy and hinder him to do what he wants in order to prevent the establishment of firm abnormal movement patterns. Do the ideas of Thelen bring us to the Bobath concept but from a different perspective? Thelen stressed that development is influenced by different parameters which, from a dynamic system approach, are very important to identify. Are the parameters of motor development different in a normal child compared to those of a CP child? According to Thelen, this question points to a need for research on early diagnosis in at-risk populations. Barbeau proposed new rehabilitation strategies to improve locomotion. He used interactive locomotor training on a treadmill with the patient (adult spastic and/or paretic) mechanically supported in a comfortable overhead harness. In this way, the patient's body weight can be supported. Initially, optimal body weight support is provided and progressively reduced until the subject can walk at full weight bearing with fewer gait deviations, coping with the adjustable treadmill speed. We think that this kind of training focuses on the interaction between locomotion and postural control. Practicing locomotion and gradually decreasing body weight support provides a possibility for such an interaction. Maybe one way of locomotor training for children with CP is to perform it in different depths of water. Barbeau declared that the application of these approaches for children with movement disorders remains to be investigated. Richards suggested that treadmill walking with body weight support could provide CP children, with missing or delayed locomotor practice, an experience needed to guide the neuromotor development. She hypothesized that enriched locomotor experience could promote neural changes, limiting the expression of the motor disorder.

Crenna elaborated on the variation in gait patterns among children with cerebral palsy. He attempted to define, in a pathophysiological profile, the components that might potentially limit locomotion in CP children. The patient's gait is consistently reproducible in this profile over a short period of time but over longer periods (1 year) dramatic changes can take place. These changes might give us a clue to the natural history of different kinds of cerebral palsy. Such a profile might enable identification of component changes that occur during treatment, after surgery, etc. The profile can also be used as a tool for differentiating etiologies of CP and as a method for individualized treatment procedures. This view raises new perspectives for assessment and evaluation.

Berger had also investigated the gait pattern of children with cerebral palsy and drew a conclusion similar to that of Forssberg. Berger, Forssberg and others state that maturation of locomotion depends on neural remodeling that includes involvement of supraspinal centers. Disorders in the gait of children with CP are partially attributable to an impairment of these supraspinal centers. The walking pattern in children with CP shows co-activation, reduced extensor EMG and enhanced monosynaptic stretch reflexes. All these signs represent a physiological stage during normal ontogenetic development. Berger also pointed out that co-contraction might be a positive mechanism to stiffen the legs and to support body weight for equilibrium control. Co-contraction is of higher energy cost, but perhaps it is an adequate way for the child to control the limbs. It is important to consider that co-contraction is a normal feature during the early stages of motor learning. A child with cerebral palsy also uses co-contraction when learning a new skill. This means that the extent of co-contraction seen in a child with CP has to be evaluated in this context.

Spasticity

Decreased spasticity is often proposed as a goal of physiotherapy. The clinical signs of spasticity are exaggerated velocity-dependent resistance to passive stretch, clonus and spread of the reflex responses to other muscles. In the reflex/hierarchical model, the aim of therapy is to inhibit spasticity in order to improve motor control and thus increase the capacity for more normal function. No conclusive cause of spasticity is known. Lack of supraspinal inhibition, release phenomenon, sprouting, enhanced fusimotor drive and also peripheral factors in the muscle itself have been suggested [Dietz, Berger, this vol.]. Many different forms of spasticity probably exists, depending on where and when the lesion appeared.

Giuliani described dorsal (posterior) rhizotomy as a method of reducing peripheral sensory input to the spinal cord and in that way decrease spasticity. Postoperatively, decreased spasticity was found, but also weakness in antigravity muscles and persistent abnormal movement patterns. Physical therapists should be aware that treatment aimed at reducing tone will not necessarily improve movement. Reducing the tone may increase the range of motion, but may unmask underlying weakness rather than underlying more normal motor control. Guiliani suggested that decreasing spasticity alone is insufficient for producing better-controlled movement. A certain period of learning is required for patients to demonstrate improved movement patterns and to use the expanded range of joint motion available to them. If there is muscular weakness in children with CP, the physical therapists should put more emphasis on strengthening exercises. Many physical therapists, especially those who follow the Bobath concept, are reluctant to use strengthening exercises for fear that spasticity will increase and hence exaggerate the abnormal movement patterns. However, several authors have reported that strengthening exercises did not increase spasticity but rather improved function [1, 2]. Richards supported Giuliani and demanded us to consider the use of different kinds of contractions during strengthening exercises. Static, concentric and eccentric contractions can be applied. If eccentric contraction is used, stretching of the antagonist muscle will be avoided. Eccentric muscle contraction is common during most movements (e.g. locomotion) and is important. An eccentric contraction of tibialis anterior after heelstrike allows a smooth plantarflexion and quadriceps is also eccentrically contracting during the early support phase when the knee is bending.

Dietz showed in his study that a large monosynaptic reflex potential is present in spastic patients. The functionally essential polysynaptic reflex response is, however, absent. Impaired polysynaptic reflexes have been found in several spastic muscles. Dietz concluded that a transformation of motor units occurs, with the consequence that regulation of muscle tension takes place on a lower level of neuronal organization. Such transformation is functionally meaningful, as it enables the patient to support body weight during gait. It becomes impossible to conduct fast active movements, however. Histochemistry and morphometry of spastic muscles reveal specific changes of muscle fibres.

Berger argued that hypertonia seems to be the consequence of these altered muscle fibre properties. Would the change in muscle fibre properties be regarded as a secondary effect of the primary CNS pathology?

Referring to Vojta therapy, Dorit von Aufschneiter expressed a different view on spasticity. She defined spasticity as a lack of 'muscle differentiation' and considered the spastic muscle to have a wrong direction of contraction, e.g. contraction starts proximally or distally. Patella alta, seen in many children with CP, is considered to be the evidence of a contraction starting proximally in the quadriceps. Leonard criticized this assumption. He was unaware of any study that has shown that a spastic muscle has a different direction of contraction. Leonard claimed that the basic problem in Vojta therapy is that the therapist elicits reflex turning and reflex creeping by cutaneous stimulation and somehow believes that these two constructed patterns can be carried over into functional activity. Leonard stated that children with motor control difficulties on the contrary should be given the opportunity to explore functionally related movements, instead of being held in these static positions.

Postural Control

Human postural control refers to the actions of sensorimotor systems organized toward contending with the force of gravity [Hirschfeld, this vol.]. The aim of postural control is to keep the center of body mass within the support base. When equilibrium is disturbed, by external (push) or internal (voluntary movement) force, this is recognized by information from somatosensory, vestibular and visual systems. Humans probably use an internal model of posture, partly genetically determined, partly learned, as a reference. It is of great importance for the child with CP to experience good sitting and standing positions during longer periods of the day to be able to build up an internal reference value in these different postures. The system/task model suggests that postural control involves an interaction between the environment and the individual. It is known that the postural responses are adapted to different parameters such as the direction and speed of the disturbance and the size of the support base. If the child is supporting himself with the arms in standing position, the postural response will be elicited in the arms and not in the legs and trunk. A child standing freely and a child holding on to a walking aid gets very different postural control practice when equilibrium is disturbed. When the child has difficulties standing freely the hands are often used to support the body. Using a standing shell, the child is given a possibility to build up a reference value for the standing position. The shell also permits him to use both hands freely in different activities. Can interaction between postural control and voluntary movements be built up in this way? In normal motor behavior anticipatory postural control is used to compensate for equilibrium perturbation induced by the voluntary movement. Thus, the anticipatory muscular activity precedes the activity in the prime mover.

In the sitting position, the same principle of training the interaction between postural control and voluntary movements could be used. If the child is supporting himself with the arms, postural responses are elicited in the arms, not in the trunk. We think that the goal of therapy should determine how training has to be conducted. If the goal is to sit at a table and write, a stable and comfortable position, where the child can control the hands and the head, is of importance. To be able to take off a sweater using both hands puts quite different demands on the postural control system. Function must be the goal, a concept repeated several times during the conference.

Interaction between postural control, voluntary movement, and locomotion was also described by Hirschfeld. Normal children between 6 and 14 years of age were studied while walking on a treadmill. At a given signal they were instructed to pull a handle. All children used anticipatory postural movements. The study suggests a continuous development in integrating postural, voluntary and locomotor activity up to adolescence. Is this kind of development possible in children with cerebral palsy or must the child be fixed in a steady position to succeed in performing voluntary movements?

Information from the vestibular system is of importance for postural control. Shumway-Cook described the role of the vestibular system in the development of motor coordination. Despite vestibular loss some children develop normally because they form compensatory strategies early in development. In children with both brain damage and vestibular dysfunction, appropriate compensatory strategies cannot be organized. Shumway-Cook questioned the efficiency of generalized vestibular stimulation to improve development globally. If therapeutic strategies instead were more specific and individualized for each patient, maybe training would be more potent.

Conclusion

The topics concerning locomotion, spasticity and postural control, presented during this session, have all elucidated a wide range of difficulties in diagnosing and treating children with CP. Several therapeutic concepts and strategies have been presented and penetrated. It is obvious that all therapists, responsible for the efficacy of functional habilitation of today, need to take part in both basic and clinical science within the field of motor learning and motor control. Frustration and uncertainty are the first steps that certainly will be followed by obtaining more knowledge and a capacity to participate in professional discussions.

References

1   Hall CD, Light KE: Heavy resistive exercise on reciprocal movement coordination of closed-head injured subjects with spasticity. Tar Heel J 1990;(Fall):12.
2   Kolobe THA: The use of upper extremity proprioceptive neuromuscular facilitation techniques with children with spastic diplegia (abstract). Pediatr Phys Ther 1990;1:186.

Eva Brogren, Motor Control Laboratories Q4, Karolinska Hospital,
S–104 01 Stockholm (Sweden)

Forssberg H, Hirschfeld H (eds): Movement Disorders in Children.
Med Sport Sci. Basel, Karger, 1992, vol 36, pp 264–271

Measurement of Motor Performance in Cerebral Palsy

Suzann K. Campbell

College of Associated Health Professions, University of Illinois at Chicago, Ill., USA

Little evidence exists in the research literature attesting to the effectiveness of rehabilitation efforts to influence the motor performance capabilities of children with cerebral palsy (CP). One of the reasons for this dearth of information is the lack of satisfactory tools for diagnosing CP and assessing problems and outcomes. The questions addressed in this paper are:

(1) What should we measure?

(2) How should an assessment protocol be structured? and

(3) What elements of a theoretical measurement protocol (tests) do we have and how useful are they likely to be?

What Should We Measure?

What to measure is determined by: (1) how we view the nature of the problems in CP; (2) which of those problems we think we can compensate for or improve with treatment, and (3) which potential outcomes are most important. If you search the research literature on the efficacy of physical therapy (PT) in the management of CP to identify the variables under study, you will conclude that the problems that can be changed include delayed development, and abnormal tone, reflexes, and postural alignment, including range of motion. Based on frequency of study, the most important outcomes are increased rate of motor development, increased stride length and increased range of motion in the ankle, all highly quantifiable [1, 2]. You will also conclude that treatment isn't very effective, and you will not know whether improvement in any of the variables studied has an effect on the child's function in the community, or on the need for assistive devices, orthotics, or orthopedic surgery.

On the other hand, if you review progress notes written by physical therapists, you are likely to conclude that the problems that can be changed include trunk/pelvis alignment, balance reactions, head control and postural tone. You will conclude that dozens of specific outcomes are important but can only be described anecdotally, and that treatment is highly effective. The literature on reliability of clinical decision making is clear on the risks of basing practice on such subjective data [3], or on results of efficacy studies that fail to measure the most critical variables. These conflicting scenarios suggest that our theoretical basis for treatment is unclear.

For a long time I have believed that the research on efficacy of PT in the management of movement dysfunction in CP lacked validity because the outcomes of therapy were misspecified by the investigators. Because of these concerns, I embarked upon two specific activities last year. The first was a study of physicians' beliefs in the expected outcomes of therapy for CP [4]. The second activity was a consensus conference sponsored by the Section on Pediatrics of the American Physical Therapy Association (APTA) at which about 100 physical therapists met to consider the outcomes of PT based on their beliefs and the research literature [5]. The data from these two activities can set the stage for determining the appropriate outcome variables for future research on PT effectiveness and can assist in the development of a clinical measurement protocol to document the most important effects of therapy.

Our research on US physician's expectations of PT for CP (197 pediatricians, orthopedists, physiatrists, and neurologists) informed us that a number of positive physical, functional, and social outcomes are believed to be likely or highly likely to occur (table 1). Clearly, these are outcomes we should seek to measure both in the clinical setting and in research on the effectiveness of treatment. Note, however, that very few of the expected outcomes suggest that PT affects the underlying impairment; most outcomes imply the use of compensatory strategies or address functional performance issues and family outcomes. Those that do reflect an expectation of decreased impairment have low levels of belief. Only prevention of contractures falls into the category of prevention of secondary impairment.

Physical therapists participating in a consensus conference exercise [5] expressed belief in similar types of outcomes, although they were not formally rated and thus might be ranked differently.

In addition to measuring outcomes believed to be important by clinicians, a second piece of the answer to the question 'What should we measure?' should come from the results of laboratory research into the neuromuscular characteristics of motor performance in CP. The hallmarks of motor performance in clients with CP of the spastic type include:

(1) Lack of selective control of muscle activation [6].
(2) Lack of appropriate force and power production.
(3) Poor coordinative structures for control of posture and movement.

Table 1. Physician's ($n = 197$) expectations regarding the outcomes of physical therapy for cerebral palsy

	Respondents %[1]
Increased independence through use of assistive devices	86
Improved parental ability to manage the physical aspects of disability	83
Improved parental ability to cope with the social/emotional aspects of disability	77
Prevention of contractures	70
Maintenance of functional abilities	69
Improvement in functional abilities	65
Increased endurance for physical activities	63
Improved ability to profit from educational experiences in school	61
Improved feeding	50
Improved postural alignment	49
Decreased influence of primitive reflexes	34
Improved selective control of movement	34
Increased rate of motor milestone attainment	32

[1] Percent of respondents who believed outcome to be likely or highly likely [Campbell et al: (unpubl data, 1991)].

Underlying these overall problems are excessive coactivation of antagonistic muscle groups, failure to inhibit primary postural reflexes, irradiation of activity in abnormal muscle synergies, failure to control reflex gain, and muscle hypoextensibility [7–10]. Although hyperactive stretch reflexes constitute the neurophysiological definition of spasticity [11], I would contend that the combination of the problems listed above represents the spasticity syndrome as clinicians describe and treat it. In the terminology of the World Health Organization's Classification of Impairments, Disabilities, and Handicaps, these are the impairments inherent in spastic types of CP that result in impaired efficiency, endurance, coordination, balance, posture and flexibility, and speed of movement [12]. Impairments are expressed as functional limitations in achievement of motor milestones (delayed development), reaching, sitting, changing positions, walking, eating and dressing. Functional limitations can translate into disabilities in mobility, independence in activities of daily living, play, learning, and communication; into secondary impairments such as contractures and deformities necessitating orthotics and soft tissue and orthopedic surgery; and into family stress and dysfunctional coping and parenting.

How Should an Assessment Protocol Be Structured?

The second question posed at the outset was 'How should an assessment protocol be structured?' If we want to measure the variables physicians and therapists think are important outcomes of therapy, and study how therapy affects the underlying impairments characteristic of CP (as well as the more functional aspects of disability), it is important to develop measurement instruments within a specific theoretical framework. The expected clinical outcomes and the neuromuscular system impairments comprise the basic outline of the constructs of interest; however, the list of outcomes and problems contains constructs at very different levels of analysis, from the organ and systems level to the societal level [13]. We need to know how these variables interact to produce disability, secondary impairments, and use of compensatory motor control strategies, and we need to learn whether therapy can influence the basic elements of impairment or only provide useful means for improving functional capabilities and preventing the development of complications such as contractures and deformities.

An organizing framework that forms a hierarchy of problems and potential levels of intervention for improving motor performance and functional outcomes can be developed based on a taxonomic system such as that of the World Health Organization [12], or a similar foundation developed first by Nagi [14] and recently elaborated [15]. Table 2 provides an example of some of the elements such a classification system might contain.

Assessment of Currently Available Tests

The third question posed at the outset was 'What elements of a theoretical measurement protocol (tests) do we have and how useful are they likely to be?' The corollary, of course, is 'What new tests do we need?' Examples of existing scales that might be useful within the framework elaborated above include the Pediatric Evaluation of Disability Inventory [16], the Peabody Developmental Motor Scales [17], and the Gross Motor Function and Performance Measures [18].

The Pediatric Evaluation of Disability Inventory is a new test for assessing functional skills in the areas of self-care, mobility, and social function [16]. The test does not, however, address issues of endurance and

Table 2. Theoretical framework (based on Nagi [14]) for measurement of motor performance in cerebral palsy

Impairment Organ/systems level	Functional limitation Potentially remediable inability to perform a task as the result of impairment	Disability Long-term functional limitation imposed by permanent impairment
Speed Balance Efficiency Endurance Coordination Flexibility Postural control	Slow and inefficient gait with poor endurance Tendency to fall	Needs ride to school and other activities limiting independence in community mobility
Subsystems: (1) Motor control impairments Coactivation Irradiation High reflex gain Reduced force Lack of selectivity	Inability to stand up from sitting Inability to reach overhead	Nonparticipation in sports limiting contacts with peers
(2) Muscle impairments Hypoextensibility		

efficiency needed for community function. Although it could be considered to measure aspects of disability that are certainly important, the limitation that scoring can be done by parent report or through professional judgment means that it will be unclear whether results indicate what a child *can* do or what she/he *does* do in daily life.

The Peabody Developmental Motor Scales might be useful to identify delayed motor development, an overall aspect of functional limitation. The Peabody has reliable subscales for gross and fine motor milestone development which were normed in 1981–1982 [17, 19]. Work by Phillips has provided a preliminary indication that the Scales provide different performance profiles for each type of CP [Phillips W, unpubl Master's thesis, University of North Carolina at Chapel Hill, 1986], so they may be useful in describing certain aspects of impairment, such as balance and fine motor coordination.

The Gross Motor Function Measure (GMFM) and its accompanying (still under development) Gross Motor Performance Measure are the only modern standardized tests developed specifically for use with children with CP [18]. The GMFM assesses some aspects of functional motor behavior such as rolling, changing positions from lying to sitting or four-point, pulling to standing, walking and so on. Skills are not, however, assessed in a natural context so the GMFM could not be considered to be a disability scale.

The Gross Motor Performance Measure (GMPM) allows for scoring 20 items from the GMFM for some aspects of coordination, including selective control of joints and segments, postural control, and balance. Not all of these aspects are tested across various levels of gross motor skill, however, so the test results confound several constructs related to impairment which may or may not need to be assessed separately. The constructs tested, however, do not include aspects of impairment such as endurance, speed, and efficiency of movement, all very important issues for clients with CP [20, 21].

In terms of specific functional skills, various means for assessing gait are available, from three-dimensional motion analysis in some high-technology gait labs to footprint analysis and other less-comprehensive clinical systems. Olney's power analyses have been most revealing in identifying impairment of power output, efficiency of movement and conservation of energy; however, her method is not practical for regular use in most clinical centers [22]. We are very much in need of research that correlates performance on clinical and community-based measures of function and disability with laboratory assessment of important parameters of impairment such as power, endurance, speed and efficiency [23].

Goniometry is one of the few well-documented means available for assessing individual joint range of motion as a feature of impairment and it should probably be used more widely than it is; however, more research on its reliability in children with CP is needed [24]. Study of the correlation of range of motion with functional skill and with impending need for orthotic or surgical intervention would tell us whether goniometry has any validity in CP.

In many clinical centers, videotapes are used to document movement problems and progress in children with CP; however, I know of none that employs this technology based on a theoretical perspective and with a specific protocol or a systematic measurement scheme. Therapists should consider the possibility of studying what types of outcomes, at which level of analysis, can be documented by videotaping and then developing a systematic protocol for filming and measuring these effects.

Conclusions

A comprehensive approach to studying and treating CP should address the dysfunction at each level of the disabling process, emphasizing those areas we believe can be changed or compensated for by intervention, and linking underlying impairments with functional limitations and disabilities.

Despite the availability of a number of new clinical assessment tools, nothing resembling a comprehensive measurement protocol exists. Few options exist for measuring impairment and disability.

Clinical tools for documenting the effects of intervention on efficiency, endurance, selective control of movement, and skeletal alignment and flexibility are especially critical to develop, as are measures of family variables and functional performance in home, school and community.

As we develop new measurement tools, we should be concerned about clarity regarding the constructs they are intended to measure. Less confounding of variables in tests would assist in identifying the specific outcomes and means by which intervention produces change in motor performance.

References

1   Piper MC: Efficacy of physical therapy: Rate of motor development in children with cerebral palsy. Pediatr Phys Ther 1990;2:126–130.
2   Campbell SK: Efficacy of physical therapy in improving postural control in cerebral palsy. Pediatr Phys Ther 1990;2:135–140.
3   Sackett DL, Haynes RB, Tugwell P: Clinical Epidemiology: A Basic Science for Clinical Medicine. Boston, Little, Brown, 1985.
4   Campbell SK, Anderson J, Gardner HG: Physicians' beliefs in the efficacy of physical therapy in the management of cerebral palsy. Pediatr Phys Ther 1990;2:169–173.
5   Campbell SK (guest ed): Proceedings of the Consensus Conference on the Efficacy of Physical Therapy in the Management of Movement Dysfunction in Cerebral Palsy. Pediatr Phys Ther 1990;2.
6   Campbell SK: Central nervous system dysfunction in children; in Campbell SK (ed): Pediatric Neurologic Physical Therapy, ed 2. New York, Churchill Livingstone, 1991, pp 1–17.
7   Barolat-Romana G, David R: Neurophysiological mechanisms in abnormal reflex activities in cerebral palsy and spinal spasticity. J Neurol Neurosurg Psychiatr 1980;43:333–342.
8   Leonard CT, Moritani T, Hirschfeld H, Forssberg H: Deficits in reciprocal inhibition of children with cerebral palsy as revealed by H reflex testing. Dev Med Child Neurol 1990;32:974–984.
9   Nashner LM, Shumway-Cook A, Marin O: Stance posture control in select groups of children with cerebral palsy: Deficits in sensory organization and muscular coordination. Exp Brain Res 1983;49:393–409.
10 Tardieu C, Huet de la Tour E, Bret MD, Tardieu G: Muscle hypoextensibility in children with cerebral palsy. I. Clinical and experimental observations. Arch Phys Med Rehabil 1982;63:97–102.
11 Feldman RG, Young RR, Koella WP: Spasticity: Disordered Motor Control. Chicago, Year Book Medical Publishers, 1980, p 485.

12 World Health Organization: International Classification of Impairments, Disabilities, and Handicaps. Geneva, World Health Organization, 1980.

13 Hislop H: Tenth Mary McMillan lecture: The not-so-impossible dream. Phy Ther 1975;55:1069–1080.

14 Nagi SZ: Disability and Rehabilitation. Columbus, Ohio State University Press, 1969.

15 Pope AM, Tarlov AR (eds): Disability in America: Toward a National Agenda for Prevention. Washington, National Academy Press, 1991.

16 Haley SM, Faas RM, Coster WJ, Webster H, Gans BM: Pediatric Evaluation of Disability Inventory. Boston, New England Medical Center, 1989.

17 Folio MR, Fewell RR: Peabody Developmental Motor Scales and Activity Cards. Allen, DLM Teaching Resources, 1983.

18 Russell DJ, Rosenbaum PL, Cadman DT, Gowland C, Hardy S, Jarvis S: The gross motor function measure: A means to evaluate the effects of physical therapy. Dev Med Child Neurol 1989;31:341–352.

19 Hinderer KA, Richardson PK, Atwater SW: Clinical implications of the Peabody Developmental Motor Scales: A constructive review. Phys Occup Ther Pediatrics 1989;9:81–106.

20 Lundberg A: Longitudinal study of physical working capacity of young people with spastic cerebral palsy. Dev Med Child Neurol 1984;26:328–334.

21 Rose J, Medeiros JM, Parker R: Energy cost index as an estimate of energy expenditure of cerebral-palsied children during assisted ambulation. Dev Med Child Neurol 1985;27:485–490.

22 Olney S, Costigan PA, Hedden DM: Mechanical energy patterns in gait of cerebral palsied children with hemiplegia. Phys Ther 1987;67:1348–1354.

23 Olney SJ: Efficacy of physical therapy in improving mechanical and metabolic efficiency of movement in cerebral palsy. Pediatr Phys Ther 1990;2:145–154.

24 Harris SR, Smith LH, Krukowski L: Goniometric reliability for a child with spastic quadriplegia. J Pediatr Orthoped 1985;5:348–351.

Prof. Suzann K. Campbell, Department of Physical Therapy, University of Illinois at Chicago, Box 6998, M/C 898, Chicago, IL 60680 (USA)

Forssberg H, Hirschfeld H (eds): Movement Disorders in Children.
Med Sport Sci. Basel, Karger, 1992, vol 36, pp 272–277

Evaluation of Sensory Integration Dysfunction

Anita C. Bundy, Anne G. Fisher

Department of Occupational Therapy, College of Associated Health Professions,
The University of Illinois at Chicago, Ill., USA

A diagnosis of sensory integrative (SI) dysfunction is made by exclusion. That is, in the absence of frank CNS damage, mental retardation, or primary sensory deficits, the individual demonstrates evidence of (a) difficulty processing and interpreting sensory information, and (b) using that information to act effectively and efficiently on objects in the environment [1–3]. Typically, for children between the ages of 4 and 9 years, the evaluation of SI functioning consists of a developmental history, the Sensory Integration and Praxis Tests (SIPT) [4], and related clinical assessments of neuromotor behavior [5].

The purpose of this paper is to examine briefly the evaluation and interpretation procedures utilized in the differential diagnosis of the various manifestations of SI dysfunction [5]. The information gathered is used for the purpose of planning and implementing effective intervention. In this paper, we will concentrate on evaluation using the SIPT, a developmental history, and clinical assessments of neuromotor behavior.

SI dysfunction manifests itself in a number of different ways. Although SI theory can be described best as a complex upward-spiraling process [3, 6], the relationships among the hypothesized constructs of the theory can be schematically represented in a linear fashion for the purpose of illustrating the evaluation and interpretation process (fig. 1). The evaluation technology related to each construct is shown in table 1. Careful examination of table 1 reveals that some tests (e.g. Graphesthesia) measure overlapping performance areas. Complete descriptions of each measure are available [4, 5].

The SIPT are comprised of 17 tests that are individually administered and computer-scored. The SIPT were standardized on a modified random sample of 2,000 children (ages 4–0 to 8–11 years) reflecting the population characteristics of the 1980 US census [4, 7]. The SIPT have been evaluated favorably for validity and interrater reliability. As a combined test battery,

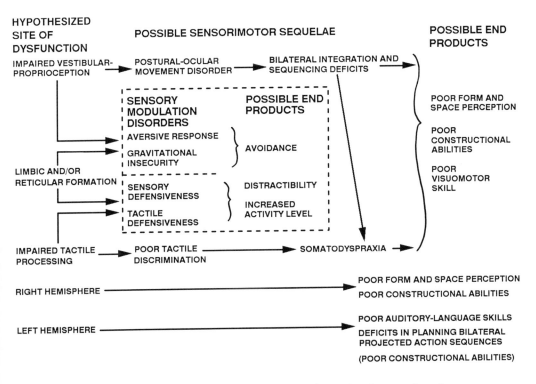

Fig. 1. Relationships among the constructs of sensory integration theory and typology of dysfunction. From Fisher et al. [5], used with permission.

the SIPT have been shown to have very high test-retest reliability (r = 0.98) [Ayres, personal commun.]. The administration and interpretation of the SIPT requires that the examiner undergoes a rigorous certification process; this assures interrater reliability.

Accurate and differential diagnosis of SI dysfunction relies on the interpretation of *meaningful clusters* of evaluation signs. That is, one or two indicators of dysfunction are not sufficient for diagnostic purposes. Careful examination of table 1 reveals that some important manifestations of SI dysfunction (i.e. postural-ocular movement disorder, sensory modulation disorders) cannot be evaluated thoroughly with the SIPT. Further, the SIPT have not been standardized with individuals younger than 4 years or older than 8 years 11 months. The accurate diagnosis of SI dysfunction in these individuals, and of postural-ocular movement disorder and sensory modulation disorders in all individuals, requires the administration of clinical assessments of neuromotor behavior and a developmental history.

Table 1. List of assessments used to evaluate each of the constructs associated with sensory integrative dysfunction. Adapted from Fisher et al. [5], used with permission

Postural-ocular movement disorder	Tactile discrimination
Standing and walking balance *Postrotary nystagmus* *Kinesthesia* Prone extension Proximal joint stability Extensor muscle tone Equilibrium Neck flexion in supine Postural adjustments Poor modulation of force Diminished awareness of body position or movement	*Localization of tactile stimuli* *Finger identification* *Manual form perception* *Graphesthesia*
Sensory modulation disorders	**Bilateral integration and sequencing praxis (BIS)**
Gravitational insecurity Aversive response to movement Touch inventory (TIE) Tactile defensiveness Other sensory modulation deficits (e.g., aversive response to sound, smell) Avoidance of sensory experiences	*Bilateral motor coordination* *Sequencing praxis* *Oral praxis* *Graphesthesia* *Standing and walking balance* (*Postural praxis*) (*Praxis on verbal command*) *SV contralateral use* *SV preferred hand use* Mixed/delayed hand preference Crossing midline of body Right-left confusion Projected action sequences Bilateral motor skills
Somatodyspraxia	**Dyspraxia on verbal command**
Meaningful BIS cluster *Postural praxis* Meaningful tactile cluster (Meaningful postural-ocular) Supine flexion Sequential finger touching In-hand manipulation Diadokokinesia	*Praxis on verbal command* *Postrotary nystagmus (prolonged)* (*Bilateral motor coordination*) (*Sequencing praxis*) (*Standing and walking balance*) (*Oral praxis*)

Table 1. (cont.)

Form and space perception	Visual construction	Visuomotor coordination
Space visualization	*Design copying*	*Motor accuracy*
Figure-ground perception	*Constructional praxis*	*Design copying*
Constructional praxis	Other constructional	Other visuomotor test
Design copying	ability measures	scores
Manual form perception		
Other-visual perceptual test scores		

SIPT test scores are italicized. Test scores listed in parentheses may be low when dysfunction is present, but low scores are not considered to be major indicators of dysfunction.

Although many clinical assessments and developmental history forms are fairly standard, and guidelines for the administration and interpretation of these measures have been published [5], few normative data are available to aid the clinician in interpreting the findings. Thus, these measures must be administered, and the findings interpreted, by an experienced occupational or physical therapist with specialized training in SI.

When the entire assessment has been completed, the therapist organizes and interprets the results. The information depicted in figure 1 and table 1 are useful in the interpretation process. In interpreting the findings of the assessment, the therapist attempts to (a) explain as many of the individual's presenting problems as possible by using SI theory, and (b) recommend a plan for effective intervention. The therapist examines the findings for evidence of meaningful clusters of test scores indicating SI dysfunction. Because some of the measures represent overlapping performance areas, the therapist must 'tease out' the best interpretation. This is done by examining the test scores associated with each of the boxes depicted in table 1, determining the best explanation for each test score that appears in more than one box, and identifying the cluster of scores that best explains the individual's clinical picture.

First, the therapist discerns whether or not there is a sensory processing basis for the disorder that cannot be attributed to a frank CNS disorder or peripheral sensory loss. That is, is there a meaningful cluster of scores suggesting vestibular-proprioceptive (postural-ocular movement disorder), poor tactile discrimination, or a sensory modulation disorder? If no such cluster exists, the disorder is not considered to be SI dysfunction. If a meaningful cluster does exist, then the therapist examines the remaining test results to determine, more precisely, the nature of the disorder.

Three primary types of SI dysfunction are most commonly identified: (a) a practic disorder of bilateral integration and sequencing (BIS); (b) somatodyspraxia; and (c) a disorder of sensory modulation. Currently, we speculate that somatodyspraxia is a more severe form of SI dysfunction than is BIS. That is, individuals who have somatodyspraxia demonstrate signs associated with BIS (i.e. deficits in planning and producing bilateral projected action sequences) and *also* meaningful clusters of scores suggesting (a) poor tactile discrimination, and (b) dyspraxia associated with planning and producing simple nonprojected, responsive movements [5].

Sensory modulation disorders are of an entirely different nature than other types of SI dysfunction. Individuals with sensory modulation disorders usually overreact to one or more types of sensory input, and demonstrate unusual fear or aversive reactions. A diagnosis of sensory modulation disorder is based on history and clinical assessment only; no standardized evaluations measure this disorder.

Although other types of dysfunction (e.g. dyspraxia on verbal command) can be identified using the SIPT and clinical assessments, these are not thought to reflect SI dysfunction. Rather, they are hypothesized to be the result of cortical dysfunction.

Interpretation of the assessment also includes reporting the findings to the client, his or her family, physician, teacher, etc.; validating the interpretation (i.e. do the client and client's family believe that the explanation is meaningful and plausible?); and making recommendations for intervention, if appropriate [5].

Some final remarks regarding the use of the SIPT in regions other than North America are warranted. First, these tests were standardized on North American samples; their generalization to other populations should be examined empirically. Second, therapists using and interpreting the SIPT are encouraged to complete the certification process offered through Sensory Integration International, Torrance, Calif. Finally, the SIPT must be computer scored in the US by Western Psychological Services, a process that may not be practical for therapists practicing outside North America.

Therapists evaluating very young children, adolescents, or adults, even in North America, are confronted with similar constraints. In our experience, we have found that the developmental history and clinical assessment of neuromotor behavior can be supplemented by other standardized tests that test the same constructs as does the SIPT, provided they are administered by experienced occupational or physical therapists with training in SI. However, there remains a need for therapists to be able to evaluate the impact of SI dysfunction on self-care, play, and school skills. Fisher and her colleagures at The University of Illinois at Chicago have piloted the Assessment of Motor and Process Skills (AMPS) [unpubl. test manual] with healthy and dyspraxic children 12 months of age and older. The AMPS shows considerable promise for evaluating the behavioral manifestations of SI dysfunction in the context of meaningful, familiar object play [8] or daily living tasks [9].

References

1   Ayres AJ: Sensory Integration and Learning Disorders. Los Angeles, Western Psychological Services, 1972.
2   Ayres AJ: Sensory Integration and the Child. Los Angeles, Western Psychological Sevices, 1979.
3   Fisher AG, Murray EA: Introduction to sensory integration theory; in Fisher AG, Murray EA, Bundy AC (eds): Sensory Integration: Theory and Practice. Philadelphia, Davis, 1991, pp 3–26.
4   Ayres AJ: Sensory Integration and Praxis Tests. Los Angeles, Western Psychological Services, 1989.
5   Fisher AG, Murray EA, Bundy AC (eds): Sensory Integration: Theory and Practice. Philadelphia, Davis, 1991.
6   Kielhofner G, Fisher AG: Mind-brain-body relationships; in Fisher AG, Murray EA, Bundy AC (eds): Sensory Integration: Theory and Practice. Philadelphia, Davis, 1991, pp 30–45.
7   Ayres AJ, Marr DB: Sensory Integration and Praxis Tests; in Fisher AG, Murray EA, Bundy AC (eds): Sensory Integration: Theory and Practice. Philadelphia, Davis, 1991, pp 203–233.
8   Jalayerian J, Fisher AG: Assessment of motor and process skills in normal and dyspraxic preschoolers. Occupational Therapy Journal of Research, in press.
9   Fisher AG: Development of a functional assessment that adjusts ability measures for task challenge and leniency; in Wilson M (ed): Objective Measurement: Theory into Practice, Vol. 2. Norwood, NJ: Ablex, in press.

Anita C. Bundy, ScD, Department of Occupational Therapy M/C 811,
The University of Illinois at Chicago, 1919 West Taylor Street, Chicago IL 60612 (USA)

Forssberg H, Hirschfeld H (eds): Movement Disorders in Children.
Med Sport Sci. Basel, Karger, 1992, vol 36, pp 278–283

Motor Assessment Tools for Infants and Young Children: A Focus on Disability Assessment

Stephen M. Haley

Tufts University School of Medicine, and Medical Rehabilitation Research and Training Center in Rehabilitation and Childhood Trauma, New England Medical Center Hospital, Boston, Mass., USA

Pediatric physical therapists have long expressed the need for a functional approach to the assessment of children with movement disorders. Current reviews of efficacy studies and measurement issues have placed strong emphasis on the importance of developing new functional outcome measures for the assessment of children with motor disorders [1, 2]. Until recently, minimal activity has been generated to develop clinically acceptable functional assessment instruments. Two main issues affect the utilization of functional assessment instruments in pediatric physical therapy, namely, the difficulty of conceptualizing and defining function in children and the limited availability of satisfactory tools to measure function. The purposes of this paper are fourfold: (1) to review conceptual issues regarding pediatric motor function; (2) to propose three measurement constructs for functional assessment measures in outcome studies; (3) to provide a brief, selected review of functional assessment characteristics, and (4) to describe an application of a new functional assessment instrument for the documentation of outcomes and recovery of children with brain injury.

Conceptual Issues

Functional activities are viewed as essential skills that are required in the child's natural environments of home and school. The most widely acknowledged conceptual framework for function is one provided by the World Health Organization [3]. In this framework, function is tied to the concept of disability, and is concerned with the restriction of integrated activities of daily living. According to the WHO classification system as applied to physical and motor function, *impairments* refer to the loss or abnormality of a motor component or process, *disability* is the restriction of a functional activity, and *handicap* is the inability to perform a social role due to motor impairments or disabilities [3].

However, controversy exists regarding the conceptual clarity of the WHO classification system [4]. A paper by Grimby et al. [5] discussed the use of the WHO classification system in adult rehabilitation and found difficulty differentiating between the constructs of disability and handicap. An alternative model of disablement developed by Nagi in the mid-1960s has recently gained attention in the rehabilitation literature. Nagi [6] introduced the concept of *functional limitations*, which serves as a bridge between the presence of impairment and the person's performance of usual roles and normal daily activities. Regardless of the specific model of disablement or the terminology used, the concept of disability and functional assessment incorporates these key concepts: (1) a child may have serious motor impairments that are not always reflected by the level of functional limitation or disability; (2) functional deficits may or may not lead to a restriction in social activities and important childhood roles, and (3) environmental factors, family expectations, and contextual elements of functional task requirements play an important role in the eventual level of disability and handicap of the child.

Proposed Measurement Constructs

Based on both the WHO classification system and Nagi's description of disability, and borrowing from recent work by Guccione [7] in the application of models of disablement to physical therapy practice, I propose a further elaboration of this model for the description of disablement in children. Note the model depicted in figure 1. This working model of childhood disablement includes three measurement constructs within functional assessment: (1) capability of discrete functional skills; (2) performance of functional activities, and (3) performance of social, family and personal roles. Advantages of this adapted model of childhood disablement are that it emphasizes the distinction between capability and performance, recognizes the distinction between discrete tasks and integrated functional activities, and incorporates both developmental and contextual frameworks into the description of childhood disability.

Capability of discrete functional skills refers to the accomplishment of tasks in either a standardized or ideal situation and represents the child's best performance independent of context. Many evaluations in pediatric physical therapy completed in the hospital or in an out-patient clinic are

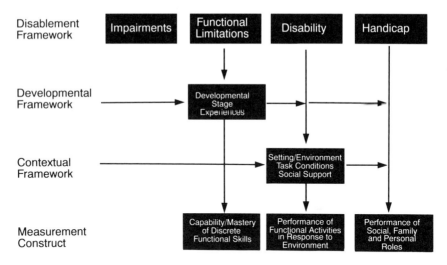

Fig. 1. Working model of conceptual framework for the assessment of disability in children.

essentially tests of the child's motor capability. As noted in figure 1, the developmental stage and experiences of the child have an impact upon the capability and mastery of functional skills and must be considered in such a model. Although there has been considerable study of the unfolding of developmental motor milestones, and, recently, motor control process in normal children, there is much less information available on the typical patterns of the development of functional capabilities in either children with or without disabilities. Tests of capability often assess functional units of behavior that are considered necessary for functional performance. For example, an assessment of mobility normally includes a number of functional units of behavior, including transfer to a standing position, balance in gait, stride length, cadence and ability to walk on uneven surfaces.

Performance evaluation of functional activities refers to the measurement of functional behaviors as they actually occur in the environment. In the case of gait assessment, this might include the assessment of locomotor patterns in the child's environment, and the amount of help needed in mobility at home or school. Recent developmental theory has called attention to how the environmental and social context affects activity patterns and the performance of functional competencies. For example, the natural environments of home and school have very different functional requirements, physical characteristics and social contexts. Thus, children's motor performance may significantly differ across settings and may be quite different from that noted in an assessment of motor capacity. Performance of motor activities is not embedded in a child, but rather is highly related to the context in which a child moves. Caregiver assistance is a dimension that is often used to measure the level of independence of motor and ADL activities in naturalistic settings. For example, Edebol-Tysk [8] at the University of Göteborg examined the concept of the care-load of severely involved children with cerebral palsy as a measure of childhood disability.

Lastly, the performance of social, family and personal roles related to physical performance and activity represents the third measurement construct. This construct is most closely related to the WHO's conceptualization of handicap. Very little work has been accomplished in this measurement area, and yet the physical ability and endurance needed for typical peer and school activities are often the most important areas of concern for children with disabilities and their parents.

A linkage exists between the three proposed measurement constructs in functional assessment and the specific mode of test administration. Two major assessment modes used in physical therapy assessments are criterion-testing (standardized test administration of motor items) and judgment-based assessment. Criterion testing is the primary mode for determining physical capabilities, while judgment-based assessment, using either professionals or parents as respondents, is a common mode of test administration for determining the performance of functional and role activities. Few, if any, standardized assessments have been developed for directly observing motor activity in a naturalistic setting.

Selected Characteristics of Pediatric Functional Outcome Measures

A number of characteristics are essential for functional assessment instruments to be employed effectively as outcome measures. Functional measures used for evaluative purposes must be structured to be responsive to clinically meaningful changes [9]. Care must be taken when choosing functional measures so that they include the range of tasks and activities typically performed by the specific group of children of interest. Functional instruments which have aggregate scoring systems must strive to clearly identify the meaning of summary score changes in both specific and concrete clinical terms [10, 11]. Although the primary purpose of evaluative assessments are to be responsive to clinical change, the analysis of recovery to age-expected performance requires a functional assessment to have a norm-referenced base. This is particularly important in estimating rates of recovery in young children with acquired injuries. Finally, relationships among motor impairment, motor capability, and motor disability and handicap measures should be explored in future outcome studies.

Development of the Pediatric Evaluation of Disability Inventory (PEDI)

The PEDI [12] is a new judgment-based functional assessment that measures the capability of functional skills and the performance of functional activities in the content domains of self-care, mobility, and social function. The PEDI was designed to provide both a standard score (mean = 50; SD = 10) based on a normative sample and a scaled score (0–100 scale; 0 = low ability; 100 = high ability) based on a hierarchical scale of functional items developed through the Rasch Rating Scale Model [13]. Data are now being collected to determine the responsiveness of the PEDI in different clinical samples and to determine its usefulness for the determination of motor recovery.

In summary, much more work in the area of conceptualization and measurement of functional motor outcomes is needed. Skilled clinicians coupled with the efforts of research scientists with strong psychometric skills are required to continue this exciting work. As we begin to clarify the constructs we wish to measure, aided both by theoretical issues and empirical studies, we will gradually work towards the effective and efficient clinical documentation of functional motor outcomes in children with disabilities.

References

1   Harris SR: Efficacy of physical therapy in promoting family functioning and functional independence for children with cerebral palsy. Pediatr Phys Ther 1990;2:160–163.
2   Campbell SK: Measurement in developmental therapy: Past, present, and future; in Miller LJ (ed): Developing Norm-Referenced Standardized Tests. New York, The Haworth Press, 1989, pp 1–13.
3   World Health Organization: International Classification of Impairments, Disabilities, and Handicaps. Geneva, World Health Organization, 1980.
4   Pope AM, Tarlov AR (eds): Disability in America: Toward a National Agenda for Prevention. Washington, National Academy Press, 1991.
5   Gimby G, Finnstam J, Jette A: On the application of the WHO handicap classification in rehabilitation. Scand J Rehabil Med 1988;20:93–98.
6   Nagi SZ: Disability and Rehabilitation. Columbus, Ohio State University Press, 1969.

7   Guccione AA: Physical therapy diagnosis and the relationship between impairments and function. Phys Ther 1991;71:499–504.
8   Edebol-Tysk K: Evaluation of care-load for individuals with spastic tetraplegia. Dev Med Child Neurol 1989;31:737–745.
9   Rosenbaum PL, Russell DJ, Cadman DT: Issues in measuring change in motor function in children with cerebral palsy: A special communication. Phys Ther 1990;70:125–131.
10 Brook RH, Kamberg CJ: General health status measures and outcome measurement: A commentary on measuring functional status. J Chron Dis 1987;40:131s–136s.
11 Guccione AA, Felson DT, Anderson JJ: Defining arthritis and measuring functional status in elders: Methodological issues in the study of disease and physical disability. Am J Publ Health 1990;80:945–949.
12 Haley SM, Coster WJ, Ludlow LH: Pediatric Evaluation of Disability Inventory. Boston, New England Medical Center, 1992.
13 Wright BD, Masters GN: Rating Scale Analysis. Chicago, Meas Press, 1982.

S.M. Haley, PhD, PT, Department of Rehabilitation, Research and Training Center, Tufts University School of Medicine, 75 Kneeland Street, 5th Floor, Boston, MA 02111 (USA)

Forssberg H, Hirschfeld H (eds): Movement Disorders in Children.
Med Sport Sci. Basel, Karger, 1992, vol 36, pp 284–296

Discussion Section V

*Anette Boll, Maj-Britt Fredriksson, Gunilla Hellberg, Helga Hirschfeld,
Monica Steen, Jenny Weibull*

Summary of Presentations

During the entire symposium several speakers stressed the value and
the necessity of measurements, assessments and evaluations for occupational and physiotherapy diagnosis and intervention. The speakers in this
session viewed it from three different perspectives.

Campbell focused primarily on clinical measurement of the movement
dysfunction in CP. She pointed out that an appropriate assessment protocol should stem from a theoretical perspective and from the knowledge
base regarding the nature of dysfunction at a variety of levels, from the
organ systems to the societal level. The protocol must contain items that
test what we want to measure and should be constructed for the types of
problems children with CP have. The protocol should provide for diagnostic capabilities and problem identification for treatment planning purposes,
as well as capture the effects of intervention. A single test cannot be used
to measure all of this, several different tests are needed. In order to
understand both the underlying impairment and its effects on a child's life,
those clinical assessments must be linked with quantitative, laboratory-
based research findings as well as with descriptions of the child's abilities in
daily activities at home and in the community.

From the framework of the Sensory Integration Theory Bundy addressed evaluation and intervention in children with *minor* neurological
deficits. She pointed out that the theory cannot be used to explain, or
help, many of the specific problems children with CNS damage (e.g. CP)
have. Some children with CP might in addition to the motor problems
from their CNS damage, also have a disordered ability to process sensory
information. For them, some of the framework from this theory can
prove helpful in understanding and perhaps solving some of their daily
problems.

She also made several comments on assessments in general. In assessments and intervention we evaluate either implicitly or explicitly based on our theories or our beliefs. The more explicit we make our theories, the more effective and efficient we are. Assessment must be guided by the problems that our patient wants to resolve, not by the problems we want to resolve for them. The following questions should rule our choice of assessment. What will I know, when I have the results of this test? How will the result of this test contribute to my overall assessment? And are those factors in agreement with what I really want to know?

Haley stressed the need for a functional approach to the assessment of children with movement disorders. We need to define, characterize and conceptualize function, in order to become better in identifying what we want to measure. One reason we lack many good assessment instruments is perhaps the difficulty of conceptualizing function. For example, in assessing mobility we have to understand the entire social context of mobility. Haley proposed that the WHO classification system can be used as a framework for defining function via its classification of impairment, disability and handicap.

He suggested that our functional assessments must vary depending upon which level of function we want to examine. To measure capability for performing functional skills, like most available tests do, we assess the impairment/functional limitation level. At the disability level, however, we might need more judgement-based assessments in order to determine what the child really *does do* in his or her natural environment. At the handicap level, the concern is with performance of social, family and personal roles and societal barriers to achieving important life goals. If we want to know about the child's function in daily life, we have to begin to get information by observing the environment and asking questions of people who really know the child, instead of only measuring the child's capabilities to perform in a clinical setting.

Different Models for Framing Assessment and Treatment

The discussion developed from two different views concerning assessment and treatment of children with movement disorders. The two models discussed were, on the one hand, the *medical* model and, on the other hand, the *skill acquisition* and *functional* models (presented earlier during the symposium).

Medical Model

In the *medical model* or the reductionist approach, the impairment is seen in perspectives of problem analysis and function analysis down to movement analysis. It is a medical explanation model. Physiotherapists, whose treatment is often directed to specific movement limitations, may have problems using functional tests concerning broad levels, e.g. Can I go to work? Can I interact with my family?

Horak asked 'Does the functional test tell us what to do in therapy?' Campbell answered that functional tests don't tell us what to do in therapy. For *that* we have to understand the components that underlie the problem. She gave an example by referring to Olney's power analysis of gait. A child with diplegic CP has a problem in gait based on the inability to create enough propulsion from the ankle plantar flexors which generate small power, often absorbed at the knee, and then use compensations in the hip muscles. Campbell's implication is that, if we learn from movement analyses such as these, we can seek new ways to improve the efficiency of their gait which hopefully will translate into more independence in mobility [Campbell, this vol.].

Haley also agreed that functional tests don't tell us what to do about the problems, but the tests help us to identify where the problems really are.

Horak continued: What a therapist has to do is to find out where the constraints are. For example, if a person has decreased ROM (range of motion) in the ankle, it might effect the movement pattern in the knee and the hip during gait. We have to find the key for the constraints in order to be effective in treatment.

Hirschfeld emphasized the need of systematic analysis during a specific task and pointed out the crucial importance of assessing in which order body segments move to complete the task. She described the push-off sequence during gait development in CP children. The force propelling the body forward at push-off in CP children is very poor. In a recent study, the cause was found not to be a decreased range of motion in the ankle joint (dorsiflexion) prior to push-off but rather due to wrong temporal sequence between hip, knee and ankle movement. The characteristic temporal sequence of normal adult plantigrade gait at toe-off is: ankle plantar flexion followed by knee flexion and thereafter by hip flexion. In contrast, CP children start with hip or knee flexion. The consequence is poor force generation around the ankle joint, at the right moment in the push-off phase [1].

For therapists it is very important to analyze the temporal sequences and movement directions of a particular task and to become skilled in observation of which body segment starts the movement and how the sequential temporal order proceeds for engagement of other body parts.

Skill Acquisition and Functional Models

In the *skill acquisition model* Gentile emphasized that we don't know much about the underlying damage of the nervous system in a child. Even if we knew where the damage was, we would not know what those structures actually do and what movements those structures permit when intact.

We cannot predict which movements *should* emerge from that child, we only know an ideal movement for a normal child. So what shall the therapist focus on? The ideal movement level or on an appreciation of the profound solution that the child comes up with and see if it works in the environment?

With functional assessment, Gentile means hard notes, quantitative, data-based movement assessment that you can use independently of the observer. We have to develop instruments of conceptualization of human tasks in human surroundings. Before developing assessment instruments you have to conceptualize and classify tasks. This has been done in developing the skill acquisition model and it is helpful.

Gordon stressed a *functional model* in which he emphasized that we have to assess ability rather than disability. We have to help the children to find the resources they have available. He calls this a nonmedical model; it is a patient-centered model or a child-centered model. The patients are the ones who are responsible for the treatment. The intervention is that we structure the tasks and the environments in which they treat themselves.

Discussion Concerning the Models
The following remarks capture the essential debate illustrating the discussion of the two models.

Campbell asked Gentile and Gordon: You talk about assessing capabilities. What would I do differently, if I were to try to assess children according to this model? I assume that when you assess for problems, at the same time you are also finding out what the children are capable of. What I use in therapy is a plan to use what they have and try to improve the things that they don't have. What would I do differently in measurement if I took your perspective?

Gentile answered; We mean that if you assess the child in your clinic, make examinations and kinematic assessments on a treadmill and so on, can you estimate his capability to cope with the environment when he comes to school, where many things change that are not measured in the clinical situation?

Gordon answered: How we look upon the child determines how we treat the child. If we look upon the child as a collection of disabilities or a collection of impairments, then we will treat the child as a passive recipient of treatment in correcting those impairments. There are times when certain impairments need to be corrected and you cannot ignore them. But as an overall framework for treatment, I don't think it is the way we want to go.

Instead we want to make the framework for treatment active with the child at the center while structuring tasks and environments so that they can use their resources.

We in the task force support Campbell's view that we need to look at both models, but we also believe that Gordon raised a very important issue. How we, in our minds, view the child determines how we treat the child. So the way we use these terms and different frameworks will have an effect on the way we work as therapist.

Richards sharpened the discussion: In an attempt to argue between Campbell and Gordon, I want to say that, as a therapist and as a scientist in creation and somebody who is trying to develop the clinical science that is to become physiotherapy, I am comfortable in the medical model. And because I am comfortable in this model, I can function in it. I can make people understand what I am trying to do. When I listen to Gordon and Gentile, I like it. It is fun. But I can't operationalize it. I have a gap in my understanding and to me right now it is a bit confusing because you are telling me something that sounds good, but you are not telling me how to apply it. You are telling me how to measure outcome and nobody has developed the conceptual framework that allows us to plan therapy in that mode and to evaluate it. Therefore, until I understand it better, I will use Campbell's approach, which is close to what Hirschfeld is saying. We as therapists have to make a decision. We must be good at one thing, and must be *very* good at one thing. Perhaps we have to define a clinical science and we have to make a decision as to what the clinical science will be. We have studied with physicians and we have learned the medical model. We have learned what we call the reductionist approach that we now are starting to reject. So what we have here is a battle between the art and the science. I understand what Campbell, Horak and Hirschfeld are saying, but I have difficulty in understanding Gentile and Gordon. *Where are we going?* (Unfortunately, this question was never answered due to lack of time during the discussion.)

In her closing remarks Horak came back to some more aspects of the models. I think both models still come down to assumptions. I think we can incorporate all of this together. I don't think it is either/or, because if you assume that you can change the nervous system, if you assume that your treatment can change the muscles and the joints, then a medical model is helpful, because you can intervene once you have identified the disability, intervene by changing ROM and the rest will follow. If you assume that it is impossible to change the nervous system, if you assume that the patient has lesions that you can do nothing about, there is a hole in the cortex and I am not going to replace the hole. Then you use the approach that says: Let us find the abilities, let us find the environment, and use what the person has to compensate for what they don't have that other people may have.

Both frameworks are helpful. We will be in trouble if we miss constraints, or miss abilities and miss the things a child can do. It comes out of our assumptions, how we use them. I think we all have responsibilities as scientists, therapists and clinicians. The scientists can give some assumptions to the therapist. They say: This is how we think the brain works. They don't know how it works. They are just giving you their ideas. They test the assumptions with experiments and data. They can change their assumptions. They come back in a year and say: I was wrong yesterday.

It is OK to let our assumptions change the theoretical framework. But we are afraid when people are questioning our assumptions, whether we can help children or not. If we really believe that we are helping children, that our intervention makes a difference, it is very important to find ways of measuring this. We have to measure in controlled, standardized clinical studies, for which the therapists are responsible, not the basic neuroscientists. And if we can convince scientists and physicians that we really are making a difference, we have to tell *them* to tell us why this is working.

Then it would be interesting for the scientists to look for the mechanisms underlying it. So we are both teaching one another. Therapy has changed the way neuroscience looks at motor control in the world, because so many therapists have gone into motor control-neurophysiology. They are now looking at complicated movements, tasks and environments which they never did when Sherrington started in 1919. But science should change therapy and we should help it do that!

We in the task force agree with Horak that it is not either/or, it is both. The experience many Swedish physiotherapists and occupational therapists have is that it is possible to combine at least part of the two models as a framework in clinical work. They don't experience a strict dividing line between the models. We need both models and they interact with each other. Might the system task model proposed by Horak be a starting point for the question from Richards: 'Where are we going?', especially if we combine it with Haley's thoughts about conceptualizing function more clearly.

Discussion on the Role of Therapists as Team Members

Fisher emphasized that each of us, as occupational therapists, physiotherapists, basic scientists, etc., have different perspectives on function. She asked: Should different therapists assess the abilities in different ways when we assess the problem? Do we assess different things or do we assess problems in different ways?

Campbell replied that we all probably assess the disability level in much the same way and there the skill acquisition/functional model is useful. We all need to know about the patient's function in their home, school and community. Then we go back to the functional limitation and impairment levels from the *unique perspective* of our own discipline to see what we have to contribute to reducing disability. It would be important to have a test at the disability level that everybody can use. A test that can be meaningful to other people, for example, parents and other professionals who are not able to understand our evaluations at the impairment level.

Haley added that it is good to have different disciplines and different professionals who look at the various problems that the child has. The primary competence of the physician is to diagnose and identify pathology and that is important information for us in terms of prognosis and for starting intervention. Physiotherapists also have capabilities that the physician does not have. We can provide meaningful evaluations in the disability, impairment and functional areas. With all these different kinds of information we can develop the competence to devise a more comprehensive approach.

During the discussion the question of who assesses function was raised. Several speakers stressed that nobody owns function; everybody in the team is working with function but in different ways.

We in the task force think it is important to know the competence of the members in the team and to listen to each other. You can get valuable information from the other members and you don't have to assess and measure everything yourself. We have to be aware of our professional role and should not try to become an 'allround therapist'. Otherwise there is a risk that we will suffer a loss of quality. Knowledge of the competence of others is important, as well as the readiness to listen to each other.

Assessment Tools

There was very little discussion about actual tests. The following tests were mentioned during the lectures, but not further discussed PEDI (Pediatric Evaluation of Disability Inventory); PDMS (Peabody Developmental Motor Scales; GMFM (Gross Motor Function Measure); GMPM (Gross Motor Performance Measure); SIPT (Sensory Integration and Praxis Test) and AMPS (Assessment of Motor and Process Skills). Many other well-known tests were not mentioned.

Videorecording, Observation, the Clinical Eye

Can we use videorecording as a reliable measurement tool? Campbell believed that it is possible to document the movement, but it is not useful unless a specific protocol or measurement scheme graded the study of outcome.

Cioni uses videorecording in notation of movements of infants following a strict scheme for what to assess. The interrater reliability was high among several persons assessing infants. In observations from video or of live performance the clinical eye is very important for identifying quality. It requires the observer to have enough theoretical background and knowledge to understand what he/she sees, not only a capacity to register.

Hirschfeld emphasized that therapists should be skilled in observational movement analysis in which the movement of the subject is observed in relation to the body and to the environment. In this kind of observation a 3 D Coordinate System is used as a reference base, similar to computerized movement analysis systems. In this way, changes between body segments (angles) as well as changes of body segments in relation to space (displacement), can systematically be observed and documented. Although the exact values cannot be received, movement direction and temporal sequence of the different body segments can be noted. In Sweden several physiotherapists and occupational therapists are using this type of analysis, but unfortunately the method is not yet documented.

Concluding Remarks

In the lectures by Campbell, Bundy and Haley, we heard a lot about tests and measurement tools. But the discussion in this session was mostly concentrated on the models and overall theoretical frameworks for measurement, rather than assessment tools. Therefore, would we, in the task force, like to share some comments and question about assessments that evolved within our group during and after the symposium.

Different Purposes Require Different Tools

Tests have several purposes. They ought to help us notice the kinds of problems we deal with, be a communication among colleagues and other professionals on the team. A good test should also be able to tell us something we don't notice in our ordinary observation.

Before using a test we have to ask ourself: What is the content I get from the results of the test? Will the result influence the intervention? What can we measure and is it relevant to measure?

Why don't therapists use the tests available today? Does it depend on the therapists or the tests? Are the tests not giving the therapist the information he/she requires or are there other reasons behind the failure to use tests? Maybe the therapist doesn't need to describe the problem in detail because he/she already has an idea of how to intervene without testing the child?

What situations affect how we work as therapists? What effects might aspects of culture, society, economy and different attitudes have upon how we as professionals focus our interventions? Even in a small country such as Sweden, these factors create different attitudes toward testing and treatment.

Most of our tests are based and validated on normal children with *normal* movements. In assessing children with minor neurological dysfunction, these tests might be helpful. But for children with CP, or other kinds of major neurological damage, we need measurement derived from knowledge about the natural history of CP.

An evaluation measure must contain relevant items and must be applicable to the population for whom it is developed, feasible to use, reliable and valid for its purpose. How many of the tests that we use fulfills these requirements? We need to be more observant of this. One example about reliability was discussed, when Bradley asked Haley if the MAI test (Movement Assessment of Infants) is a reliable test. He replied that not all items were reliable. The items with voluntary movements were most reliable.

Our need of assessment tools can be addressed from the following two perspectives:

(1) Patient-oriented assessment tools for:

Screening – to decide which children need further comprehensive examination and possibly intervention.

Diagnosing – identifying functional problems on different levels.

Intervention – planning, focused on ability-disability.

Evaluating treatment effect.

(2) Research tests:

Laboratory-based research, for instance, with the goal of describing children's motor function in specific, repeatable and measurable situations. To gain knowledge about group differences between, e.g. normal and CP development, or age appropriate development.

To develop the professional body of knowledge for different diagnostic groups, our theoretical base for treatment.

We also need tests at different levels for problem analysis, functional analysis and movement analysis, corresponding to, e.g., the WHO classification.

To be able to measure treatment effects, we need different functional tests, because it is the child's functional capability in his/her daily life that we must try to have an impact on with treatment. But in order to know how we should plan our treatment, we often need a more reductionistic test to determine the underlying problems that prevent the child from accomplishing the function efficiently and successfully. Knowing the child's abilities is also important, because it is at the edge of ability that we can help the child expand to his/her functional capabilities.

Bradley accentuated that how we measure is important, for it has to be engaging for the child and still valid. She gave an example of an investigation measuring pronation and supination. When the test situation was altered in a more playful activity, the child's functional ability drastically changed for the better [2].

In a comment to the discussion about how functional tests don't tell us what to do in treatment, Bundy suggested that most assessments we use today have not been developed by therapists. This might be one reason why they don't give us information about the function itself and the factors that allow us to accomplish that function. We need such assessments.

Research Areas in the Future

To know what a child *can do* is not the same as what the child *does* because function has to do with the child's capability to plan the movement and adjust force, as well as the temporal and spatial aspects of movement. If the child needs to do two things at the same time, he might not be able to perform as well as when he does each thing separately. There have to be tests that reveal whether the movement assessed in the clinical setting is useful in ADL, social communication or learning situations. Today we do not have those instruments. If, in future development of assessments, we use the 'system task' model presented by Horak, we might be able to better understand the underlying constraints for certain tasks, and thereby find a solution to this type of problems.

Cioni focused on the natural history of CP. He said that he agreed with Campbell that we can't use the framework of normal child development as a guideline for children with CP. He believed that we should not even talk about cerebral *palsy*, but cerebral *palsies*. There are different kinds of CP and we must collect data in the framework of the natural history of the cerebral palsies if we want to be able to measure motor performance and to judge treatment. Cioni pointed out that treatment is an attempt to make some change in the natural history. Sometimes it can be a good change; unfortunately, sometimes it can be a bad change that we provoked. Cioni continued, we have to collect data about the natural history of CP and he thinks that the Bobaths did a great deal years ago, when the panorama of CP was different from the kind of CP we have today. We now have the tools to try to establish the natural history of CP because we can identify lesions in the beginning. In this we need the unified efforts of doctors, physiotherapists and people in the intensive care units. He emphasized that we will never improve, if we work separately.

Do We Need Other Research Methods in the Future?

Very little time was spent on discussing what kinds of research methods we might need to be able to generate more knowledge about treatment outcome for the patient. Campbell touched on this subject when she described the discrepancy between what researchers, on the one hand, have thought to be valid measures of treatment effect and how therapists, on the other hand, describe the child's changes in their progress notes. Those findings can't be described in numbers, only words. Maybe we also need to look outside the neurobiological scientific research methods if we want to be able to collect data that is important to our specific professional body of knowledge, like the judgment-based assessments that Haley mentioned.

We need separate tools for basic research and for clinical evaluation for treatment planning. The reason is that the strict reproductional test situations, which are necessary for basic research, can very rarely take into consideration the child's maximal motivation, concentration and other psychological behavior. These are things that are bound to influence the everyday functional performance.

This is the same problem as Gentile pointed out, that kinematic measurements of preschool children might not be valid, as a child in a more natural situation is acting dynamically with his environment and is, in fact, environmentally dependent.

This is the risk in the basic research laboratory setting for specific purpose that the task has become transformed in the process to actually measure something else than what the researcher had in mind in creating the measurement instrument. One example is the situation of research on a treadmill: Is toe off on a treadmill really the same type of movement initiated in the same way as toe off on a stationary surface?

One documentation system or method that was discussed by several persons during the symposium was structured videorecording that could be analyzed. It is important to have strict protocols with specific items, employing very clever camera settings operated by persons, who are experienced in the purpose of recording. Furthermore, therapists must invent relevant and measurable items. Because videorecording only gives us a two-dimensional illustration, we also have to be aware that it can be difficult to see the details in the quality/character of the performance.

Most children with CP or other movement disorders belong to highly heterogeneous groups, and the underlying problem for the same observable dysfunction may vary from child to child. Research methods like 'single-case studies' and 'life quality assessments' might prove to be more useful for documenting intervention effects under these conditions. The intervention may have led to a different strategy that made it possible to perform the task better, which in turn increased life quality. Intervention effects are not always measurable in increased motor function. We need better and quantifiable assessment tools, but can all assessment components important for our therapeutic intervention be quantified? An essential element of our therapeutic professions is the 'clinical eye' based on our theoretical knowledge and professional experience. If we try too hard to quantify data, important aspects might be lost. Are there any risks that this will affect our professional development in a direction we have not been able to foresee?

Collaboration between Clinicians and Researchers
We in the task force definitely agree with the statements that we practitioners must become better at finding ways of objectively collecting important data about the patient, especially when we believe that our treatment is effective, but we don't understand why! Basic research might shed some light upon it if we can define the problem well enough.

Today's problem is not only that we don't have the assessment tools we need we also don't always have enough theoretical knowledge of what is most important to measure. We have to become better in identifying for ourselves the theoretical framework and hypotheses we use in our clinical work.

In her discussion, Campbell stated her belief that the disciplines of occupational and physical therapy have a current status similar to the one that the various fields of psychology had before the time of immense growth in psychological tests and measurements. Many opportunities exist for both clinicians and researchers. According to Campbell: 'They can indeed, no, they *must* contribute to this enterprise.'

Bundy suggested that we must become better at determining in what it is we think we can change, what aspects of the child's problem we think our intervention can effect, and then set the goal in terms of real-life abilities. Maybe this is a starting point for us to demonstrate effectiveness to ourselves, to patients and to our colleagues.

In our group we are now looking forward to the continuous growth in our professional area. With good assessment tools that tap into what we believe to be the underlying causes of a child's problem, as well as assessment tools to measure treatment outcome in the same perspective, we eventually can know more about how and why our therapy has an effect.

So we have a long, but interesting way ahead of us, in which occupational and physiotherapist clinicians become involved in composing and developing relevant assessment tools.

References

1   Leonard CT, Hirschfeld H, Forssberg H: The Development of Independent Walking in Children with Cerebral Palsy. Dev Med Child Neurol 1991;33:567–577.
2   van der Weel FR, van der Meer ALH, Lee DN: Effect of Task on Movement Control in Cerebral Palsy: Implications for Assessment and Therapy. Dev Med Child Neurol 1991;33:419–426.

Anette Boll, OTR, Habilitering, Barnkliniken, Huddinge Hospital, S–141 86 Huddinge (Sweden)

Subject Index